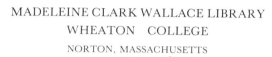
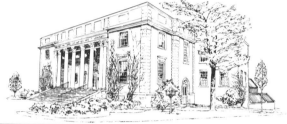

The Age of Immunology

The Age of Immunology

CONCEIVING A FUTURE IN AN ALIENATING WORLD

A. David Napier

THE UNIVERSITY OF CHICAGO PRESS / CHICAGO AND LONDON

A. David Napier is professor of anthropology and Dana Faculty Fellow at Middlebury College and director of Students of Human Ecology, a nonprofit organization that combines academic mentoring and community service. He is the author of *Foreign Bodies: Performance, Art, and Symbolic Anthropology*, and *Masks, Transformation, and Paradox*.

The University of Chicago Press, Chicago 60637
The University of Chicago Press, Ltd., London
© 2003 by A. David Napier
All rights reserved. Published 2003
Printed in the United States of America

12 11 10 09 08 07 06 05 04 03   1 2 3 4 5
ISBN: 0-226-56812-1 (cloth)

Library of Congress Cataloging-in-Publication Data

Napier, A. David.
   The age of immunology : conceiving a future in an alienating world /
A. David Napier.
      p. cm.
   Includes bibliographical references and index.
   ISBN 0-226-56812-1 (cloth : alk. paper)
      1. Ethnology—Philosophy.   2. Intercultural communication.   3. Self.   4. Change.
5. Immunology.   I. Title.

   GN345 .N36 2003
   305.8′001—dc21

                                                                    2002012926

♾ The paper used in this publication meets the minimum requirements of the American National Standard for Information Sciences—Permanence of Paper for Printed Library Materials, ANSI Z39.48-1992.

For Andrew, Harriet, and the future M.D.

Objects in mirror are closer than they appear

Contents

Acknowledgments

"You are what others make you," a doctor once told me when I asked how he could have worked for so many years among the homeless. We are each of us no more or less than a reflection of the experiences we have shared with those who affect us. On this the conclusion of the Feast of All Souls, 2002, one might well feel more overwhelmingly than at other moments the presence of those dear friends here and gone.

To list the many people who have influenced this book over the three decades during which its subject matter occupied my thoughts is not possible, for their numbers are legion, and many must by the nature of ethnographic practice remain anonymous. Still, to let this book go to press without some specific acknowledgments would be unacceptable, even if I risk not attending to everyone who helped form it.

As an anthropologist, I feel bound first to acknowledge my peers who patiently critiqued my presentations and papers and who read and commented on all or part of the various manuscript fragments. These colleagues include Michael Adelberg, Conerly Casey, Susan DiGiacomo, David Eaton, Lee Miller, Bill Mitchell, David Nugent, John Palmer, and Don Pollock, as well as several members of the Harvard Medical School's Department of Social Medicine who helped me give shape to this enterprise during my years as a fellow in medical and psychiatric anthropology. Most notably among that group I would like to thank Byron Good, Mary-Jo DelVecchio Good, Chris Heggenhougen, Arthur Kleinman, and Joan Kleinman; but I should also like to acknowledge the close friendships of my office and soul mates, Jon Sugar and Don Vereen, who were an ongoing source of inspiration and good will.

Elsewhere in the Medical School, I am especially grateful to Matt Liang, rheumatology director of the Multipurpose Arthritis Center at the Brigham in Boston, a researcher and clinician whose intellectual interests extend far beyond the mysterious world of autoimmunity.

As always, I remain grateful for the unflagging support of my Oxford mentor, Professor Rodney Needham. Though he played a less direct role in the research and writing of this book than in previous projects, I have benefited immensely from his incisive clarity of thought, his intellectual rigor, and his personal loyalty. Jonathan Benthall, too, deserves special thanks for encouraging me years ago to be the first anthropologist to put the cultural construction of immunological knowledge into print. Though I passed up that opportunity, Jonathan's annual reminders allowed me to retain a modicum of self-confidence in the darker periods of this enterprise. Likewise, Paul Sender not only encouraged me to persist in my work with the homeless in Great Britain but, as a doctor, anthropologist, and friend, read my drafts and patiently helped me through some of my more liminal intellectual moments. I wish him the best in his newfound love for Afghanistan and its beleaguered people.

If there is any single social cohort that sensitized me to the potential utility of liminality it would have to be the homeless themselves, a group of individuals I engaged as research subjects, and then as friends, for a decade and counting. Among them I should single out for thanks Reginald Young (a.k.a. Terminator 24) for his extraordinary insights about life on the edge, and Nnamdi Monnorman for his perceptive critique of social interactions in public places. Here, also, I would like to acknowledge the good-spirited and tireless efforts of Paul Dionne in collaborating with me on the documentation of homeless life. In providing, over the years, friendship, remarkable conversation, and a meeting place for countless encounters with the homeless, I include my thanks to the doctors of the Wytham Hall Sick Bay and the surgery at Great Chapel Street in Central London. The hospital's director, David El Kabir, OBE, and its administrative assistant, Ms. Jane Ball, were most helpful in making it possible for me to meet the homeless without invading what little privacy these people can find on the street.

Whatever moments of perceived epiphany I have enjoyed in this project, many are the outcome of days of talk and a voluminous correspondence with Francis Huxley, a friend and raconteur who possesses perhaps the most consistently startling mind I know. Other intellectual genies include Michael Adelberg (neurophysiology), Deborah Doniach (autoimmunity), Max Essex (herd immunity), Subhash Kak (information theory), Emily Martin (gender and stigma), Richard Forman and Grace Spatifora (the cell colony), Bruno Latour (network theory), Andrew Lemert (the bell curve), Mary Midgeley (neo-Darwinism), and Edward Steele (evolution). To these individuals I owe thanks for providing signal moments where my thinking was shaped by a re-markable suggestion.

Of the many researchers and bench scientists to whom I am indebted, I at least want to single out for thanks David Warrell, my Oxford allergist (who went on to become professor of tropical medicine and a leading malaria re-searcher), and John Bell for some early conversations on lupus that helped me to steer my course of interest in the experience of autoimmunity. Though there are many other Oxford friends and colleagues who gave their time and creative insights to this work, I must thank Sir Crispin Tickell for inviting me to be a founding fellow at the Green College Centre for Environmental Policy and Understanding, and Green College and All Souls College for fellowships that provided me with that crucial chemistry of time and intellectual colloquy.

Other scientists who contributed to the shaping of my thoughts include Matt Dick and Chris Watters of Middlebury College, and Melvin Cohn and Rodney Langman of the Salk Institute in La Jolla, California. As the man whom many consider the dean of theoretical immunology, Mel Cohn probably helped me more than any single scientist by taking the time to write lengthy and compelling responses to what has become chapter 7 of this book. Given the closed-shop mentality that constitutes so much of American bench sci-ence, his patient and careful input stood out as so much more than generosity.

While French academic life may be dominated by similar academic net-works and a mandatory allegiance to one's intellectual équipe, this environ-ment also produces interdisciplinary work of a sort I have witnessed nowhere else. Here, I would especially like to single out for praise and thanks Anne-Marie Moulin—philosopher, medical doctor, social historian, and activist. To her unique combination of diplomacy and native intelligence must be attrib-uted the extraordinary symposia on immunology and vaccinology in which I participated under the aegis of L'Institut Pasteur and the Fondacion Marcel Merieux. One wonders how, without such people, true interdisciplinary work would ever be possible.

At the level of clinical practice, I want to state my admiration for the scores of primary caregivers with whom I have worked in my role as director of Students of Human Ecology, a nonprofit organization devoted to mentor-apprentice teaching in the areas of medicine, environment, and culture. I should also like to single out my Middlebury colleague, Sandy Martin, for his years of work on programs that enabled me to meet and interview dozens of professionals who are devoted both to managing complex immunological problems and to advocating in general for the needy individuals they tirelessly serve.

At the level of this book's production, I owe special thanks to Robert Churchill, Helen Reiff, and Lisa Jasinski for illustration and research assistance. And though I cannot count all of the students who have assisted in the various research projects that have been folded in one way or another into this book, I do owe special thanks to those students who both assisted directly in part of this research and who were also my thesis advisees. The weekly tutorials I held with each of them were deeply important to my remaining engaged in this project in the face of an increasingly market-driven educational workplace. Of this group, I would like to acknowledge Laura Cohen, Angel Diaz, Paul Dionne, Leslie Fesenmyer, Lisa Janicki, Ryan Kelty, Jennie Klintberg, Andrew Levinson, Doug Rogers, and Mark Vail. I would also like to thank David Brent of the University of Chicago Press, for it is rare that one can find an editor who has a keen interest in immunology and is also an accomplished philosopher in his own right. Likewise, my reviewers deserve credit for providing support and useful suggestions in the revising of the text, as does my copyeditor, Richard Allen, for his carefulness and rigor.

Finally, I should thank the many patients who are anonymously quoted in this book. Their words speak for them even if I have vowed to withhold their identities. Though the dozens of patients I interviewed in clinical setting must, by agreement, remain anonymous, I am able to thank by name those whose long-term professional and personal friendships allowed me to know them primarily outside of domains governed by the human subjects protocols to which researchers rightly subscribe. These include, in particular, the late Andrew Duff-Cooper, the late Bruce Dakowski, the late Annette Weiner, and the very much thriving Paul Stoller. Might the rest of the world attend to adversity with such dignity as they have.

To conclude a list of acknowledgments without some recognition of those who gave most to the project in human terms would be wholly inappropriate. Here, I would like to thank Elizabeth Napier for her love and caring for our two children, Andrew and Harriet, during the many years of part-time travel that this project required, and Margaret Donlon, who more than anyone else encouraged me to see this project to completion.

He who is unable to live in society, or who has no need because he is sufficient for himself, must be either a beast or a god. —Aristotle, *Poetics*

OUTSIDERS

The Caribbean writer C. L. R. James once said that "a man's unstated assumptions, those he is often not aware of, are usually the mainspring of his thoughts" ([1963] 1983, 63). The idea, from *Beyond a Boundary*, was based on James's observations of how enthusiastically his own colonized society had embraced the English game of cricket; for James loved the sport immensely, even while hating the colonial "playing field"—the foreign set of rules—that he had culturally assimilated and grown personally to value.

These "assumptions"—the things that set guidelines and boundaries—are what social anthropologists call *cultural categories of thought*; they are the basic cognitive maps that we individually obey, modify, ignore, or misread in an attempt to find meaning and value in the living of life. The categories, amorphous though they may appear to those using them, are a big part of life's picture, the other big part being how we relate to them, what we do with them, where our use of them leads us—in other words, what variety we bring to an otherwise stereotypical or essential experience of life.

For those living life at society's complacent center—for those wedded to the status quo—these categories can often go entirely unrecognized. But when they limit what is possible, or position us in ways that seem hopeless or unfair, we sometimes just stop playing cricket; we make, that is, the conscious decision to step outside of the normal rules of behavior that govern the commerce of everyday relations. For James, this move to "step out," this going "beyond a boundary," was always ignited by the inner conflict of his radical political views and his deep love for biblical morality—the merging of Marx and Trotsky with Moses and Jesus. Being colonized (inoculated, if you will, by things foreign) had made him aware of—had sensitized him to—certain dimensions of biblical thought that had escaped his more dogmatically inclined colonizers.

Indeed, many biblical stories even seem designed to encourage us to think of the importance of transcending social boundaries. I sense, for instance, that the day Jesus stormed into the temple to chase out the money changers he had given up on cricket. Intoxicated by his own anger, he had, like the hard drinker, finally left the playing field of "their" rules for a world of excess somewhere beyond the boundaries that normally guide daily living. For how else could the embodiment of self-sacrifice and compassion be so thoroughly given over to his own passions? No doubt this Jesus was deeply alienated; above all else, he feared being ignored. Like a writer with no audience, he felt some deep spiritual need for change in a complacent and unresponsive world.

Viewed this way, the parable of the money changers is less about righteous anger than about the frustrations of having one's message to others fall on deaf ears. For Jesus was an outsider—one given over not only to the recognition of himself as "different" but to the understanding that his new message to the world might easily go unrecognized. It is a feeling we are all familiar with: you know for yourself what is the right thing to do, but you fear you may never figure out how to implement what you believe in. Being "outside" has sensitized you to a certain social "need" but not necessarily to how that need might be addressed, let alone brought back to society's center. It is the age-old dilemma of wanting to change the world you live in but of not knowing if there is a place at all where you might intervene. You're at your crossroads, the place of transition, of potentiality, of unallocated power. But where to go?

Why do we so often have this feeling—of sensing what is right but not knowing how to achieve it? Though the dilemma has perhaps always characterized human indecision, why, somehow, should it seem so prevalent today? Is it the outsider's fear that society's "center" has forgotten about the need to risk anything new? Is it simply that complacency conditions us to be more complacent—that indecision leads to yet more indecision? What role can being on the outside play if the outsider's importance remains unrecognized—if his mission gets whitewashed by false kindnesses and polite language? How might "outsiders" respond to what they see as society's basic ignorance of its own degradation? Are there alternatives to storming the temple?

INSIDE OUT: A PITTSBURGH ALLEGORY

Let us begin at the beginning.—Terminator 24 (a.k.a. Reginald Young)

I was born in Pittsburgh, Pennsylvania. Even Charles Dickens, chronicler of the appalling working conditions of Victorian England, was perhaps never so horrified as by his single visit to Pittsburgh. He called it "hell with the lid off." The Pittsburgh of my childhood was not hell with the lid off, but it had its moments. During World War II, this single town produced more steel than Germany and Japan combined, and its rivers were the busiest—and the most polluted—in the world. By the 1950s it had become an environmentalist's nightmare (figure 1).

But while the city's filth made it the first place in the world to pass real anti-pollution laws, the environmental movement hardly existed. The Environ-

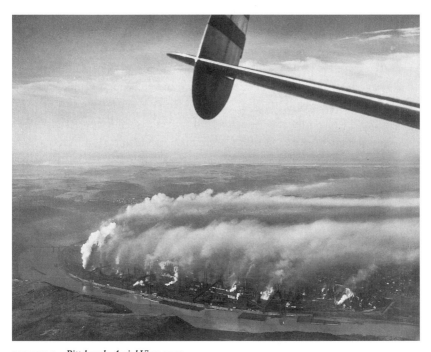

FIGURE 1. *Pittsburgh, Aerial View,* **1955**
Perhaps no place on earth more clearly represents the realities of the industrial revolution—the consequences of progress—than does the city of Pittsburgh, Pennsylvania. Charles Dickens called it "hell with the lid off," but its extreme environmental degradation also gave way to the first antipollution legislation in the world. (Photo by Margaret Bourke-White. Reproduced courtesy of Carnegie Museum of Art, Pittsburgh; gift of Carnegie Library of Pittsburgh.)

mental Protection Agency had yet to be created in response to public demand. Though my grandfather's company, begun in the early 1930s to help purify the region's contaminated water, was certainly America's first "environmental" consultancy, the words "water treatment" spoke more directly to the needs of his era than would have the environmental language now in fashion; for it is hard today to imagine the degree to which this city was industrialized. The Monongahela (how many can say they know of this Algonquian river?) was the world's busiest waterway, and the masses of miners and "mill hunkies" who went to their graves from chronic lung disease were all in "blue collar" because their work did not allow them the time taken by their white-collar bosses to change shirts at midday. The productivity of the region was ultimately reflected not only in its human and environmental degradation but in the fact that several of America's greatest fortunes were made there: Carnegie, Mellon, Scaife, and Frick were all Pittsburghers; and the discovery of oil in the nearby village of Titusville meant that other industrialists, like Rockefeller, weren't far off. Pittsburgh epitomized the "pollution" of the natural world by the invasive agents of culture and progress.

By the 1950s most of Pittsburgh's flight capital was in New York or in tax-free havens abroad, and its remaining production had been, or would soon be, either shifted to plants in Gary and Birmingham or simply eliminated. The smaller, but once lucrative, family-run mills, like those of the Swiss Heppenstalls, had already closed their doors. Pittsburgh after the Second World War became as interesting for what it was not as for what it was: it was not a cultural melting pot (though it claimed more ethnic organizations than any city in the United States); and it was not made habitable by any extraordinary civic initiative (although in recent decades it has become a better place to live). In fact, corporations like General Motors were literally taking the city apart by actions such as buying and shutting down the company that made replacement parts for the city's electric trolleys. Pittsburgh was to become a better place to live mainly because people were getting out in droves, while those who stayed, stayed put. As late as 1990, and even in 2000, Pennsylvania was the only state in the East that had once more undergone a population decrease. At the same time, those who remained, remained in the same homes longer than anywhere else in the nation. It's still not, it seems, an especially fashionable place to live, despite the fact that its industrial heritage also gave us spectacular art museums, our Carnegie free libraries, our first serious public television, and the nurturing views of adolescent socialization that would change how all American children would be taught. Of these, it was this last fact which, for me, proved crucial.

I spent the first several years of my life in a poor but still relatively stable neighborhood. And it was into that world that Dr. Benjamin Spock, along with his graduate students from the University of Pittsburgh, brought their experimental nursery school. Like building a medical school in a ghetto, there was significant social reciprocity. Spock and his students got their studies done; we got a remarkable refuge from reality. Even today the Arsenal School (it was formerly a Marine hospital) is magical—its white colonial interior, its all-wooden toys, abstract paintings, and the near total absence for over forty years of anything plastic, all mark it as a site where these intellectuals attempted to refigure society's diminished center.

And they really did try. As a preschooler there, I was so interested in building that I was given an entire room (my three-year-old's "laboratory"—for, after all, my grandfather chemist had his own) in which to construct my endless projects. This school seemed flawless in our very flawed local world, even though in some ways it was too magical; for its only oddity was the fact that all of its rooms, including the lavatories, were walled with one-way mirrors. Needless to say, I didn't grow to like mirrors in public restrooms. I still don't (figure 2).

So they watched—the "they" being not only Spock and his students but also visitors like Erik Erikson and the indefatigable Fred Rogers. Yes, Mr. Rogers also came to our school to glean ideas from Margaret MacFarland, the school's director, for his new television program, *The Children's Corner*, which ran locally from 1954 to 1961. My father has distinct memories of talking with her about the then-new programs and what she thought they should be. But, like Rosalind Franklin's contribution to understanding DNA, Margaret Mac-Farland's important thoughts were never really acknowledged. She was far too busy, anyway, thinking about our welfare and how she might generate enthusiasm for experimental psychology among participating families; for whole families contributed—not just to the upkeep of the school but to the psychological research and even to this new thing called educational television. One of my uncles hosted what must have been the first educational live-animal show for kids (we remember him driving through town with a full-grown lion in his car). Another uncle, my mother's brother, used his skills

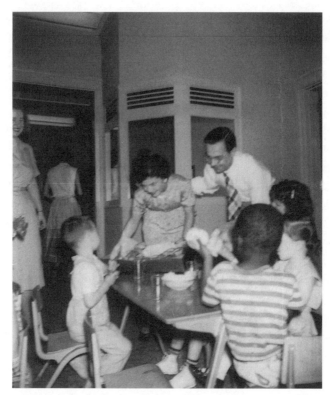

FIGURE 2. **Hall of Mirrors: An Immunological Allegory**
Arsenal Preschool, Pittsburgh, Pennsylvania. Children who attended Benjamin
Spock's experimental preschool soon learned that the mirrored walls (seen
here in the background) concealed viewing rooms for Spock and fellow
psychologists. Adults spied on children, while their subjects were "schooled"
in viewing self as other, and other as self. (From author's collection.)

as a barber to cut Mr. Rogers's hair. Erikson and Spock even requested that my
parents allow themselves to be studied as an "ideal family." Fortunately, they
refused.

The problem was not simply that they studied us; it was that they studied
us covertly, and in so doing broke the most sacred responsibility that a social
researcher can have to a child—for children in particular are psychologically
vulnerable to covert research (Homan 1991, 19), especially in classroom settings where they are "unlikely to decline to do what [is] asked of them" (123).
But we also looked at them, by looking at ourselves through the glass, for at
three one learned rather quickly about the curious anterooms, which were of-

ten left open and empty. I now know that this glass—like Alice's looking-glass—sensitized me to a lifelong interest in philosophy and art and to a fascination with ways of seeing. For the mirror effect, as Lasch once said, "makes the subject an object; at the same time, it makes the world of objects an extension or projection of the self" (1984, 30).

The mirror is also, as Genette so incisively notes, the perfect symbol of alienation.[1] At four, like many boys my age, my hero was "the masked man," the Lone Ranger. My father even convinced a store manager to sell him a larger-than-life cardboard Lone Ranger that stood in our basement until I reduced it, in battle, to debris. Perhaps it is too easy to justify that anger, as well as the alienation created in preschool by those architectural "masks"—those one-way mirrors in which one mistook another for self.

Although I never paused long enough then to think reflectively about masks, more than two decades later, when I came to write my Oxford D.Phil. on the cultural construction of personhood in non-Western societies, masks (and mirrors) became the focus for my theorizing about human behavior. It is easy, also, for me to see why I would one day become interested in theoretical immunology, for no book can be written on the topic without some firm sense of how self and not-self can be distinguished, of how pathogens blur that distinction and wear us down by masking.

Any armchair Freudian can chuckle over the developmental uncertainties that such concerns signal. But, as I will argue in this book, we cannot speak glibly about "normality" when an entire era becomes characterized by a conscious reassessment of Kant's famous questions:

1. What can I know? (metaphysics)
2. What ought I to do? (morals)
3. What may I hope? (religion)
4. What is a person? (anthropology)

In a world in which people are highly self-conscious, these questions become immediate and even threatening—a far cry from that smug satisfaction a psychiatrist may feel once he or she has got a label for something. To name—like calling an opponent in a medieval joust—is to control and even destroy someone. This is why in so many societies naming is a powerful and often dangerous activity.

To live with the paradox of potential psychological or personal transformation is far more problematic, uncertain, and, indeed, creative, than to label, to atrophy by typologizing. Accepting uncertainty demands that we admit to the possible benefits and to the real disasters that genuine change can effect. This is one of the reasons why creative people so often experience moments of existential crisis or outright clinical depression, why anxiety (as Szasz [1961] argued some time ago) is as much a sensible response to an insensible age as it is an illness as such, and why the deviations of actual phenomena from psychoanalytic categories—that is, behaviors that don't fit our models—present greater possibilities for "curing" than do those conditions that may be readily categorized.

True, there was something awfully immunological and violent about those mirrors (to which I often look for some understanding of my turbulent and pugilistic childhood), but the school itself was a wonder and a great creative stimulant. For even three-year-olds can enjoy, as Lewis Carroll knew too well, such illusory games—though I certainly had no idea at that age of how seeing "self" for "not-self" in the one-way mirror into which I gazed would later become paradigmatic of the antibody seeing itself in a mirror behind which an antigenic "other" silently waits.

A 1994 news article, addressing the then-aging Dr. Spock at the time of his publishing his last book, described him as *the* most influential living American. After all, except for the Bible, his study of children was the best-selling book of all time; he could claim, save for the Lord himself, to be the most widely read author ever. Yet I still think of him as the man who dug our sandpit with my father: on that day, they found worms for fishing; in those years, we students found the basis for the immunological imagination. Just what I mean by this is my answer to why I have written this book; for the 1994 article also described Dr. Spock as "troubled." His late despair over violence, the deterioration of the nuclear family, and the inability of many people to construct meaning in life provides a fair inventory of the destructive tendencies of modern culture; however, the other half can be creative. Rats confined to impossibly cramped quarters do attack and eat one another; but chimps suffering from like conditions—like people stuck in elevators—will often show unusual deference to the sociospatial anxieties of the group—if, that is, they have been collectively socialized in advance.

This, of course, is that same crucial "if" that keeps them from simply abandoning their babies during hard times. To put it on the sociopolitical level, our contemporary obsession with the presumed inalienability of life, liberty, and the pursuit of happiness desensitizes us to the fact that social stress—like rigorous exercise—is also adaptive and conditioning. Bad homes cause pathological lifestyles, but some wonderful people have withstood and outgrown horrid living conditions. Good people sometimes do overcome appalling childhoods and social environments. Yet, we fool ourselves into thinking that dangerous confrontations with "not-self" are always and only harmful. This assumption is undeniably wrong-headed.

Though part of this book concerns the practice of the medical science of immunology, I also in other ways use the word "immunology" quite liberally. In fact, I have intentionally applied its basic assumption—that we survive through the recognition and elimination of "nonself"—as a fundamental category, and perhaps the dominant premise, of modern life. In what follows, I have applied this assumption to the popular and erroneous expectation that change should not be painful or difficult, and to the equally unacceptable idea that "otherness" ("non-" or "not-self") can be celebrated at an appropriate and politically correct distance, or, conversely, by virtue of an assumed and unearned familiarity.

Thus, one of the central convictions that guided the writing of this book is that the language of enforced multiculturalism is actually a foil for never engaging difference, for never having to negotiate with someone who might actually be the catalyst for a real change—a period of profound uncertainty—in one's own life. In short, our assumption that we are entitled to be what we are without labor or pain positions us very poorly in the social world by suggesting to us that we can get through life—even that we are entitled to get through life—without having to earn our identities.

Indeed, we sometimes today even flaunt our ignorance of "not-self," as if an absence in the skills of human diplomacy was actually a sign of knowing who we are. My argument, in turn, is that the degradations of contemporary life are actually only signs of a moral condition, not the necessary cause of the world's social ills. An unwillingness to work, and a disrespect for those willing to risk personal change, are actually the more basic problems that need to be recognized; for it is here where the apparent coming apart of culture in this immunological era can be met by some creative response. Benjamin Spock, like Dickens before him, may see "hell with the lid off" wherever he looks; but, as Twain once said of Wagner, if you listen with a different ear, "he's not as bad as he sounds."

Introduction

Isn't it nice to know things? —Bertrand Russell to Julian Huxley

"Actors, taught not to let any embarrassment show on their faces, put on a mask. I will do the same. So far, I have been a spectator in this theater which is the world, but I am now about to mount the stage and I come forward masked." These words, one may be surprised to hear, are not those of a twentieth-century master of disguise, nor the literary ruse of a Beckett or a Pirandello, but those of René Descartes, the father of modern thought, about to embark upon his great metaphysical meditation on the origins of consciousness (1964, 10:213).

Already, Descartes knew well that the best way of understanding how the "enemy"—the pathogen—functions is to engage in some kind of intercourse with it. The best way of producing an internalized defense—an "antibody"—that can neutralize and destroy an enemy is (as anthropologists are often told in tribal settings) to marry that enemy: to devise a way (in Descartes's case, a mask) by which one can encounter that danger, produce a mild form of its infection, and thereby arrive at a method of distinguishing, and thus protecting, a "self" from an "other."

Such protective methods are, of course, essential to all masked ritual; but they also form the basis of what we now call "immunity"—where "other" becomes the "nonself" that must be identified and eliminated. Unlike the performer of a masked ritual, whose purpose in engaging "otherness" is to facilitate personal change, Descartes's sole objective in imitating "nonself" was to deconstruct (even to destroy) it. Self-consciousness, in this line of thinking, becomes not a mode of transformation, a creation of something new, but a device for inducing stasis, a surface modification that, as it were, "cheats" change by attacking difference. This, of course, is why it is so difficult for most of us to use the word "mask" in any other than a pejorative way.

It is not coincidental, then, that Descartes immediately follows his methodological confession with another: "In my youth, when I was shown an ingenious invention, I used to wonder whether I could work it out for myself before reading the inventor's account. This practice gradually led me to realize that I was making use of definite rules" (1964, 10:214). Descartes, in other words, had thought of his mask not as "inventive" (as a means of "creating") but as "innovative" (that is, as a way of "modifying an existing creation"). What he did, put simply, was engage in a trial of what patent attorneys today call "reverse engineering"—a process by which one controls another's creation by breaking it down and reassembling it. And the outcome? The Enlightenment, the Age of Discovery, the homogenization and elimination of difference that has brought us from this hoary past and into our "immunological" world.

Instead of effecting his own transformation, Descartes became—in the language of microbiology—"another's virus." For this is what viruses do: they put on masks, enter another's world, and engage in reverse engineering. Or, to be more accurate, they *are* the masks—genetic codes or templates that come to life when they are, as it were, "worn" by a cell: protein and protean, still and mutable, dead and living.

In what follows, I intend to describe how contemporary attitudes and fears about transformation and change are articulated in the theory and practice of virology and immunology, disciplines which, as Sir Gustav Nossal (1969) pointed out long ago, either stand or fall on their ability to distinguish "self" from "not-self." I hope in the process to illustrate how metaphors of immunology both reflect and are symptomatic of contemporary cultural terms within which change is or is not made possible—to illustrate how immunological metaphors influence the way individuals dynamically engage that condition of "not-self" which we call the "pathogen," and how pathological encounters are, and are not, understood.

I would like, in other words, to build upon Descartes's paradigm of the conscious relationship between "self" and "not-self" in order to provide certain examples of how cultural is our understanding of the relationship between pathogenicity and transformation—of how cells are personified and treated as volitional agents, as adversaries, as negative transformers.

Thus, although this book is about the science of immunology, it is also about immunology as a cultural paradigm; it is also, moreover, about racism in the sciences. In fact, its central argument is that immunological ideas now provide the primary conceptual framework in which human relations take place in the contemporary world. It, therefore, openly accepts that a certain metaphor of science also now dominates the social interactions in which human relations are rhetorically negotiated and described. In making my case, however, I will not accept that life follows science, or even that science has led the way to a more modern way of life; rather, my argument is that a central paradigm has found its way into our lives, and that the power of that way of seeing may be evidenced in various personal and professional domains, including—because they focus on "well-being" and its absence—the medical sciences.

This study, therefore, may be characterized as an analysis of the ways in which "self" and an *internalized* "nonself" function: culturally, medically, scientifically. Though using self and other to construct boundaries may be essential to what we call identity, the increasing *internalization of difference* within a presumably autonomous self may, arguably, be what distinguished immunology from other time-honored techniques for dealing with difference. Indeed, its medicalization may, as a scientific practice, be all that separates immunology from simple demonology. But it is an important distinction, for it makes possible new forms of living that, while echoing the past, will nevertheless set the stage for the coming millennium. It is this scientific demonology, therefore, that forms both the sine qua non of immunology and the essential metaphor for modern life.

Broadly speaking, immunology—the attempted elimination of the internalized "other"—is projected everywhere. So, why favor a "scientific" conceptualization of immunology rather than a cultural, a metaphorical, or even a mythological one? Why look at science at all when the central metaphors of immunology are not the exclusive property of the medical discourse that has crystallized around them—when what scientists say is so frequently obfuscated by the esoteric language of its priesthood, when scientists who began reading the opening paragraphs of this introduction may already have closed this book?

First, because the science—its theoretical basis, its history, the way it is practiced—can be studied. By its language and its practice science has increasingly contained and isolated itself as a body of knowledge. Its presumed strength is, in other words, also its weakness; for, in its smug refusal to say much of anything simply, it has become vulnerable and limited. Immunology stands or falls on a few very fundamental assumptions; as an important medical science, it is quite recent; and its youth has led it to describe itself openly, and to be practiced, in ways that are sometimes stark, startling, and even at times innocently prejudiced. Though its main defense is to argue our ignorance, we will see that its paradoxes are not inescapable, and that they can be understood by anyone patient enough to unravel them.

Second, in examining both the science of immunology and its cultural content we can see just how much these domains of esoteric knowledge are in fact dependent on the same cultural values that are everywhere else at work— to wit, how the relational paradigms of cellular biology have made consistent, but limited, use of the heroic constructs we so deeply value at the social and religious levels. If Darwin's survival through competition is understood as the hero epic which certainly it is, there must of necessity be a concluding episode (scientists beware) in which, as Lord Raglan (1936) once prophetically demonstrated, the hero dies out—alone, ignored, in isolation, even untouchable.

Although I will not presently provide an overview of my entire project, I will, for purposes of debate, broadly review my line of thought—as much as a way of orienting readers with respect to what will follow, as a way of summarizing my argument.

First, I believe that humans fundamentally admire change (especially growth)—organic, social, religious—but live in fear of it. Likewise, I believe that much of our attention to change (developmental, evolutionary, morphological) is actually directed toward its opposite—namely, toward stasis. Here, anthropology provides a perspective that, to modernists at least, seems counterintuitive; for the worldwide evidence concerning processes of transformation indicates that lasting change is almost always orchestrated not through slow growth, but—problematic though it may seem—through what I have elsewhere called "selective dissociation" (Napier 1992). By selective dissociation I refer to the processes of deindividuation, inversion, and catharsis that mark worldwide the threshold crossings we associate with traditional rites of passage.

I believe, similarly, that the function of self-consciousness for the process of transformation is largely preventive—that is, self-consciousness serves to disrupt (in both positive and negative ways) the embodiment of the dynamic preconditions of change. Self-consciousness, in other words, is preservative; it helps us to control and not be controlled by the cultural values that unselfconsciously govern our daily lives—to separate a sense of self from what anthropologists call "covert cultural categories." Perceiving others to be swayed by "popular opinion," in other words, is just like choosing stasis over change: it may save one's identity, but it may also stop one from growing. Like Descartes's mask, self-consciousness helps us to understand in advance, and thereby to limit, the "other," the "outside" forces by which we might have been, under different conditions, transformed. It directly stalls transformation. Here, I would point to the basic conundrum of psychoanalysis—how is it possible self-consciously to become unselfconscious about one's inner demons?

Second, I believe that the Age of Immunology is not only a result of the extreme self-consciousness that characterizes modernity, but a coded parable (a story) about identity stasis. On the microbiological level, Descartes's mask has its analogue in the virus that only comes alive when it is "worn" by a cell—becoming a cell that looks like its prey. The viral cell is, as it were, the "product" of self-consciousness: it perpetuates its own stasis by donning your appearance. It looks like you. It fools you in order to "reverse engineer" you. In this way, viruses are no different than Descartes's mask, since his self-conscious motives are structurally identical to the pathogenic behavior of viruses. Descartes's act of "possessing" the other is the same act that accounts for our fear of being virally possessed.

Third, I believe that the "Age of Self-Awareness" (from Descartes and the Enlightenment onward), eventually creates a deceptive rhetoric of "not-self" that is largely defensive. Here, in concepts of diversity and in socially acceptable speech, the rhetoric of acknowledging difference allows for a kind of cultural potluck dinner at which we each bring a different dish but all eat by the same rules. We invite the Balinese as long as he doesn't eat with his hands; the Indian can come if he doesn't belch; and the Greek of old may have his lamb, but he may not sacrifice it first. The potluck, in other words, uses a rhetoric of difference to destroy what is genuinely "not-self"—to eliminate those habits that, to extend the analogy, "make us sick." The microbiological parallel here is the selective medium, the petri dish, in which a culture is engineered to encourage a particular life form from a diffuse, unspecified field—to limit certain kinds of growth and to promote others. And let us not forget that in the lab, as in life elsewhere, an ideal culture of cells is one that has a single pro-genitor—one that is cloned from a quite conservative ideal. Like those cells, we too employ a rhetorical acknowledgment of diversity in order to avoid en-counters with that which is *different.*

Fourth, I believe that while the potluck dinner has as its hidden agenda the preservation of "self," the direct result of having defused unequal or danger-ous "not-selves" is, simply put, that we unlearn or actually forget how to ne-gotiate subtly with difference; in fearing the pain, we forget the pleasures that such negotiating can bring. Now in our petri dish we see how cells at the cen-ter of our "culture" are the most complacent (the least dynamic, the least ca-pable of adaptation). The evidence for this ignorance is to be found in all of the salvage operations that we exercise on that "other"—that "not-self"— once it is no longer a threat. It is the old story of not knowing what you've got until it's gone. Teddy Roosevelt invents the national park system once all of the wildness has been mapped; he and J. P. Morgan subsidize the encyclope-dic recording of Native Americans (by Edward Curtis) once all of their belli-cose forms of life have been eliminated; today, we fight for the rights of tribal peoples and glorify their lifestyles once we have finally pacified those who fight most—when, furthermore, not a single group of traditional peoples stands capable of sustaining our top-heavy ecological programs. Alas, we fuel the rage for "environmental studies" even at the very moment when no part of the world remains uninfluenced by our industrial errors, and I must watch while my students all flock to this field, and embrace every cliché about tribal peoples as noble anachronisms, while there has not been a single long-term success in managing traditional resources through the deployment of what the foreign service community has hideously labeled "cultural capital."

The list is endless, but the scheme whereby the soul of the unknown or un-knowable is destroyed, and its corpse tamed and revivified, is fairly consistent. Here, Mary Shelley's worst nightmare of a reconstructed "other" may be commonly evidenced in the many editorials in which even blue-blooded racists will argue for cultural diversity on the grounds that the sparing of tribal peoples is necessary not for humanitarian reasons but in order to preserve a diversified gene pool. The cells at the center of the petri dish have, alas, vaguely sensed the potential consequences of their own complacency, even if they have fully unlearned the necessary role that difference plays in their own survival.

Fifth, I believe that the result of protecting ourselves from transformational encounters with "otherness"—our desire, as it were, to be at the center of the colony—is a social hysteria wherein the absence of an awareness of the "differences" that can only be experienced at the boundaries leads us to repeat in ever more banal ways our culturally valued narratives of change (hero epic for most of us). Like the repetitive actions of an autistic child, or of a mouse repeatedly washing itself when confronted by a cat, these narratives are incessantly reenacted through the media and through life itself in ways that become increasingly facile, as if to remind us of a connection that we think we should have but that we cannot verify locally. As Bill Buford claims, in his horrifying and graphic account of British soccer hooliganism, the behavior of the most violent hooligans is basically an exaggeration, an "ornate version of an ancient [working-class] style, more extreme because now without substance":

> But it is only a style. Nothing substantive is there; there is nothing to belong to, although it is still possible . . . to belong to a phrase—the working class—a piece of language that serves to reinforce certain social customs and a way of talking and that obscures the fact that the only thing hiding behind it is a highly mannered suburban society stripped of culture and sophistication and living only for its affectations: a bloated code of maleness, an exaggerated embarrassing patriotism, a violent nationalism, an array of bankrupt antisocial habits. This bored, empty, decadent generation consists of nothing more than what it appears to be. It is a lad culture without mystery, so deadened that it uses violence to wake itself up. It pricks itself so that it has feeling, burns its flesh so that it has smell. (1991, 264–65)

One need only replace Buford's working class with the multicultural society to see how the banal celebration of diversity also becomes more grotesque as the supposed differences honored become less substantial.

Sixth, I believe that this incessant repetition of the simplest forms of hero epic, from Pasteur's magic bullet to Clint Eastwood's, is our best evidence of our cultural autoimmunity, our culture at war with itself—of a social and psychogenic shock where peripheral circulation shuts down in an attempt to salvage blood for the brain in the form of the narratives of transformation that society values most, and where the subtle negotiation of our boundaries gives way, first, to a preservation of the body's core, but, eventually, to the production of its own pathogens, to its own anaphylaxis. This is what I mean when I call ours an Age of Immunology.

WHY NOW?

> *Everything is falling into place. It can't be too long now. Ezekiel says that fire and*
> *brimstone will be rained down upon the enemies of God's people. That must mean that*
> *they will be destroyed by nuclear weapons.* —Ronald Reagan

Anyone who grew up in the United States in the postwar era knows how little cultural awareness was necessary for survival. It is also easy to remember how little time was devoted to reflecting on the fact that success was plentiful: I don't think I can remember a single child my age whose father had not easily eclipsed the financial security of the previous generation. Though everyone in the middle class was not wealthy, every parent came from a family dominated by silent sufferers of the Great Depression, who, themselves, were easily stupefied by the mere absence of true suffering. When I think of all of the brash parents (and silent grandparents) that I knew, I cannot believe that everyday people never stood back and questioned this obvious social reality. Nobody seemed much alarmed by the fact that it took something like an idiot to bungle the economic and egoistic opportunities made possible by the era that brought us the material excesses of the 1950s and 1960s. That's how overt the expression of ego can be.

It is hard, except nostalgically, to excavate the uncritical sentiments that dominated that era—partly because criticism and self-doubt are central paradigms of our (not their) age. "There must be something right about what we're doing if the outcomes are what we now experience." This is a view not only made explicit in Calvinism; it was an embodied principle of capital enterprises in America at mid-century. Surely, the period between—and including—the wars was deeply difficult; but self-doubt was, itself, far less frequently thought of as a virtue: reality was, as it still largely is, justified by the living out of the heroic narrative in every small space in our great landscape.

Simply stated, we have now reached a different chapter of that epic in which the heroic obsessions of that generation will either bring the world down within their lifetime in Reagan's self-fulfilling Armageddon, or the world will learn how to look back upon that time as one of unexamined excess—in which those obsessed with their own heroic portrayal start looking as crude and overstated to us as do the "boats" in which many of them rode to the office (see figure 3).

Why, then, we now find ourselves at this cultural juncture is as much a function of the way we embody these heroic narratives—how they become

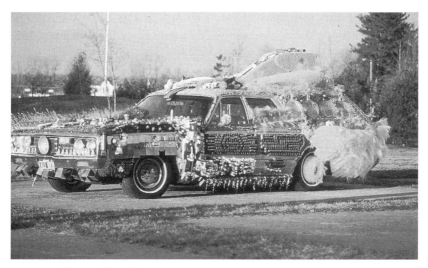

FIGURE 3. *Town and Gown Car*

In the work of Californian car artist David Best, the waste and excess of American culture is visually represented by the dramatic violation and demystification of a cultural icon. In a surrealist's worldview, Americans of the postwar era might have more honestly and openly reveled in the excessive display of familial fetishes and cultural totems, for excess was itself idolized. (Photo by Candice Wilhelmsen.)

somatic stories—as it is a function of the domains of experience that we label "political," "social," or "economic." One argument of *The Age of Immunology* is, therefore, that we are obsessed by a sequential notion of history that encourages us to play out our hero epic over the brief life of the single generation that can appropriate this myth and embody it. We not only create our own history by attaching events to a deeply entrenched heroic narrative, but we become trapped by that narrative, fulfilling the role that has imprisoned us, a "Children's Crusade" where our consuming ends in being consumed.

Today, there are lots of people who are suffering this way—people whose parents were quite happy to have our culturally prescribed "hero" epic unfold in their own lifetime. I can't think of anyone I grew up with whose father did not have more opportunity than either his Great Depression parents or his post-1960s children. In that "suburban" generation one had to be a true sociopath (or someone without civil liberties) not to be able to own a house, buy a new car regularly, afford a family vacation, or provide basic familial needs. Even minimal wage-earners could send their kids to college and find a way to make it work financially.

One need not exaggerate this point to see that those who survived the pains of the Second World War were poised for the first time in recent history to embody within their own lifetime the heroic myths our society had worked for centuries to realize. Clearly, the biggest baby-boom wound is the one created by growing up as a character actor in the hero epic of one's parents: the postwar era was in America a time of unlimited resources; a time when we created modernity and filled our museums with it; a time when a last generation of respected intellectuals lived out their university careers and sent their own graduate students off to drive taxi cabs for a living. These are not so much facts as they are deeply accepted perceptions: as history makes clear, the sons and daughters of "heroes" almost never amount to anything, for they are given no value outside of the subsidiary role provided them by parents who were actually tempted to believe that they had been selected by the hand of God and that they deserve such rewards.

Loved though these children were, their role was clear: to participate in the epic narrative of their parents. There is lots of evidence for this: the most grotesque example is Reagan's private belief in Armageddon—the belief not only that he was a culture hero (the once-voiced opinion that the country was "inside Mr. Reagan"), but that the world was never as good, and could never again be as good, as it was in his lifetime. How convenient to have a religion that also predicted that the world would end just about when he would.

Although in some ways this generation of Americans may have been kind, it is abundantly clear (and will become clearer as the years go on) that it was a generation that did not believe in a future because it was too self-absorbed to know how to want one. Even when it is financially more advantageous to disperse family assets, many Americans with six-figure incomes (and seven-plus-figure estates) die allowing the state to take what they will not give to their own children. Compare this to the Hindu view—in which to die without plowing back one's shares is the greatest form of evil—and you get by contrast the picture of our culture (as one that has no concern for the perpetuation of its lineages), and certain traditional cultures (that value this continuity deeply). Hercules is our he-man; let us not forget that he also ate his own kids.

Looked at epically, we find ourselves in an "immunological" era perhaps now poised to reopen Lord Raglan's neglected, majestic study of the hero; for there we can discover not only how much our homogenization of human difference has caused us to simplify heroic narrative, but just how much that homogenization has led us to unlearn certain crucial elements of what makes epic narrative meaningful. These being, in particular, the fact that, though the hero may be the son of a god, we know almost nothing about his childhood, and that, though his children are positioned to succeed him, they almost never do so with success—either because of his own egoism, or because of their own impotence.

In either case, what is clear—and this is the crucial point—is that *his children are raised to be vicarious participants in his life*, and that they themselves, despite the real anguish and torment they may experience, never amount to much. In fact, their world becomes characterized by the rejection of self. It becomes "autotoxic"—whether this cultural autoimmunity is the consequence of the Tarzan-like suppression of hero epic's less palatable features (of its being performed in simpler and simpler involutions), or whether the cultural autoimmunity, the entrapped self-hatred, that we see played out every day in American life is an inevitable consequence of the pioneer mentality that induces us to abandon those parts of self we can no longer sustain, to run off in search of something new because we can no longer tolerate the place that should be "home," to escape into the mountains in search of purity.

Given the potential pessimism of these observations, the task of writing this book has not always been a sanguine one: to talk openly about the age of immunology risks inducing terrific depression, as well as the wrath of those who hide behind whatever ideological problem affords them comfort. Still, there is enough of a directive in an anthropology of immunology that, one hopes, some practical benefit can be had; moreover, I do believe that these difficulties can be overcome, painful though the process of so doing might be. If anything, immunology's recognition and elimination of "not-self" embodies at the emotional level the deferred human contact that we have come to live with and, alas, accept. Immunology provides the right metaphor for appreciating what must be addressed in transforming the apparently hopeless isolation of contemporary life into an outcome we can treat creatively if not wholly admire. For Americans who feel that they are entitled by birthright not to suffer, the investment of energy required to transform may be more than they are willing to risk. Such people will temporarily comfort themselves in that "ornate" style made more extreme because it is now without substance. They will, in other words, choose to huddle together like cells at the center of the colony, to don the darkened protective spores that signal their fear of change (see figure 4).

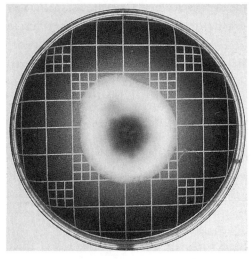

FIGURE 4. **Cell Colony, Species of** *Aspergillus*
Usually a disease-causing opportunistic pathogen, *Aspergillus* is also used commercially (e.g., in the fermentation of soy sauce and in the production of citric acid). In this colony we see death at the colony's center in the form of the darkened spores created by cells to protect themselves. Though cells living on the edges of the colony are in real danger, their lives are much more vital and dynamic. (From *A Photographic Atlas for the Microbiology Laboratory*, by Michael Leboffe and Burton E. Pierce [Englewood, Colo.: Morton Publishing Company, 1996], 125. Reproduced courtesy of Morton Publishing Company.)

Finally, as a more optimistic act of faith, I believe that psychological transformation and human change are creative ventures, that they occur when one encounters difference and finds some space in which the net result of an encounter with a genuine "other" is greater than the sum of the parts of that encounter—where "taking a chance" (i.e., deciding deliberately to step over the boundary—from what can be consciously articulated into what must be phenomenally sensed) facilitates the creation of something genuinely "new." Now in our petri dish we see not only how static and complacent cells become at the center of our "culture," but by contrast, how those at the periphery of the colony—where toxic wastes do not collect in high concentrations—tend to have access to the nutrients of change and, therefore, to be the most vibrant. Remember, cell colonies are cultures that are engineered not only to promote certain types of growth but to limit others.

This study, if such an exploratory treatise can be so called, is in some places closely argued and in others expansive. The former occurs mainly where another has taken up an important detail (e.g., in describing an illness experience, or a scientific research strategy): in such instances my relatively close commentary is meant both to isolate what I take to be essential to a general view of what immunological thought gives rise to, and to indicate why certain elements of another's overall thesis cannot be readily discounted. Elsewhere, I try to make the argument as directly as a former autistic can, and to make it, so far as is possible, accessible. The project was taken up for those who are not afraid of generalities, and its flaws I ask the reader to anticipate with this objective in mind. Writing something general about disciplines that deliberately obfuscate is always dangerous. My justification is that immunology is a symptom, not the cause, of the kind of simplifying—the dumbing down—that we have allowed to dominate, and sometimes to defeat, our creative inclinations. What are the real costs, in other words, of our obsessive denial of difference?

The book is also based upon a fundamental bias regarding creative life: I say openly that today's world relies heavily on innovation (the streamlining of an existing art) rather that on invention (the creation of novel ideas). Despite exponential population growth, we have produced no more Edisons, Bells, and Einsteins than did previous generations. We have, in fact, produced fewer. The Age of Immunology relies heavily on innovation for survival. It is, regrettably, a paranoid view of the world seen not through McLuhan's rear-view mirror, or Carroll's looking glass, but over one's shoulder. In lab science it actually results in an obsession with reverse engineering—with trying to dissect the means by which something was put together in order to see if it can be modified into something that legally qualifies as "different." This is one grotesque consequence of worshipping in Darwin's chapel of innovations; it is also an end to a certain conceptual scheme of productive life.

The drawback to identifying a cell only by its surface receptors is, to extend the biological metaphor, that you can't distinguish the antigens from the antibodies. It is easy, in other words, to be "for the environment," and easier still to appear to be morally responsible by simply laying claim to an understanding of another's suffering. Having the luxury *not* to form human alliances may, as in any mannerist age, leave us unaware of just what is to be gained by making them.

Part I Anthropology

What do you do when you have the deep sense that you are just not making it? As the only son of a family with four daughters, for me there might have been little in the way of contestation, or, perhaps, everything was contested. My godmother, my father's sister, had five boys to whom I became an older brother. Her husband, my godfather, was an ex-Marine (in fact and in spirit) who worked for my father. Four of those boys became fighter pilots; I chose anthropology.

As an anthropologist, one freely describes the particulars of everyday experience among one's subjects; but vanity normally keeps us from considering ourselves exemplary of much of anything. So, why should I introduce this unsensational information? I think because it is a conundrum for me, an example of one curious notion of ego that I find deeply "immunological." Let me explain.

When I was a child I insisted on dressing only in black. I would have nothing else to wear because black allowed me a place where options were real: I defended Indians; I felt duty bound to defend almost anyone; I fought constantly; I loved nature; I took the name of Francis when I had to be confirmed. My primary sport—swimming and high diving—left my Mediterranean complexion enough "black" that I spent many summers in urban Pittsburgh and rural Appalachia being called "nigger." In the parlance of psychology these inclinations would be distressing.

Yet, what is the origin of psychosis? Is it found in the photograph of me as a child playing Elvis songs on a guitar at age three? Or the hours, days, years I spent in autistic, percussive spasms that had me rebounding off of walls and chairs and couches? Maybe it is located in a congenital spinal problem that complicated simple body functions, or its pain which created a need for constant motion—like some Hindu pilgrim for whom meaning becomes embodied in a kind of repetitive visceral swooning?

*Perhaps it is more common still—like the wallowing in dirt that every child recog-
nizes as the most primordial form of ecstasy.*

*Were I that child today, I would certainly be diagnosed as having some attention deficit
disorder. I would be "medicalized" and labeled. I would be contained from completing
whatever private rite of passage these dissociative episodes kept trying to make happen. The
pain of knowing that one can grow out of hardship but hasn't raises the question of whether
we gain new strengths of character when change occurs. Is it any wonder that so-called
"depth" psychologists—whose notions of ego are inherited from Descartes—found me and
my kind strange objects of fascination? After all, where else could they turn for their
wilderness children, their little savage monsters who would cry while pounding at the earth
during a heavy rain, or who would be deeply grieved by the simple event of forced bathing?*

*I raise these episodes to make clear my view that there is a commonness to the other
we fear. After all, nothing described here is very novel or extreme, even if excising the
strange from the normal, exaggerating it, made the psychologists who peered at me
through one-way mirrors feel very fulfilled. The experiences I relate, in other words,
are not especially edifying: they neither contribute to a refined notion of what it means
to be human, nor do they allow me to establish any control over a specific rhetorical domain, to speak to people here and now about "the other side." I relate them to illustrate
how* uncommonness *is located for us in the common—how for each of us life becomes
a struggle to recreate one's past in a world that tries to label the uncertainty of transformation as "other"—to overinscribe ("I had a problem") experiences that should
not be so quickly named, labeled, and codified.*

*And is it not mere codification—inscribing, naming—to which we all pay hom-
age anyway? Man is a namer, the Bible tells us. Nobody wants to read a text that
cannot be appropriated, expropriated, transcribed, and inscribed onto another experiential domain. And, yes, I was aware as a child of the degree to which I had become a
spectacle for the Spocks of this world; for there was the director of our school, the gen-
teel and self-effacing Margaret MacFarland, who provided the ideas for the likes of
Benjamin Spock and the ubiquitous Mr. Rogers—that man who, as a graduate student, visited our school in search of ideas for our nation's first programming in what
was then called "educational television." Indeed, there were many (including Erik
Erikson) who saw in our preschool enclave a fertile ground for inscribing themselves
on the history of an "enlightened" world of adolescent psychology. Finding a black
"other" inside a white exterior, that was the reverse engineering that made them so
very "enlightened."*

*Stigma and naming—making psychology out of the peculiar manifestations of
cultural categories of thought: this is what I would now like to explore.*

1 | Anthropological Inoculations

all the people that you made in your image, see them starving on their feet 'cause they don't get enough to eat from God. . . . —Andy Partridge, "Dear God"

LOCAL KNOWLEDGE

In 1974, on a very hot Virginia day, I accidentally drove a scythe into a nest of hornets while clearing a farm pasture. Caught in the swarm, I received numerous stings and enough venom to make my entire body swell into a leathery second skin, a grotesque version of Descartes's mask. I was beginning to experience anaphylaxis, the basis, one might argue, of our modern understanding of immunology (Moulin 1989). Had I been able to consider my condition abstractly, I would have described the feeling as quite literally "superficial," as if the tingling sensation were occurring to another body, or on the surface of a rubberized diving suit. My rapid breathing and irregular heartbeat combined to produce a sense of profound disorientation—indeed, a near complete state of dissociation. People appeared to me as if in a dream, a semi-conscious state.

The strangeness of the experience of anaphylaxis, though, was far less unsettling than were the fundamental ways in which this experience changed my life. I am still not clear about all of the cultural implications of coming of age as an immunological participant-observer, but let me outline a few of them.

Because my experience took place not very far from one of the best teaching hospitals in the United States, my treatment became an education not only for me but also for the up-and-coming doctors who stared down at me that day while one of them hopelessly tried to find a place to insert an IV. The resident in charge proudly informed them that this was the real thing: all of the other localized vespid swelling they had previously seen was not indicative of the systemic reaction they were now witnessing. I will never forget that day: not so much the physical sensation as the lecture I received before leaving the hospital. Indeed, the description of what had happened to me was perhaps even more disturbing than the experience itself; for, though shock is frightening and strange, it is not exactly painful, and, in any case, I was not in a position at the time to reflect in any systematic way about what was taking place. Now I was being told that my body could not recognize itself—that a reaction designed by nature to save me (by limiting peripheral circulation in a moment of trauma) had taken its morbid turn; that my body (me?) had misjudged itself because some of my cells had mistaken "self" for "nonself." I also learned that certain antigens had had the privilege of reading Descartes.

Finally, the prescriptive lecture: avoid bees assiduously, but, if you do happen to be stung, remain calm at all cost. Otherwise, you may die. The classic double-bind: as in seeing a road sign and trying not to read it, I felt bound by a prescription that could not be implemented. "But am I actually allergic?" I asked. After all, hadn't I received a rather large dose of venom? The problem, of course, was that I had been sensitized; the only way of knowing whether or not the next sting would be lethal would be to experience it.

In the era of HIV, it's hard to imagine how much less glamorous a discipline immunology was prior to the epidemic. After all, for those educated in the postwar boom, the eradication of major illnesses was the stuff of which scientific heroes were made (Moulin 1996). Ultimately, I am grateful for my anaphylaxis because it thrust me as an experiential observer into a discipline that, though today flooded with *heroi iatroi* (hero-physicians), was then, at least at the local clinical level, the refuge of those doctors who (so their colleagues thought) could not make it professionally in the rough and tumble world of surgery or in the competitive world of research dedicated to the elimination of major diseases. I raise this point not so as to claim any kind of ethnographic authority for my experience (though anthropology, like medical science itself, had yet to find immunology glamorous in 1974), but more to help emphasize how rapid and recent has been immunology's rise both as a science and as a domain of popular discourse (Moulin 1989).

So, there I was, a soon-to-be anthropologist intent on carrying out research in tropical Southeast Asia, being told about prevention: that I was to avoid contact with bees; that the next sting might have no effect whatsoever, it might kill me; but that, were I stung, I should remain calm (since reactions, though not themselves psychosomatic, could be so influenced) and find my way immediately to a specialist. Despite the reverse engineering that was taking place in my body, I decided to do fieldwork anyway.

I don't need to invoke here the many double-binds that I lived out in the following years, or recount the unrealistic treatment scenarios that they gave rise to when I contemplated my epiphany as taking place during one of my stays in some remote part of the world. Rather, I would like to move on to a second example, of, as it were, "the inoculation of an anthropologist," because it offers a much better sense of how Descartes's mask already signals the immunological conundrum—this being, how can you get close enough to a pathogen so as to know it, while distancing yourself from its morbidity enough so that it becomes possible to achieve a state of immunity? How can one remain unmoved by a potential danger—a negative transformer? Here, the social manifestation of the vaccine—the medium by which we introduce a pathogen of lesser virulence—can be examined cross-culturally. This is particularly important if what we hope to understand better are the ways in which the theoretical problems of contemporary immunology are socially constructed and personally understood.

THE CROSS-CULTURAL DIMENSION

"Experience," as Herman Melville once said, "is the best judge," except, he cautions, in cases of genuine transformation. I ask, therefore, that the reader permit me one more autobiographical example; for it gives some indication, as Latour (1987) has argued for the ethnography of science, of the need to follow an idea wherever it leads, regardless of what boundaries it crosses. In my case, this search has meant following the one-way mirrors of my childhood: first, to an interest in personification (1986); second, to the creative arts and a study of the cultural assimilation of "otherness" (1992); and now, to the visceral assimilations (creative and destructive) of the masked or monstrous other.

Some years after my encounter with anaphylaxis, I went to Bali with the idea in mind of looking at how the Balinese employ ritual—especially masks and trance states—to negotiate socially with their own pathogens. Such a task could not be accomplished without, at some level, examining how trances are used in Bali as an arena of somatic negotiation. Though I still cannot profess any special understanding of this phenomenon, I can readily demonstrate the relevance of cross-cultural studies for reframing immunology by showing why good animists (like the Balinese) make, in general, the best "immunologists." To do this I will put forth some concrete cases of animism in action, and, later on, show how this animism better positions individuals not only to respond to the naive international health propaganda that they are fed, but to adjust through novel ways of thinking to whatever new dimensions of human suffering they face.

There is no doubt that polytheists (and, in particular, those good animists who expend much effort negotiating with harmful demons) are already highly sensitized to immunological concepts—in fact, much more sensitized than the average bench scientist. In Balinese ritual, the conceptual framework for immunity (for understanding why one would inoculate a modified virus as a preventive measure against negative transformation) is already highly developed through negotiations with a diverse and diffuse range of pathogenic agents; indeed, immunity from demons—the social prevention of undesirable transformations through interactions with the "other"—more or less defines what ritual is all about.

Ritual, therefore, tells us something about how transformation can be dynamically negotiated at the peripheries of what can be known about "self," rather than only telling us about how the assumptions of who we are, and our expectations about what will happen, can be preserved. Ritual becomes the major vehicle for addressing social and individual diseases, and particularly in so-called "polytheistic" contexts; for recreating well-being in the presence of something pathogenic is largely accomplished by orchestrating powerful symbolic stimuli—by creating hyper-real contexts in which some kind of visceral embodiment at least becomes possible. Disease, like religious experience, is a site of transformation—a space that is uniquely created, off limits to outsiders who may want to represent it, full of both uncertainty and potential. Anthropologists have noted this phenomenon worldwide. Most often it is seen in the way that illness leads to transcendence,[1] but even where real illness is not the catalyst for becoming a healer, mentors may intentionally sicken their initiates to sensitize the transformational moment.[2]

Here are some "social" examples of what I am suggesting. None of these will strike those with a clinical fix on health as necessarily "medical"; however, all of them are "sociosomatic" in the sense that they have important consequences for our understanding of human change. They also show how the "everyday" world of experience is not, as many anthropologists argue, the primary site of "real," lived meaning, but a place that actually has meaning because it can be affiliated with the more-than-real ritual domains in which symbols come together as powerful, super-real transformers:

A man about to partake in a well-known and often-observed Balinese trance ritual puts on a mask and suddenly runs out of the temple and into the jungle. We follow him to a graveyard, where he speaks in tongues from beneath a holy cloth about the specific misdeeds of those present. The entire temple festival is reorganized in response to the god's dissatisfactions.

A friend returns from a festival with laments. He is sorry another ritual obligation had prevented me from accompanying him to his mountain village, for a deity was so impressed with the dancing that it announced that no one would ever again be allowed to dance in the ancient sacred mask that had been worn. After an initial shock, the villagers built a shrine for the old mask and asked the local carver to make a new one for next year. The priest would consecrate it, and the festival would continue with an additional ceremony at the new shrine.

On the eve of an important temple celebration a group of villagers take their sacred mask in the middle of the night to a powerful temple in a spiritually quite dangerous seaside location. Everyone is terrified, but all recognize the necessity of these actions for attracting a particularly powerful force to the mask. We wait in fear for a few hours. Occasional outbursts of violent trance heighten the silent anxiety. Suddenly a young girl begins to speak in the god's voice. "But she could not possibly," all agree, "be the vehicle for such a powerful force." A brief silence (that seems endless) is followed by uproarious laughter. Later accounts would confirm that a petty demon had entered this unprepared youth and was using her as a vehicle to impersonate the invited and more powerful spirit.

The first point that is made obvious in these examples is that there is no such thing as a "typical" catharsis, and that pathogens and their illnesses, like the rituals employed to negotiate with them, are never and can never be "typical." Second, there is a lesson here for what we have come to call "actor-focused" anthropology—that is, the form of the discipline which maintains that significance can be located as much in the examination of the minor everyday encounters of a specific ego (e.g., Bourdieu) as in major cathartic orchestrations, where change takes place when actors deploy specific strategies in the face of new or novel phenomena, and where actors deliberately, if not altogether self-consciously, challenge the tyranny of "the system." What "immunology" in the field makes abundantly obvious, however, is the need to distinguish between boundary maintenance and the requirements of transformation—the former of which is *innovative* (preservationist and adaptive), while the latter is *inventive* (transformative and cathartic).

Inoculating a modified virus as a preventive measure against a negative transformer is first and foremost a *social* activity, as the Latin *immunis* (a release from reciprocal social obligation) indicates; for a physical force can have no meaning unless it is contextualized, and ritual (a word our biologists have ruined by limiting its meaning to repetitive, dysfunctional behavior) provides the only setting in which dynamic consensus can be phenomenally achieved—where dissociation allows for the possibility of real change.

According to the practice-based view, however, a study of daily routines—the lived experience, or practice of daily events, that has become the current vogue in my field—is meant to illustrate how cultural meaning is embodied in minor activities, which, as Ortner puts it, are thought to "embody within themselves, the fundamental notions of temporal, spatial, and social ordering that underlie and organize the system as a whole" (1984, 154). In such circumstances, however, the prospect of missing the forest for the trees is real. It is not that "culture" is absent in the everyday world, but, put most simply, that one has to leave in order to come back—that the powerful settings we call "rituals" are the conduits for the most transformative kinds of embodiment.

So, why do social theorists undermine the importance of ritual in favor of the everyday? Why tear down the delicate phenomenal theaters that others have constructed, unless only because we ourselves have been desensitized to how common grounds of performance can be artfully rendered and carefully utilized? Although attention to the "self" may be universal, the actual "localization" of self-interest may be, as we will see, only a major Enlightenment theme in which heroics are measured by the successful neutralization of difference. Focusing on the workaday worlds of those who live within other systems of thought may be what one would expect from those whose own moral horizons have descended to pedestrian levels, but such focusing in no way reflects the diverse moral domains that anthropologists purport to study.

Much, of course, depends on how we define or measure what is "normal" and what is "anomalous"[3]—that is, on how individuals see the relationship between their personal actions and the range of socially tolerated behaviors available to them. The distinction is especially telling, since "practice," by definition, implies innovative responses to acceptable forms of social engagement. To our focus on "actors," therefore, Ortner adds other central conundra: these being, first, the issue of "whether in fact all practice, everything everybody does, embodies and hence reproduces the assumptions of the system. . . . How, if actors are fully cultural beings, they could ever do anything that does not in some way carry forward core cultural assumptions. . . . Whether divergent or non-normative practices are simply variations upon basic cultural themes, or whether they actually imply alternative modes of social and cultural being" (1984, 155). Indeed, culture *is* embodied in minor activities, but the way that individuals work with those meanings is, as we will see in the following chapter, rarely conscious. Second, there is also a conundrum in thinking of culture as a system against which individuals act, since "major social change does not for the most part come about as an intended consequence of action. Change is largely a by-product, an unintended by-product, of action, however rational [that] action may have been" (175).

I would go further still: in downplaying anthropology's more traditional focus on ritual, we fail to recognize the mechanisms by which major change— i.e., transformation—is facilitated. For while transformation requires an initial intention to change, the actual change itself nearly always (I am tempted to say *always*) results from the willful depersonalization, deindividuation, or dissociation that individuals are, by definition, at a loss to articulate in advance. There is, put simply, no other means by which one can at all positively project an intention into its outcome (one's past into one's future) so as to become what one is not. And it is here where ritual offers the best chance to engage one's dissociative condition with powerful cultural narratives that have been brought into collective focus; it is here, in other words, where real change becomes possible, even if, or precisely because, it cannot be guaranteed.

Thus, in the following chapters, we will see how this attention to individual action—as the locus of cultural meaning—is, in part, a direct consequence of a desensitized and sensuousless world for which anthropology is sometimes an unwitting apologist. We will also see how the so-called "postmodern"— with its focus on individualized uncertainty—may come to be viewed as a very minor chapter in the history of Enlightenment thinking.

So, we begin with a group of Balinese who have already been highly sensitized through ritual negotiation to immunological concepts, and we then ask how they fare in the world of cosmopolitan medicine. As one would expect in any tradition that has maintained its vitality, indigenous healing practices must themselves respond to the exigencies of modern life if they are to be

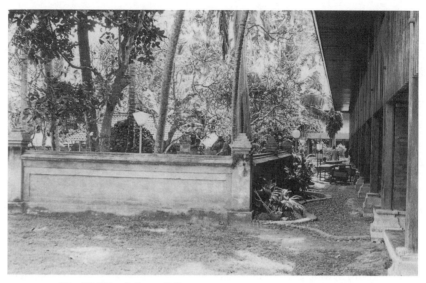

FIGURE 5. **Hotel Bali Beach, Sanur, Bali**
Tourists staying at Bali's only high-rise hotel are unaware of the fact that the hotel was laid out so as to avoid having to relocate a local temple. Tourism and tradition coexist in such close proximity that tourists regularly assume that temple events are "staged" for their pleasure. (Photo by author.)

successful. They must be responsive and adaptive to new forms of knowledge, to new kinds of illness, and to the new dimensions of human suffering that these illnesses give rise to. This is why some powerful Balinese ritual practices get cultivated right at the center of modernity. One might today, for instance, walk to the center of Bali's busiest tourist hotel and discover, face-to-face with the plate glass windows of tourists' bedrooms (literally less than ten feet away), a temple that could not be moved when the hotel was built, and around which, therefore, tourists perform their profane endeavors in complete ignorance of the fact that this monument was not placed there as a decorative accoutrement (figure 5). Only when the Balinese turn up to sacrifice pigs for the temple's birthday are sunbathers treated to a visual display that is rather at odds with what they might have anticipated when opening the drapes of their rooms!

This is one example (and we will see more) of how unfamiliar ways of treating "nonself" result in relational models that are at odds with immunology's obsession with elimination—how even these models may offer us new ways of conceptualizing how scientists interpret what they see in their microscopes. Within these unique ways of dealing with difference, in other words, are preserved quite novel and useful ways of understanding how danger may be accommodated. Let's take a closer look.

Today in Bali the modernizing of traditional demonology means, of course, formulating an indigenous response to AIDS. However, unlike many of the neglected and impoverished nations now struggling with AIDS, Bali is a country of two million people overwhelmed by several hundred thousand tourists each year, many of whom—especially those Australians and Japanese for whom it is nearby—think of the island as something of a promiscuous paradise. One need only recall that Bali is Sydney's closest tropical Eden, and that Sydney has had one of the industrialized world's worst problems with HIV, to sense the potential peril. If that weren't enough, Balinese tourism is regulated and its profits enjoyed by Javanese, and now Western, investors. While the Balinese call themselves a Hindu island in a Moslem sea, for non-Hindus Bali is a lucrative investment—a cultural Disney World of bizarre and scandalous customs that, nonetheless, make profits. Predictably, all sorts of problems on Bali are played down, as much by those who have invested in tourism as by the Balinese Hindus, who shield themselves from tourism by defining outsiders as ineffectually liminal (as opposed to spirits who may be both liminal and dangerous).

The difficulty does not end with the downplaying of illness: paradoxically, any study of pathogenicity in Bali will prove to be both much simpler and much more complex than one would imagine. This is because every bodily disorder is discussed in a metaphorical language liberally populated by invasive agents, much (at least in this respect) like the language of microbiology: every intrusion of the body is, as it were, a personified pathogen (*buta-kala*), a demon. The idea of a slow virus so parallels existing traditional explanations of black magic, of how one becomes ill, that the initial complexity for the Balinese first came in trying to recognize AIDS as something new and different. It was, and in some respects still is, entirely proper for a Balinese to respond to an inquiry about AIDS with a smile of recognition and the claim that this is something that has been understood for many generations. Although today the discourse on AIDS in Bali, as elsewhere in the world, is a rarefied blend of indigenous explanation and international rhetoric, it must be remembered that only a few years ago the Balinese response was, at the level of explanation, culturally quite well informed—indigenous concepts, that is, served very well to "explain" novel infectious agents.

Thus, the rhetorical battle that is so frequently waged between various forms of public-health discourse and what are claimed to be unacceptable local models of pathogenicity exemplifies for us how destructive it is to assume that their "unenlightenment" must be tempered by our "enlightened" awareness of "what is really going on." In other words, this smile of recognition (which we find so uninformed) might in itself be the very thing that could allow us to replace the inadequate metaphors that currently dominate microbiology. Indeed, just how important anthropology may one day prove for immunology can be readily demonstrated both historically and epidemiologically. As Chase (1982), for instance, points out in his study of the history of vaccination, what differentiated Jenner from his fellow researchers was less his clinical skills than his willingness to be a good anthropologist. Although it was common knowledge that deliberate inoculation with the smallpox virus conferred immunity to reinfection on the survivors,[4] Jenner was the one to take note of the fact that "the men and women who milked cows never again got cowpox. Nor, if rural farmers, milkmaids, apothecaries, doctors, naturalists, and mothers of many farm children could be believed, did any person who had ever had cowpox catch smallpox" (1982, 46). Jenner's "discovery," in other words, was as much a function of his attention to folklore as it was the result of inductive thought.

The point to be made here is not that traditional wizards have cures for modern epidemics (though, indeed, they may well have some), but that just why these and other techniques were either unknown or undeveloped was, we must acknowledge, *an entirely social matter*—as was the fact that Jenner's discovery did not lead to the swift eradication of smallpox in England and Europe. Jenner, Chase argues,

> not only unwittingly started the science of immunology, but he also scored a historical precedent: In the act of immunizing James Phipps against the then and still medically untreatable disorder of smallpox, Jenner had become the first person in history to transform a clinical disease into a wholly social or societal disorder. That is, he turned smallpox into the first major disease to be made completely preventable by massive societal intervention. (46–47)

Yet, as any anthropologist knows, transforming a clinical disease into a social disorder—thinking of health as "well-being"—more or less defines both what we call ethnomedicine and the field of medical anthropology (see, e.g.,

Kleinman 1988a; Martin 1990, 1994). For, like the Gloucestershire peasants of Jenner's day, most indigenous peoples continue to treat what we call clinical diseases as cultural ones, and, in so doing, utilize different pathogenic models. One important avenue for assessing the potential significance of anthropology for immunology, therefore, certainly rests in studying ethnomedical systems, but perhaps it rests even more in anthropology's serious treatment of other models of pathogenicity. For once we transform a clinical disease into a wholly social disorder—one made preventable by massive social intervention—we must also define just what social entity is meant to intervene (see, e.g., Brandt 1987), and, of course, to do that means starting back at the beginning with the defining of culture itself.

It is for such reasons that diverse notions of pathogenicity are worth studying in their own right, even when (or, actually, *particularly* when) they are—like unique psychological conditions—so difficult to define and categorize. Here's a Balinese example.

There was a farmer (I will call him "Nyoman") who lived in a Balinese town in which I was residing in the early 1980s. Though he tended his rice fields faithfully, he would return home each midday and, instead of taking the customary refuge from the tropical heat, position himself on a promontory outside of his house. From this elevated position he would speak in tongues. Nyoman was genuinely *gila* (mad) and had been so for some time. He had a number of voices that he utilized to yell at passers by, and, so far as I could tell, villagers simply ignored him. One day, after feeling comfortable enough to ask, I inquired about his condition, and was told the following: "We don't yet know what demons have possessed him; but when we find out, he'll be all right."

At first the response mystified me; soon, however, I understood its brilliance. Since he had been genuinely taken over by demons, it stood to reason that, once the demons could be removed, he would return to a more socially agreeable state. Whether or not this condition was brought on by his own karmic misdeeds, or by the extraordinary magical skills of another, what mattered was that we get rid of the demons, not that we relieve ourselves of responsibility by casting blame, establishing his weakness, or in any other way exonerating our sense of social guilt by saying it's his own damn fault. Furthermore, the fact that we could not determine which demons had possessed him—because, that is, we were incapable of establishing the right strategy for their removal—did not mean that we would never cure him.

The problem was ours as much as it was his: everyone would just have to live with this nonsense (alas, the poor man most of all) until *we* (and I emphasize the collective pronoun) could transform this situation into something good, into some positive social outcome. After all, Nyoman had actually never hurt anyone, and he was, in fact, a good farmer. His sociopathology was perceived, that is, in entirely sociosomatic terms, and his "cure" was enough *our* "cure" that the stigma of his illness was ours as well. Get rid of the demons and you have a normal man, not someone with lifelong guilt and a record that would prohibit him from getting a job or being trusted. That we had yet to cure him was an enigma, a conundrum, a social challenge to the community. His illness was, that is, *anomalous.*

Sociosomatic illnesses require social creativity—hence the need for rituals (such as Balinese trances) in which unlikely elements can be creatively superimposed into new associations, into novel solutions to age-old problems that (like an antigen/antibody match) present themselves uniquely each time they reappear. And just as proteins are constantly refigured across a veritable sea of DNA, so too do Balinese live for the benefits that they obtain when first going, via ritual, to the peripheries of what can be known, and, later, returning and assimilating socially those experiences. These "advance-guard" (*avant-garde*) activities are thus not only "medical" but deeply social. They are, as it were, the Balinese equivalent to the Lakota vision quest in which the challenge experienced individually by personal trial at the periphery of things has meaning only when its content is brought back for group examination of its transformational moment. These events are, thus, *not* those of actors having "personal" experiences in light of a tyrannical system, but settings in which individuals willfully dissociate in the interest of constructing social responses that are creative and new.

The Balinese—indeed, Hindus in general—are in some crucial ways (at least for us) unique in their approaches to pathogens; for they realize both the importance and the necessity of negotiating with these agents if they are to arrive at a working notion of what an organism is—and especially some idea of when and how a body gives way to its environment (e.g., Wikan 1990). Unlike Boccacio or Dante, who escaped to the countryside to avoid the plague, you can no more describe that which you don't know than you can transmit that which you don't have. Know it a little. Transform it and be transformed.

The Balinese are more French than American here, more "avant-garde," more aware of the need to know the opposition (of the need to negotiate what the French understand as the body's *terrain* [L. Payer 1988]), the organism's landscape in which antigen and antibody interact. The Balinese, that is, have a deep sense of the benefits that can be obtained both by going to the peripheries of what can be known, and by returning and assimilating those experiences socially—so much so that the "going out" and the "return" are visibly facilitated by the assistance offered by those not in trance.

Because of their acute awareness of the value of liminality and anomaly, the Balinese are also less likely to experience the lethal social shock that occurs "anaphylactically" when an organism, unaware of "otherness," experiences its first pathogenic inoculation. For the Balinese can exorcise pathogens across a sophisticated body-image boundary through tools that have been developed by *cultivating approaches* to otherness, rather than by cultivating *avoidance*. Because of this, they are, I would argue, much more likely to offer the world revised metaphors of immunological or viral transformation than we ourselves are. For in the Balinese view, we do not contract cancer when pathogenic cells gain control; we all have cancers which must be negotiated or they become pathogenic. The Balinese are, in other words, more aware that to inoculate means, according to the dictionary definition, not only to graft, implant, or "inject a serum, vaccine, etc. into (a living organism) . . . in order to create immunity," but "to introduce ideas . . . into the mind."

The argument starts to unfold: the answer to the question of how the Balinese use structure to achieve embodiment is to be found through what we pejoratively call "ritual," not so much through what we might label "self-awareness" (the dwelling on one's individual condition in a social and psychological vacuum). Because for the Balinese the world is motivated by any number of conflicting forces that must be stabilized, the need for "health maintenance," and for what we would call "preventive medicine," becomes self-evident. And the most unique forms of clinical encounter, therefore, are not those of individuals working against a system, but of individuals working in hyper-real consort to systematize an inherently chaotic world.

Now, we can look at some "lived experience"—specifically, some modern motoring events—to see how ritualized embodiment has, or could easily have, "clinical" implications. Motoring, ethnographically speaking, is a key experience in Bali—not only because of the legendary visceral dangers of these events, but because the traditional invocation that one control one's balance by moving slowly is seriously challenged by the chaotic dangers of walking or driving on any highway.[5] Here are a few examples:

An American friend is crossing a busy intersection in Denpasar, Bali's capital. She is knocked down by a vehicle—a hit and run. She lies on the pavement bleeding profusely from the head, while many Balinese avoid her. After a long wait, one man helps out. Those who avoid her do so because of the belief that her misfortune has a "cause," and, therefore, that she is emanating bad and contagious karma. Yet, in this culture some person does eventually step forward. This person may be one of the rare Christians or Moslems who inhabit Bali; but, if they are Balinese, they have (for whatever individual reason) perceived some need to extend the circle within which they will respond to danger—from the family, through the social, to the foreign. Such initiative is itself dangerous and may have disastrous results; for it involves behaviors that should only be engaged in by powerful people (*wong sakti*) who have ritually prepared themselves, or by those who for reasons of their own bad karma feel the need to take an extraordinary risk. The volitional act, in other words, is less an individualized form of praxis, a personal elaboration of how a rule works, than it is a strategy for realigning individual actions with powerful social archetypes.

I am riding down a busy highway with a Balinese friend when suddenly our vehicle is hit from behind. We stop immediately and notice that we are the final strike in a chain reaction, a bumper-to-bumper pile-up. The vehicles in the primary collision, being the worst hit, are badly damaged. My friend's apparently actor-focused response is to take in the scene, say simply "not me," and proceed immediately to a vendor where offerings may be purchased. What would, by any outsider, be interpreted as a personally focused—even self-centered—response to calamity is actually a response to pathogenicity that has a collective focus; for the comment "not me" referred to the fact that the gods were, relatively speaking, not so displeased with him as they were with the other drivers. He responds by reciting mantras, blessing the two of us and the vehicle, and only then continuing the journey. His actions are the result of his awareness that he has been warned about some ritual oversight, and his reaction to this warning is to perform some act that he recognizes as a minor, less efficacious version of what he and others might (and now will) engage in under the more auspicious circumstances of a visit to a priest, a temple, or a family shrine. In a world concerned with balancing conflicting superhuman forces, the intentions of actors are important, but they are always a subset of events that have "more meaning."

A minibus in which I am riding strikes a cyclist. The young woman is knocked down and looks hurt. The driver smiles, gets up, and exits the bus.

The woman is now on her feet and is also smiling. They exchange pleasant remarks, including the driver's willingness to assist her, for this is the appropriate individual response to extraordinary karmic danger. The driver returns to his bus still smiling. On taking his seat, however, he finds that some of the occupants are not willing to suppress their views. One older woman (who, by her age, is entitled to be more outspoken) expresses her anger—not at him, but at the girl who carelessly drove in front of him. Though still smiling, he indicates his agreement with her assessment. Later he will wonder about his response to stress—not so much his initial reaction (which was admirable), but his allowing himself to participate, even indirectly, in the older woman's display. His concern, in other words, will have more to do with his belief that his individual response *falls short* of a "more meaningful" cultural performance than it will with his awareness that his minor aberration is more "meaningful" *because it is unique.*

I must say it amazes me that those who specialize in making predictions about issues of international health feel confident about measuring the prevalence of HIV in Bali; for the Balinese are quite quick to protect a body-image boundary that can be so readily influenced by the possessive, and for them "cannibalistic," possibilities that arise when bodily fluids are removed for tests, exchanged in surgical procedures, or "polluted" by inoculations. Where "sampling" bodily fluids implies owning, controlling, and possibly destroying another person, who would step forward and offer themselves up for medical testing or admit to another when they have been taken over by an infectious agent?

I am also amazed that researchers would not see immediately how such cultural hypersensitivity would lead the Balinese, almost of necessity, into orchestrated social engagements (i.e., into *rituals*) through which pathogens could, as we might put it, be "clinically tried." Ritual, in other words, is not the locus of mere repetition, but a way of creatively establishing a new and vital language, a common ground. It is anything but the categorical opposite to lived experience that many of us would make of it. Seeing ritual as structured and emotionally "dead," therefore, is itself a commentary on the self-centered, "Enlightenment" values that Westerners find inescapable.

That is, conversely, why it is both acceptable and proper for Westerners to prohibit openly the precise forms of selective dissociation that in other arenas enable individuals to accommodate real difference, approach that which is dangerous, risk failure, and be creatively fulfilled. Meanwhile, some allusion to the need for creative public engagement on the part of "ill" individuals—

and especially those who search for meaning in modern medical settings—should be noted here. For those who represent the illnesses of others (medical counselors, therapists, writers—i.e., all who claim to have awarenesses that are "experience-near") are so often involved in claiming knowledge of, and codifying, the experiences of sufferers, that they rarely see just how "being sick" can have highly creative outcomes.

Although the examples I have provided do have meaning in the sense that they are "lived," make no mistake: for the Balinese, they are not exemplary. Because meaning in Bali is most powerfully expressed—as it is in so many non-Western settings—in domains that are creative and hyper-real (i.e., in the kind of orchestrated embodiment that is characteristic of ritual), the individualized experiences that define "actor-oriented" forms of meaning tend to be *devalued*. In Bali, although one's personal experience does have meaning as evidence for, or as an expression of, some basic truth, what we know individually will always remain a rather pedestrian manifestation of some more highly focused ritual truth. Indeed, a central argument of this book is that the dynamics of ritual social engagement are at the foundation of how humans creatively respond to what they sometimes viscerally perceive to be the tyranny of having one's identity self-consciously and inescapably fixed by daily circumstances that are sometimes punishing.

Today, the evidence for this tyranny is nowhere so powerfully apparent as it is in the science of "not-well-being" (i.e., modern medicine), and, specifically, within immunology's metaphors of alienation. This is precisely why so many non-Westerners are better positioned than bench immunologists to offer new models of antigen/antibody relations; for, in the modern world, the stigma of being chronically ill leaves little room for interpretation, and those who offer diagnoses so rarely provide much more than a concept of illness that entraps and limits sufferers as "patients."

But, while the Balinese are relatively more "sensitized" to the way in which spiritual and physical "landscapes" coexist as a balance between the harmful and the helpful, they are never frivolous about the dangerous nature of encounters with the unknown. On the contrary, like the modern-day AIDS phobias that keep Americans from having their teeth cleaned by the local dentist, the Balinese are extremely cautious about random physical contact. Indeed, their response to an immunological universe is perhaps even more cautious than ours. They try actively—*outside of ritual settings*—to avert contact with pathogens: don't have unsafe contacts with others, and, above all, don't let them have any part of you that could be magically manipulated. Be sure that your neighbor does not possess any of your personal belongings, for these could be used as catalysts in black magic. Above all, never have your blood taken by an anonymous physician.

In what way, then, are Balinese fears of the foreign different from ours? While the Balinese may appear even *more* cautious than we are during every-day encounters with the foreign, they are not so as the result of believing that pathogens may be permanently eliminated. Their caution stems from an awareness of how engaging difference is the mainstay of what they accept as the "flow" of life. Relating to pathogens is inevitable. This is also why the Balinese may be better positioned to think creatively about their interactions with pathogens—why their rituals, as events designed to deal creatively with alien forces, are more fully cultivated at the social level than are ours. And the Balinese are not at all unique in the cultivation of such sensitivity. Throughout West Africa, for instance, divination is employed as a mechanism for locating misfortune and revealing to those endangered by it the ways in which it might be contained or transformed.[6]

For modernists, on the other hand, individuals make themselves; we abhor the notion that we might be defined by the events that we experience. Yet, at the same time, even in modern societies that are dominated by cults of the self, individuals undergoing profound illness transformations will frequently create public settings in which to contextualize (i.e., to socialize) their transformations—settings in which at death's very door one insists on the need to "inoculate" the mind with some new version of what we are or are to become. It's simply that we are less likely to recognize and value the degree to which our very identities are realized socially, and therefore we are that much poorer at treating such transformative moments in an artful manner.

In the end, though, control in the face of chaos is, for all of us, essential, because illness is, beyond pain, a shamanic trial that ultimately empowers or disempowers each of us. Confronting illness is, in other words, less a matter of minimizing its tragic consequences (Harris 1994) than of facing the real transformative dimensions of one's illness experience. When filmmaker and gay activist Marlon Riggs was interviewed about the influence of his HIV diagnosis on his sense of self, he responded provocatively:

> I hit the jackpot with HIV. I knew I simply had to use it. When you're dealt
> what might be considered a bad hand, you've got to transform it in such a way

that all that is considered a handicap becomes a virtue, a means of empower-
ment. For me, as a cultural worker with certain explicit ideological and political agendas, it's not only empowering in helping my community, but also in
helping me deal with those demons inside. . . . The process was cathartic.
(Vaucher 1993, 80)

In another setting, Riggs could easily be speaking about what happens in the
transformations of great artists. Here, though, his statement reads like a ver-
batim translation of what the Balinese so often say about the creative dimensions of trance; for, in Riggs's case, "the cathartic" bringing of his illness to a
public stage was the single most important way of transforming a life that had
formerly been characterized by, in his own words, "self-effacement, pretense,
masquerading, concealment, and indirection" (80).

From a Balinese perspective, what Riggs is doing is using a social form of
ritualized illness experience to effect a personal catharsis, a transformation.
To play down the ritualized, public, collective nature of Riggs's experience as
superficial and not "lived," or as the glamorization of suffering—a confession—is just nonsense. And to claim, by extension, that one is anthropologically engaged in an "experience-near" activity because one can claim to
understand human suffering through the dissection of another's agony is only
to say that one is really not experienced—that one has not had enough experiences to construct any rule or generality about a phenomenon, any *form* of
living that one is willing to bring creatively into a negotiated world of "super-
charged" collective meaning. Is not the very act of conducting fieldwork—the
passive observer who becomes other—precisely parallel to the dormant virus
that restructures its victim by taking possession of its cellular vitality? This is
also where studying another way of life becomes, hauntingly, the intellectual
equivalent of the bizarre disorder called Munchausen-by-proxy—where
someone effects an illness in another (a parent in a child, a nurse in a patient)
in order to participate in a therapeutic encounter.

A world in which individuals wander in search of another's experience to
appropriate and be empowered by—or where they merely follow the sign-
posted footpaths set out by previous travelers—will necessarily lack the sensi-
tivities that ritual creatively depends upon. Here the sin of ignorance has the
effect of killing off, even unknowingly, the very difference, the diversity, that
is publicly heralded. Such a world—where difference is diffused into an
agreeable clone—has formally, categorically, and, indeed, truly achieved an

autoimmunological state, where so-called "self-awareness" has the effect of producing ontological ignorance, and where an increasing focus on interiority starves both the "other" and the "self." Does this cultural autoimmunity, which is now so much a part of cosmopolitan life, signal something of a twilight of the Enlightenment? Well, how could things be otherwise?

So much, at least at this moment, for the cross-cultural applicability of the metaphors of microbiology. On the more practical epidemiological front, how do you describe something that is not "curable" in cosmopolitan medicine (say, AIDS) to someone for whom the symptomatology of AIDS is already well known in the traditional demonic system? How do you respond when someone reacts to your simplified World Health Organization description of AIDS with a comment like: "Oh yes, my grandfather had that"? How do you explain the concept of a slow virus to someone for whom an illness that blossoms late more or less epitomizes the most successful forms of black magic?

While the consequences of HIV for Bali will be ghastly, one must realize that on the cultural level the cognitive issues—and, hence, the public health issues—are extraordinarily different than they are for cosmopolitan medicine. For the Balinese, the conceptual problem presented by AIDS is not that it is something new and unknown, but that *it is too much like other things that are already known*. In fact, the Balinese will have much less difficulty in conceptualizing AIDS (and even in giving meaning to its horrid effects) than will most Westerners; and thinking about this not only leads us to consider how much better prepared the Balinese may be to revise old ways of doing things, but it also leads us to reverse our inquiry (and here's where Descartes returns): why in the post-Enlightenment, cosmopolitan world, focused as it is on the integrity of personality and on an entirely phobic concern with a negatively transformative loss of self, should such a "demonology" (of the body *invaded* by alien agents) prevail both in popular description and at the vanguard of science itself? What is it about modern life that has called for such a "sensitization"? To this question the core of what follows will be devoted.

NEO-CREATIONISM

In order not to patronize women, I speak negatively. —Terminator 24 (a.k.a. Reginald Young)

We know that Asclepius, the father of medicine, was trained by a centaur (a "wildman"); and we may even come to accept that the continuity and fluidity of life creates the possibility that "illness" might be a kind of "well-being"—a creative moment when the prospect of real tragedy shows a different face. At the least it is clear that our distinction between self and nonself—and between what we call health and nonhealth—are based, as they are for the Balinese, on a fear of the outsider's world. But there is, for sure, a crucial difference: for us, otherness, in the absence of a means of approaching it, should be eliminated; for the Balinese, engaging the foreign through ritual provides some knowledge of what can be known at the limits of experience.

And if we have not the means to approach the outside, the outside will not provide such a means for us; for genuine outsiders confound what is socially prescribed. A homeless man once explained this to me in an eloquent description of why he had intentionally abandoned his subsidized housing:

> Like, when I was homeless again last week. . . . They asked for a position on my case, and I never defended it, and I'm so glad I never defended it. . . . So I purposely made myself homeless. . . . There was a list of grounds, of reasons why [I was being evicted]. And I could have defended myself against those reasons; but if I defended myself against those reasons, I felt I would have been guilty of those reasons. By not defending myself, I felt that I was innocent. . . . There was a list of reasons: they said my behavior was unacceptable. I don't know who "they" were, but I found their behavior unacceptable.

We know that outsiders, because they do not participate in our fears of alienation, are both more vulnerable to the forms of destruction that a society can generate and, paradoxically, more immune to danger. We respect and fear these outsiders because they can change our complacent world, our collective culture, and they can also somehow transcend it. Gandhi is a good social example; cancer cells a good biological one.

We also know full well that life on the edges of modernity's social "petri dish" is not kind to liminal people—that for every one of them who becomes a transformer of life there are thousands who die anonymously—for every Gandhi who can create the world's largest democracy, there are thousands who die unknown or who are crucified for their efforts to change society's center. If they appear weak, we either go all out to destroy them or afford them some clinical diagnosis that enforces their hopeless dysfunctionality.

Anyone who has ventured outside of the still and complacent center of social life knows that a decision to return can bring destruction to those making

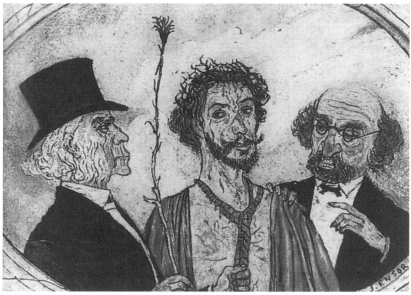

FIGURE 6. *Ecce Homo, or Christ and His Critics*
In this small cartoon Ensor portrayed himself as the liminal Christ surrounded by the status quo, here depicted in the form of two of the artist's most hostile critics. In Ensor's world the artist was, like Christ himself, an inhabitant of society's extreme periphery—a figure of loneliness living at the edge, one always mocked and misunderstood. (James Ensor, oil on panel, 1891. © 2002 Artists Rights Society [ARS], New York/SABAM, Brussels.)

the journey from outside in. Indeed, is this not the very meaning of the Crucifixion? Is not the crucified Christ an emblematic honoring of the millions who try to change the center but who are destroyed in the attempt (figure 6)? Is this not the deep meaning of Christianity, the Creationist's truth, the inventive reality that cuts through the static complacency of modern life?

| # Thinking Immunologically

> *Examine language . . . what is it all but Metaphors, recognized as such, or no
> longer recognized? —*Carlyle, *Sartor Resartus*

METAPHORS OF DIFFERENCE

In a commentary about what we would today call self-awareness, Mark Twain
once noted that the first duty of every human being was "to think about himself until he had exhausted the subject, then he is in a condition to take up
minor interests and think of other people." Twain's sarcasm about our occasionally indulging ourselves in another's well-being was, of course, directed
toward what he thought to be the crude self-interest that characterizes life in
general, but it might as well have been a metaphysical judgment of the reflexive entrapments of the post-Enlightenment world, in which one falls repeatedly toward oneself in the mirror of self-concern.

Yet to be overconcerned with the self, one has to assume some awareness
of it; and immunology—precisely because it focuses on that area where "self"
and "not-self" become ambiguous—provides our best scientific illustration
of the amorphous space of negotiated realities in which the distance between
subject and object is not absolute. Setting aside common self-indulgence and
the idiotic cant by which we are meant in earnest to refrain from speaking
for the "other" (because all we can actually know is a reflexive "self"), for most
of us "self" and "other" daily function as practical, rhetorical devices for attending to a multitude of inchoate experiences of which the living of life is
constituted—experiences wherein self-interest is mitigated by the necessary projections and dissociations that enable us to challenge difference by
"embodying" otherness. Through mimesis and imagination we experience
precisely the uncertainty of just why another ought to be construed as "different"; and cultural categories or academic disciplines that focus on how a no-

tion of "self" arises from this socially articulated dynamic deserve to be studied comparatively and in some detail.

There is, of course, an enormous literature in anthropology that is devoted to the comparative study of "self" and "other," one originating in the work of Durkheim, Hertz, Hubert, and Mauss, and focusing on what we call "the category of the person." Yet, oddly, while such concerns have helped shape the anthropological enterprise both academically and in the field, we have fared far less well in the looking glass of cultural practice. Immunology provides the perfect case in point. Here is a domain of scientific inquiry that by its own definition exists specifically in order better to elucidate the biological influence of "other" on "self"; and though immunology is now a very complex, subtle, and sophisticated science, it is essential to remember that it is, and always has been, a science of "foreign bodies," one where "self" and "not-self" are specified on the molecular level in the paradigmatic battle between antigen (foreign invader—i.e., *anti*body *gene*rator) and antibody (defender of self—i.e., *anti*-foreign *body*). Yet, despite the advent of the AIDS pandemic and some understanding of the supposed viral basis of certain cancers, this once obscure domain of scientific inquiry has yet to receive the ethnographic attention it deserves. We have, for instance, few studies that document the recent and widespread assimilation of immunology into popular discourse (e.g., DiGiacomo 1987; Haraway 1989; Martin 1994). And, though some of its concepts go back to the last century, we should not forget just how recent a science immunology is.

By the early 1970s the idea that there was something called an "immune system" was just beginning to take root in general practice, having only first appeared in the scientific literature in the mid-1960s (Moulin 1989, 221–22). The change was subtle but important, for the science of immunology moved away from an earlier, reactive definition of itself to one now characterized by maintenance and balance; although my anaphylaxis was not, as scientists had once thought, "the unavoidable preliminary step in the production of immunity" (ibid., 232), the experience certainly sensitized me, at an important moment in the history of science, to the uncertain emergence of this domain of research. Since that time, I have watched both closely and from a studied distance while the metaphor of "the body at war" became transformed into a very real social conflict—one that today involves, through AIDS, the potential collapse of systems of health care worldwide. At the same time, immunology has stepped forward from relative obscurity, bringing its questions of "self" and "not-self" to the forefront of medical practice and, along with them, its popular narratives of alien invasion in which the "self" is assaulted and taken over by "outsiders" or (in autoimmunity) by those mistaken for such. What is most intriguing here is the fact that these battle metaphors were fully developed in immunology well before the AIDS pandemic; so it is not accurate to argue anachronistically that AIDS actually brought these metaphors into the popular imagination.

Although military language has always been a part of microbiology and of Darwinian "fitness" in general, "self" and "not-self" become much more problematic in immunology and virology, especially once the notion that there is a *system* to eliminate not-self takes hold. This *systematization* of im- mune responses is further complicated by the attribution of *volition* to viruses which, strictly speaking, are not even alive; left to itself, a virus is inert: it can- not grow, it cannot move, it cannot reproduce, and it has no power unto itself. If viruses are thus understood, why do we talk about them as if they are voli- tional and intentional beings? Why do we say that they appropriate, mask, in- vade, deceive, enslave, destroy, and reproduce?

One answer is that what we are really doing here is using a microscopic parable to reconfirm our cultural predilections regarding just what it is that makes a person (figure 7).

Determining what in such storytelling actually constitutes a "self" be- comes much more than a matter of science. This is why social anthro- pology—as the discipline that looks at "self" and "other" cross-culturally— has emerged as the arbiter of what would otherwise be a "mere" scientific problem. Yet, despite its major agenda having become preeminent in the lan- guage of scientific inquiry, anthropology itself has not focused in any thor- ough way on the question of what might be gained either by a better understanding of what immunologists actually think, or by a clearer sense of how immunological thought becomes embedded in daily discourse. Although anthropologists are often accused of embodying the very vices they elsewhere observe, it is hard to see just why the study of "self" and "other" in less exotic, but culturally valued, disciplines has been largely neglected. It's not that we've gotten it all wrong; we simply haven't gotten very much of it.[1]

Since my encounter with anaphylaxis more than twenty years ago, I have made it a habit to follow the growth of the concept of the immune system in medicine and in popular discourse, but, most importantly, in the language used by doctors and by those who popularize scientific concepts for the rest of

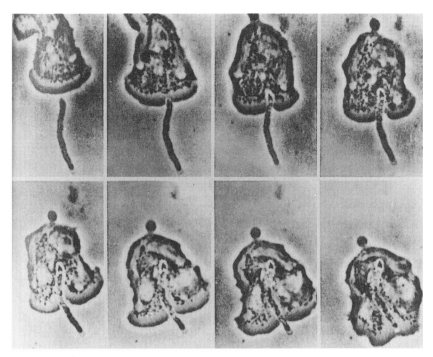

FIGURE 7. **Phagocytosis**

Engulfment and ingestion by a human phagocyte of a chain of cells (*Bacillus megaterium*). It is not only in the popular literature where cellular transformation is described anthropomorphically. Even in medical texts phagocytes are described as scavenger cells that devour foreign matter, earning them the label of gluttonous micro-warriors. But phagocytes engulf inanimate matter as well, so that they no more do battle with the foreign than each of us "kills" the food on our dinner plate by ingesting it. (From *Biology of Microorganisms*, by Thomas D. Brock, Michael T. Madigan, John Martinko, and Jack Parker, 7th ed. [Englewood Cliffs, N.J.: Prentice Hall, 1994], fig. 11.26. © 1994, reprinted by permission of Pearson Education, Inc., Upper Saddle River, N.J.)

us. I wanted to know more about how patients came to terms with the idea of a "body at war with itself"; about how this concept was employed in doctor/patient interactions; about how it was used in causal blaming.

To achieve such an understanding involves, first, some awareness of how metaphors function as conveyors of cultural categories of thought, and, second, how immunology becomes a dominant medium through which those categories are variably embodied. It is only then that we will be in some position to discover how the tyranny of being subjected to the powerful negative transformers of immunology can be handled more creatively. What, we will ask, are the ways in which we might more constructively embody those non-propositional aspects of immunology that are not reducible to the sorts of expressions we use to name them, and that are not, furthermore, always and everywhere "self-conscious"?

"DRESSED TO KILL": THE FUNCTION OF METAPHOR

Men kill the thing they love. —Oscar Wilde, "Ballad of Reading Gaol"

In his compelling work on metaphor, Mark Johnson (1987) argues that nearly all traditional semantic theory is dominated by a kind of objectivism in which imagination is thought to be completely irrelevant to the specification of meaning. Because of such an analytic focus on semantic content, we tend, Johnson argues, to ignore or at best to undervalue the sort of semantic phenomena that are central to metaphors, or to any other sorts of "nonpropositional and figurative structures of embodied imagination" (xxxv). A number of philosophers concerned with the nature and function of metaphor (e.g., Hesse 1987; Hausman 1989) have likewise argued that metaphoric thinking is not always reducible either to rational propositions or to literal concepts, and that what is ignored by such reductive thinking is precisely the way in which embodied structures of imaginative thought actually influence human behavior. As Johnson puts it, "imagination seems to exist in a no-man's-land between the clearly demarcated territories of reason and sensation" (xxix).

Johnson is, of course, using the concept of metaphor in an expansive way—one that cuts across traditional semantic distinctions by not necessarily isolating metaphors (i.e., indirect comparisons), from similes (direct comparisons) or analogies (resemblances, parallels, functional similarities). What he is actually focusing on is the practice of using one thing to stand for another in negotiating meaning—on relations which at times seem loose and "meaningless" in the strict sense, but which, nonetheless (or, perhaps, because of this looseness) become central to the phenomenon of transformation, of paradox, of the *perception* of change (Napier 1986, chap. 1). These are phenomena which, because they are not easily specified, are of necessity eliminated from descriptions of semantic content.

To sense the scope of metaphor's significance, Johnson argues, it is necessary to question that objectivist account of metaphor which asserts that meaning is reducible to "a series of literal concepts or propositions" (6). Metaphor is not a background against which meaning is set, but is the vehicle for embodying meaning: metaphor, that is, is itself "not reducible to the propositions we use to name it" (7), and its embodiment, as Bourdieu has argued of embodied understanding in general, must remain "beyond the grasp of consciousness" if an effective transformation is to be made. This is not a dreary argument against the ability of language to describe the phenomenal world of experience. It is also not laying claim to domains of experience that cannot be described.[2] Attributing "meaning" to metaphor, in other words, is not merely to engage in mystifying that which is already ambiguous. On the contrary: when one actually observes how metaphor functions in negotiated meaning—how our visceral responses to them have quite specific consequences for what we understand—one can see that Johnson's conclusions are ethnographically significant.

Let us examine a passage Johnson utilizes to illustrate his argument. It is an excerpt from Timothy Beneke's disturbing book, *Men on Rape* (1982). The voice is that of a San Franciscan law clerk:

> Let's say I see a woman and she looks really pretty, and really clean and sexy, and she's giving off very feminine, sexy vibes. I think, "Wow, I would love to make love to her," but I know she's not really interested. It's a tease. A lot of times a woman knows that she's looking really good and she'll use that and flaunt it, and it makes me feel like she's laughing at me and I feel *degraded*. I also feel dehumanized, because when I'm being teased I just turn off. I cease to be human. Because if I go with my human emotions I'm going to want to put my arms around her and kiss her, and to do that would be unacceptable. I don't like the feeling that I'm supposed to stand there and take it, and not be able to hug her or kiss her, so I just turn off my emotions. It's a feeling of humiliation, because the woman has forced me to turn off my feelings and react in a way that I really don't want to. If I were actually desperate enough to rape somebody, it would be from wanting the person, but also it would be a very spiteful thing, just being able to say, "I have power over you and I can do anything I want with you"; because really I feel that *they* have power over *me* just by their presence. Just the fact that they can come up to me and just melt me and make me feel like a dummy makes me want revenge. They have power over me so I want power over them. (Beneke 1982, 43–44; in Johnson 1987, 6)

Johnson argues that a traditional analysis of the semantic content of the law clerk's statement assumes that "the meaning of what he [the law clerk] is asserting can, in principle, be spelled out in a series of literal concepts and propositions" (6). The primary assumption of such an "objectivist" account is that there is "a core of publicly accessible meaning reducible to those literal concepts and propositions, together with various functions or speech acts performed on those propositions. Whatever else might play a role in our understanding of this text is ignored as not included in the *meaning* of what he says" (6). Much as actor-oriented anthropology assumes a directed, self-interested, even intentional, actor, the objectivist account of this passage assumes that the intentions of the speaker are embedded in a florid discourse that is reducible to certain logical propositions. But to eliminate the metaphorical content of the passage, Johnson argues, is to undermine our understanding of its meaning. To say, "The man wants to have intercourse with the woman," or "The man wants the woman to submit to his desires," undermines the way in which the meaning of the passage is both embodied culturally and employed rhetorically; for our grasping the clerk's statement requires that we make certain connections that consist "partly in our understanding of shared metaphorical projections, partly in 'folk' models our culture provides for various aspects of reality, and partly in a broad range of schematic structures that develop in our nonpropositional embodied experience" (6–7). All of these, he continues, are "part of our understanding of the passage in question—they are part of its meaning. They are not merely background conditions for understanding" (7). Reducing this passage to a series of literal propositions, Johnson argues, results in the total loss of the collective meaning that is embodied not in the circumstantial peculiarities of the actor's "lived experience" but in the dominant metaphorical structure: Physical Appearance is a Physical Force. To wit: "She's *devastating*. He is *strikingly* handsome. She'll *knock you off* your feet. He *bowled* me *over*. She's *radiant*. I find him so *attractive*. She's a *bombshell*. He was *blown away* by her" (7). And in the passage quoted above: " . . . she's *giving off* very feminine, sexy vibes. . . . I'm supposed to stand there and *take it*. . . . the woman has *forced me* to turn off my feelings and *react* . . . they have *power over* me just by their presence. . . . Just the fact that they can come up to me and just *melt me*. . . . " Although metaphor—the "mapping of a structure from source domain (physical forces) onto the target domain (physical appearance)"—is clearly at work here, Johnson is quick to point out that the proposition he uses to label that structure ("physical appearance is a physical force") is "merely a name for the complex web of connections in our experience and understanding"—that (to repeat) "the metaphor is not reducible to the prop-osition we use to name it." Physical Appearance is a Physical Force is the metaphor that carries the shared cultural meaning of the law clerk's passage, regardless of the precise label one attaches to the actual words.

Now, while a reader may be quick to argue that Johnson has clouded his case by alluding to complex sociocultural factors and assumptions about shared categories of thought, I would like to point out that what Johnson argues is ethnographically verifiable without alluding to nebulous structural relations or to "bad metaphysics." In fact, I have tested Johnson's basic argu-ment in several settings (lectures, discussions, and interviews with patients) with specific reference to the function of metaphor in immunology, and I have concluded that the veracity of his basic argument may be evidenced in four phenomena that I have repeatedly observed.

The first is the surprise that many listeners exhibit when the actual met-aphors (in this case, of Beneke's informant) are isolated. Within American cul-ture individuals are so used to hearing about people being "knocked out" by each other's looks that they *respond viscerally* to the passage without being at-tentive to the violent categories that function unconsciously, if not (one is tempted to say) covertly. It would be odd not to be affected by the law clerk's words.

Second, all listeners profess to an awareness of the prevalence of this vio-lent language—its "reality"—once it is pointed out. No listeners stand up and profess not to know what is implied by hearing others commonly describe a person he or she likes with words like "devastating," "striking," and "knock-out." In fact, the realization of the prevalence of these categories—brought about simply by calling attention to them—is for most listeners embarrass-ing, in part because they have so embodied the idea that it can be said publicly and repeatedly without notice.[3]

Third, the realization of the fact that the metaphor has wide social cur-rency is, except in cases of defiant sexism, always followed by denial: "Yes, these concepts are basic to our culture—I know they are real—but I don't em-ploy them, and neither do the kinds of people I associate with." In other words, people begin to challenge the authority of metaphor, and perhaps even to modify it, as soon as it is brought to consciousness: their disgust and anger at what they hear—even if they don't actually *hear* the words "bombshell" or "blown away"—results in an immediate response, a challenging of the metaphor's universal authority. This is what I call the "not me" syndrome—i.e., "*yes, but* not me or anyone I associate with." The "yes" and "but" here are nearly simultaneous.

And fourth, the bringing of metaphor to consciousness can actually result not only in "not me" but in a *creative* revision of that collective meaning, if—and this is essential—those actively modifying the metaphor are aware both of the inevitability with which metaphors convey cultural meaning, and of the dissociative domains in which those metaphors have social currency—i.e., they *accept* that metaphors *do* have power. What is important, in other words, is not to denounce the functioning of those metaphors as "unjust," nor to focus on the "lived experience" of an individual actor working against the hegemonic tyranny of "the system," but to recognize that this "living" is carried out in *response* (as a *reaction*) to what Durkheim would have called a shared category of thought, a "social fact." And seeing how such shared categories are individually negotiated tells us *both* about the real power of these categories (including the traditional, anthropological need to study and understand them) *and* about how dynamic individual responses are formulated by bringing metaphors to consciousness, by revising as an individual the social meaning that each metaphor embodies. No students to whom these realities are demonstrated ever again hear the words "knocked out" in the same way.

METAPHOR AND STEREOTYPE; OR,
WHAT IS A CULTURAL CATEGORY?

Everything means something to someone, even if it's only a habit. —Gertrude Stein,
Everybody's Autobiography

It doesn't take a great deal of insight to realize that the cultural meaning that is carried by metaphor finds its way into both archetype and stereotype. Nor does it take much empirical observation to see that, individually, we have been culturally conditioned to run from collective ideas, to deny, modify, or otherwise revise our personal relationship to a collective category once it is brought to consciousness. Indeed, the very specificity with which we rigorously determine what can count as meaningful encourages us to eliminate the elusive and sometimes sloppy domains in which metaphors, and the stereotypes they can perpetuate, prevail. Yet, as the previous example illustrates, the empirical evidence for how people utilize and respond to metaphors suggests that some collective category *is* being shared. It is hard to argue against a pattern of collective thinking in the following: "She's dressed to kill . . . He's strikingly handsome . . . She's devastating . . . She'll knock you off your feet . . . She bowled me over . . . I'm blown away by her . . . She's a bombshell . . . " The list here could go on. I now notice, for instance, that, when a man is flirting with a woman, my students say, "He's hitting on her." And when they are drinking (which is now the precondition of being personal), they describe what they are doing as "getting hammered." I don't want to belabor the point, but the empirical evidence cannot be brushed aside as meaningless because it does not lend itself easily to precision. At the least, we are entitled to recognize that our language of gender relations is extraordinarily violent; most American youth would be at a loss to understand what an Englishman means by "chatting up," which is an English equivalent of "hitting on." There is certainly a world of difference between what is connoted in "chatting" and in "hitting."

In addition to this simple awareness, we are also entitled to the empirical observation that individuals modify their relations to stereotypical constructions when they are brought to consciousness—that the more intellectually oriented of us deny outright the "meaning" of metaphor as imprecise. And, finally, we are entitled to the observation that, when metaphors and the stereotypes they promote go unaddressed, they tend to prevail. These observations are evidenced not only in the ways in which metaphors are utilized and revised but in the ways that individuals manipulate and respond to stereotypes.

How are stereotypes utilized? Propaganda is a common mode. Within popular media one thinks immediately of Nazi-era anti-Semitic film, or the way in which *Birth of a Nation* incited the rapid growth of the Ku Klux Klan in America. In such cases, stereotypes are used to criticize, isolate, or even eliminate those who are thought to threaten a given form of group identity. Used in this way, propaganda is understood as an entirely *negative* manipulation.

However, stereotypes are actually much more complex when viewed phenomenally, rather than in retrospect. Take humor, for instance. Did those who viewed the films of the Marx Brothers in the 1930s laugh because their stereotyping of Jews, Italians, and idiots were so ridiculous as not to be believed? Or were viewers laughing because the behaviors they viewed confirmed some deeply felt racist suspicion? And do contemporary filmmakers who set out to address stereotypes (e.g., Spike Lee in *Do the Right Thing*) actually promote them through the codification of the parodic forms they are hoping to undermine? The empirical problem with humor, in other words, is that, although the whole audience is laughing, and you are fairly sure of *what* they are laughing at, you don't know *why* they are laughing. Humor, therefore, can result in *a negative or a positive* manipulation; indeed, sometimes these types of manipulation are coextensive.

Given these ambiguities, the ways in which victimized individuals formulate responses to stereotypes are varied and complex. In other words, these are responses to the fact that the cultural construction of the stereotype presents a no-win situation for those who are victimized by the stereotype—when its negativity and/or inevitability makes possible only a limited number of options. What follows are some ways in which responses are constructed. The list is tentative, but it makes possible a few basic distinctions.

Option 1: Passing. Passing is a management strategy first described in detail by Erving Goffman (1963). Here one manages discrediting information by not challenging another's misperception—as in the popular film *Imitation of Life*, where a light-skinned woman of African descent allows her friends to think of her as white. Since the basis of passing involves merely allowing another's misperception to flourish, it functions in a much wider range of phenomena—as, for example, when an individual silently allows others to think that the name they may share with a well-known public figure is familial rather than coincidental. Flirtation, as one might expect, is the bedfellow of passing.

Option 2: Affiliation (re-identifying the stereotype). Here, someone decides that a stereotype with which they have been affiliated is so problematic that they seek out another one that they feel they have a claim on—when what appears to be an inevitably negative characterization of a stereotype leads an individual to seek out another social category that seems more viable. Examples of this response are common among blacks in America, where the identity of "black" or "African American" is so dependent on its "otherness" that assimilation is ruled out from the start. When "black" is defined as "not white," an African American individual who affiliates himself with anything considered "white," such as academic achievement, is denied his ethnic identity and labeled a sellout, an "Oreo." Blacks achieving in a white world exemplify how realigning affiliations can result in victimization. Indeed, the victimization can be so extreme that life in a particular setting becomes intolerable: the American writer James Baldwin went into self-imposed exile in Europe; the filmmaker Marlon Riggs finds, as we have seen, that the only reconciliation of his "black" and "gay" identities is in contracting HIV, where he "hit the jackpot."

In fact, the impossibility of success may be so extreme that entire groups, or even generations, find themselves so stereotyped—that is, so closely identified with a given stereotype that no moderating response (such as passing or new affiliation) is allowed. Here, culture creates the very conditions of stigma from which one cannot escape—conditions where, as Gramsci and Fanon argued, the experience of being represented and dominated allows for only one role for the dominated. This kind of relationship is, as we shall see, not restricted to cultural or political oppression but also obtains within cultures, within families, and within individual relationships. In fact, it obtains at the deepest level in any setting in which heroes require friends, family units, or individual offspring to play supportive roles in their personal narratives of success. Why, then, should this "hegemonic" pattern take its clearest form when applied to the oppression of minorities? Because here the obvious level of social injustice allows for a moral posture that implicates us least. In general, though, the case is more complex.

It is hard for me to forget, for instance, the numbers of my students who grew up abroad (in such places as Germany and Japan) who have said, categorically, that they didn't know what it was like to be a "minority" until they returned to the United States. What could such a comment mean? For bell hooks (1994), minorities must find a way of identifying themselves that does not reiterate the structure of oppression that, in turn, codifies that "minority" identity—one which separates and stigmatizes at the same time. Note, for instance, the Darwinian tone of the National Association of Black Social Workers, the very people devoted to the social well-being of blacks: "Black children belong physically and psychologically and culturally in black families where they receive the total sense of themselves and develop a sound projection of their future. . . . Black children in white homes are cut off from the healthy development of themselves as black people" (McRoy 1989, 152). If only life were so simple, the trap set by this otherwise laudable position would not be so fatal. For Marlon Riggs, the possibility of participating in some "healthy development" was precluded from the outset by the stigma attached to both his gender preference and his ethnicity. This is why the argument posed by *The Bell Curve*—namely, that minorities are less socially successful than their white counterparts—is so controversial; for difference, by definition, must be located at the categorical peripheries of the norm, the rule, by which it may be recognized and distinguished (figure 8).

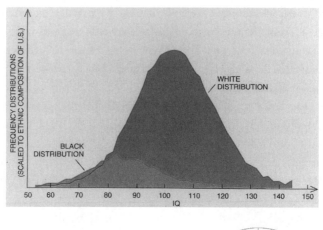

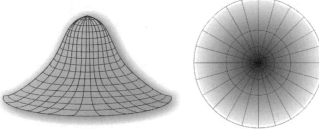

FIGURE 8. **The Bell Curve**
As a controversial linear model of intelligence—i.e., read from left to right (*top*)—
we find African Americans, as a group, pooling toward the lower end of the IQ
range. As a three-dimensional model of social conformity, however, the bell curve
betrays itself as none other than a fitness landscape at whose dense center success is
measured by conformity (*bottom left*). At the periphery of this second model, we
find liminal people of all ability ranges. Commonly used as a device for rational-
izing the less frequent social successes of minorities, the bell curve reminds us
hauntingly, when viewed from above (*bottom right*), of the petri dish and its cell
colony. The bell curve is thus as much proof of discrimination against African
Americans (who have been marginalized) as it is a measure of their intelligence.
(*Top:* From "Blind Spots," by Leon J. Kamin, *Scientific American* [February 1995],
100. Copyright © 1995 by Scientific American, Inc. All rights reserved. *Bottom:*
Drawings by author.)

Option 3: Exaggeration. Exaggeration takes place when people deliberately
take on a negative stereotype or stigma in order to threaten or ridicule those
who stigmatize them. Examples of the exaggeration of stereotypes are commonly seen in popular media: shaft films (in which black "studs" pose as sexually threatening); "rap" musicians posing as "gangstas"; the homeless person
who responds to an intelligent question with the response, "Don't ask me, I'm

a bum." These are all examples of how the victims of an alienating stereotype respond through exaggeration. In the film *Portrait of Jason*, a black male prostitute goes so far as to work for white folks as a "houseboy"—making whatever money he can scrape up by "cooking chicken" for those who think that all blacks do this well. Exaggeration is, however, especially dangerous; not only does its nihilism alienate the antiheroes who take this route, but the result may, as in humor, undermine the intentions of those who exaggerate. In the popular film *Do the Right Thing*, Spike Lee uses ground-level and wide angle shots of blacks on the street to throw them into the viewer's personal space. The exaggeration of the stereotype, however, can backfire when both white and black viewers express fear and discomfort with the stereotypes Lee is portraying.

Option 4: Impersonation. Outright impersonation can take place when someone sets out to change his or her identity by adopting a personality associated with a more viable or successful social category. Here, the no-win situation of negative stereotyping causes a radical identity shift, even in the face of stigma (e.g., as when psychiatry attacks such individuals as having entered a state of complete denial, or when their friends see them as having "gone over," having "fallen off," or having "lost it"). Examples are not hard to find: con artists, tricksters, individuals with multiple personality disorders, impostors—even so-called "Voguers" (where gay blacks dress and pose as *Vogue*-like models). It is far too easy, however, to use flagrant impersonators as cultural scapegoats. We should not allow ourselves so readily to participate in the alienation of such individuals, since impersonation can also function as a primary catalyst in successful transformations. The actress Anna Deavere Smith, for instance, has made a profession of embodying the behaviors of those who find themselves participants in widely publicized tragedies. For this black actress, the fact that she perceives herself as "not looking like anybody" enables her "to create the illusion of looking like everybody." Indeed, many of those who act professionally find that the activity allows them the only exit from a victimizing stereotype. Any successful foreign language student is familiar with the relationship between impersonation and transformation.

Nearly all of these examples have, as one can easily imagine, dangerous and destructive elements—not only because of the ways in which society at large alienates such individuals, but also because of the ways in which members of the very category they are trying to transform will do the same thing: those who are not brave enough to challenge and transform the cultural construction of their identity will commonly turn on their neighbors—on the "Oreos"—who attempt to change.

Option 5: Positive manipulation (revising a damaging stereotype). Now, it stands to reason—since positive manipulation may be the most promising kind of response to ethnic and cultural stereotyping (i.e., to "immunological" aliens)—that we should be able to find many examples in which the inevitability of a particular stereotype is undermined or challenged. Since positive manipulation provides the only response that is *not ambiguous or racist* (humor, propaganda), and that is *not potentially destructive*, one would expect to find it everywhere. But here too it seems that social pressures (from without and from within) work aggressively to discourage those who might otherwise transform a stereotype. Evidence for these pressures can be had simply by looking for cases in which the *inevitability* of a prevailing stereotype is directly challenged. In short, they are few and far between. Here is a personal example: A class assignment in a course I have given on ethnic stereotyping produced *no* examples (at that time, at least) in all of the popular American films about Latinos in the United States that did not include references to illegal immigration and gangs. As one student put it:

> It was very difficult to find a film portraying Latinos that did not deal with gangs and immigration. The Latino men in these films dressed and spoke the same, regardless of whether they were of Mexican, Cuban, or Peruvian descent. The gang "uniform" of gold crosses, hairnets, bare chests, and low riders prevailed in these films. . . . A theme of violence runs throughout all of these films. Stereotypes of Latino women (Latinas) were harder to come by, as most of the films dealt with gangs. The women played the roles of mothers and girlfriends left behind wondering what would become of their sons and boyfriends.

Wrote another:

> The prevailing stereotype associated with Latinos in modern film is one of violent and often sociopathic behavior . . . portray[ing] Latinos as potentially cunning and always violent criminals. Latino characters are seen defacing and destroying property, physically abusing others, and often committing cold-blooded acts of murder.
>
> These degrading stereotypes are propagated and perpetuated by the seem-

ingly endless films about Latino gang violence and criminal activity, though other stereotypes are presented in modern film. For example, Latino characters are frequently associated with vigorous energy, which is often used destructively. . . . These stories do little to raise the image of Latin Americans, however.

Visual media increasingly illustrate Latino characters as unintelligent, downwardly mobile individuals obsessed with outlandish fashions, dances, and material objects. Medallions, low riders, and gang fashions are repeated time and again and comprise a portion of the largely depreciative cult of personality associated with the Latino.

Indeed, not only did we find that there were no filmic initiatives afoot to revise creatively popular stereotypes about Latinos, but we were also troubled to discover that this ethnic group was consistently being constructed in a non-varying, one-dimensional way. Moreover, it was clear that the "master stigma" previously associated with blacks in America was shifting; in Latino films, that is, blacks are often cast in mediating roles, as individuals who, for instance, have given up a life of crime, who are *contrasted* with the Hispanic immigrant who is shown to be immature, violent, and, above all, an *outsider*. Like the "master illnesses," which invariably become the focus of public discourse about suffering, specific ethnic stereotyping seems also to characterize the anxieties of social groups at particular historical moments. Indeed, even the films that self-consciously set out to counteract negative and racist stereotypes are often themselves found to advance negative and racist sentiments among viewers. Compare the aforementioned ambiguity of Spike Lee's *Do the Right Thing* with the film *Guess Who's Coming to Dinner?* (in which a black surgeon meets the parents of his white girlfriend). Spencer Tracy and Katharine Hepburn, the parents in the film, were famous not only for their own real-life affair (which for Tracy, as a married Catholic of the era, presented real problems) but for their earlier famous portrayal of gender liberation in *Adam's Rib*. Whether one loves or hates *Guess Who's Coming to Dinner?* is irrelevant to its forthright attempt to revise a number of then-prevalent stereotypes—an attempt that any informed viewer of the period would have been well aware. Although these last two films are regularly criticized, they offer rare early examples in which gender and ethnic stereotypes are overtly revised.

Do individuals, we must ask, shy away from modifying negative stereotypes because they feel defeated by, or simply do not recognize, those stereotypes? Or, we must ask, is the act of recognizing a stereotype itself part of the codification of the very negative image that such recognition tries to displace? To test our hypotheses about stereotypes, students in the class already described actually dressed in the manner in which various stereotypes were portrayed in film. The students met with insults, stares, contempt, and outright anger: one student who imitated the filmic attire of young, streetwise Latinas was consistently harassed by passing motorists as she walked to and from classes. Is the stereotype a mere "straw man," a polarized "other" against which cultural values are contrasted? If so, do stereotypes fare better in more reflective and presumably responsible intellectual or academic settings? Not necessarily. In fact, to evidence the utilization of unexamined ethnic stereotypes in scholarly research we need not delve into the ancient past of phrenology; for only a few years ago *Scientific American* could publish unblushingly a serious article in which the "origins" of the AIDS pandemic included unsubtle allusions that linked the spread of AIDS to blacks engaging in unnatural acts with monkeys. And the case, though dramatic, is not exceptional: any contemporary public health journal in which ethnic attitudes function as a research control will almost de facto develop a research strategy around specious ethnic assumptions. Today the oversexed wildmen of the world are less frequently African and increasingly Latino. Here is an example. It is from *Family Planning Perspectives*, a serious medically oriented public health journal that has published a good bit on AIDS and AIDS-related behavior. We get the stereotype right up front:

> To understand the incidence of multiple sexual partners among Hispanics, cultural factors must be examined. Traditional Hispanic culture is characterized by a male-centered view in which men tend to prove their virility by having multiple sex partners. The Hispanic notion of machismo may perpetuate traditional sex-role stereotypes and double standards. These *traditional* attitudes may result in a greater number of unprotected sexual contacts, and thus an increased risk of HIV infection among Hispanics. (Sabogal and Faigeles 1993, 257; my emphasis)

The study then goes on to explain just how much higher are the rates of both hetero- and homosexually acquired AIDS among Hispanics than among other groups. The statistics among homosexuals are, we discover, not reliable because of the traditional stigma attached to homosexuality among Latinos, but the rates for heterosexual transmission of HIV are ten times higher among Hispanics than among non-Hispanic whites.

So far, there is nothing in this study that does not conform to the broadly accepted stereotype of a macho male culture, one that researchers and social workers are faced with on a daily basis. But the authors then proceed to their final discussion:

> In all demographic categories studied, Hispanic men were considerably more likely to report having multiple partners than were Hispanic women. In general, Hispanic men were almost five times as likely as Hispanic women *to report* having multiple partners. Hispanic men who were unmarried, highly acculturated and had a higher income were more likely than other Hispanic men to have multiple partners.
>
> Hispanic emphasis on masculine pride may encourage traditional Hispanic men to have multiple sex partners, to be womanizers, to frequent prostitutes, and to search for women constantly. Within this traditional value system, "the better man is the one who has the most girlfriends." (Sabogal and Faigeles 1993, 261; my emphasis)[4]

What's wrong with this argument? In the first place, it takes a serious imaginative leap to advance from the finding that "Hispanic men who were unmarried, *highly acculturated* and had a higher income were more likely than other Hispanic men to have multiple partners," to the conclusion that "Hispanic emphasis on masculine pride may encourage *traditional* Hispanic men to have multiple sex partners, to be womanizers, to frequent prostitutes, and to search for women constantly." Is it, then, *tradition* or *acculturation* that is the catalyst for Latino womanizing?

Certainly given their data, a more reasonable conclusion would have been that, in acculturated settings, the absence of traditional constraints on machismo and on male aggression toward women (e.g., family pressures, agrarian lifestyles, or simply the unavailability of women) make possible a more unrestrained, even at times grotesque, living out of a cultural theme. Is active womanizing, in other words, a traditional activity, or is it rather a traditional *mytheme* that tends to *get realized* in acculturated, even cosmopolitan, settings? From the standpoint of cultural identity, the distinction is, of course, crucial: one point of view suggests that Latinos in traditional settings engage in unrestrained sexual activities; the other suggests that Latinos in acculturated settings engage in unrestrained sexual activity. Needless to say, what the study does not indicate (nor even suggest as feasible), is that there are numerous ways in which some male Latinos revise, undermine, negotiate, and creatively manipulate these collective categories. What we are left with, in other words, is at best a deductive fallacy, and, at worst, a perceived scientific confirmation of an unexamined stereotype. Second, the fact that Latinos have higher rates of both hetero- and homosexually transmitted HIV suggests that whatever is taking place is not stereotypical womanizing, but unrestrained sexuality. If this is so, why should the stereotype persist as an analytical category?

Now, the reason for focusing on metaphors of gender and ethnicity in a study of pathogenicity—for examining metaphor and cultural stereotype in a study of the recognition and elimination of "not-self," for casting immunology as a broad cultural phenomenon—is, I trust, abundantly obvious: If the only way one's identity is articulated is through claiming that one "is" what one's neighbor "is not," how can a framework for creative social interaction ever be located? And if stereotypes are changed by finding a space where one can build something new—where one can stop living behind clichés—why do we have so few examples of this actually happening? Because both the medical and clinical domains of immunology are built fundamentally upon the distinction between "self" and "not-self," we can effectively address these questions through examining the framework within which its metaphors unfold, and through analyzing exceptional cases in which these metaphors are creatively manipulated—by those who suffer from immunological disorders, by those who treat sufferers, and by those who define those illnesses scientifically.

BODY-CULTURE: THE SOCIAL WORLD OF MICROORGANISMS

Virus: A genetic element containing either DNA or RNA that is able to alternate between intracellular and extracellular states, the latter being the infectious state.
—*Biology of Microorganisms*, 7th edition

From antiquity, and in the written word at least from Plato onward, the body has been described as a sociopolitical unit, and sociopolitical units have been described as bodies. The universality of this analogy, however, never seems to prohibit us from being surprised by the particular forms it can take. When stigmatized groups are described pathologically—as bacteria, as tumors, or as viruses—the ugliness of our organic view of society may temporarily embarrass us into trivializing the connection, but we never have desisted, and probably never will desist, in describing a collection of people as a body. This is why the sudden rise in medicine of a self-conscious science of "not-self"—that is, immunology's direct and overt critique of the body's eliminating identity—demands no small attention.

Though immunology has increasingly become an eclectic domain of esoteric knowledge, it is important to remember that its disciplinary legitimacy has always stood, and for now still stands, on a fundamental distinction between "self" and "not-self." Self-recognition is central—and, in fact, crucial—to the understanding of antibody formation (Nossal 1969); and despite the recent trend to include immunologists in the widespread scientific habit of mystifying everything, we must remember that immunology's focus on identity has given centrality to the fundamental autotoxic metaphor of *the body at war with itself*. Even medical school courses bear titles such as "Identity: Microbes and Defense." As one text puts it:

> While normally acquired immunity is carefully regulated so that it is not induced against components of "self," for various reasons, when this regulation is defective, an immune response against "self" is mounted. This type of immune response is termed *autoimmunity*. . . .
>
> In many cases, exposure to foreign substances results from clinical situations in which tissue is transplanted or blood is transfused from one person to another. . . . Rejection of the transplant or transfusion is not a manifestation of some force of nature designed to frustrate the physician and the patient. Rather, such rejection occurs because of the central tenet of acquired immunity—recognition and elimination of "not-self." (Benjamini and Leskowitz 1988, 10)

Identifying allies defines for immunology a condition of well-being (i.e., of health), and its converse (misrecognition) neatly defines the discipline's domain of inquiry (i.e., of immunological disorders). As currently understood, immunology cannot exist without the recognition and elimination of threatening cells—i.e., without battle—and, in autoimmunity, without a body that wages war on itself. It is for this reason that the discipline is also characterized by a highly *volitional* and florid language in which cells exist as intentional beings—in which survival is understood as a function of *recognizing, scouting, tricking, discovering, alerting, evading, sensing, recruiting, mobilizing, prodding, masking, defending, scavenging, attacking, invading, adapting, appropriating,* and *killing.* It is a domain, moreover, where the "dumb" cells lose and the "ingenious" ones win; where cells become "committed" to certain activities. Not only, moreover, do we have a full range of intelligence among cells, but, like humans, some cells are psychopathic: "antigenic suicide," for example, is a social event involving activities such as cooperation, deletion, and sacrifice (see, e.g., Roitt [1977] 1980, 305).

The language of war is everywhere in immunology, but perhaps most prominently in the mid-level, popular literature for the scientifically minded. Here is an example from *Science News*; it is typical rather than exceptional, but in isolation it speaks for itself:

> When *faced* with a *foreign invader,* the immune system *mounts* either of two *defenses.* One, humoral immunity, involves primarily B cells. These white cells *recognize* a particular antigen, then make antibodies that bind to that molecule. The other depends heavily on T cells—not *helper,* but cytolytic CD8 T cells— that can *destroy* tumors or cells infected with viruses or bacteria. These *assassins,* including *natural killer* cells, become part of the cell-mediated immune response.
>
> T *helper* cells are the *sergeants* that roust T or B cells into action. As *helpers* form in the thymus, each becomes *sensitive* to just one antigen *trigger.* They *drift* in the bloodstream or *hang out* in lymph nodes *in a "naive" state* until they *meet* the antigen they were primed to *recognize.* At that moment, a *helper cell's fate* is sealed as either a TH1 or a TH2, or so some researchers think. If it becomes a TH1, the cell then *readies* cytolytic T cells to do *battle,* generating the TH1 response. As a TH2 cell, it *initiates* humoral immunity.
>
> "Essentially, it seems like in the Western world, the condition of health is linked to a strong TH1 profile," explains Mario Clerici, an immunologist now at the University of Milan in Italy. These *beneficial assassins* can *destroy* a cell that has been *tricked* into *harboring pathogens* where antibodies and TH2 components *can't get at them.* (Pennisi 1994, 121; my emphasis)

Immunology thus is warfare made small, and, as we shall see, hero epic writ large (figure 9).

But how entrenched, as it were, are the metaphors of warfare within immunology? How resistant are they to change? Why are they so dominant

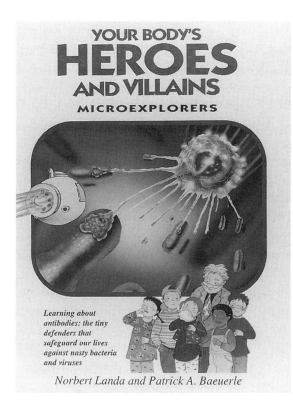

Learning about
antibodies: the tiny
defenders that
safeguard our lives
against nasty bacteria
and viruses

Norbert Landa and Patrick A. Baeuerle

FIGURE 9. *Your Body's Heroes and Villains*
A common example of the military metaphors that dominate our notions of immunity. While no one would doubt that cells do destroy one another, such interchanges account for only one kind of cellular interaction. In fact, such micro-relations run the entire gamut from wholesale slaughter, to cellular "self-sacrifice," to assimilation, to symbiosis and interdependence, and, of course, to peaceful coexistence. (Permission to use this book cover granted by Useful Books S.L.)

today? These are the socially significant questions to which the following discussion will be devoted.

Just how deeply seated are military concepts and metaphors of battle in the field of immunology? A quick perusal of medical texts in the field illustrates the fact that scientists are no less "immune" to this language than are sufferers who cling to these metaphors in the hope of giving their illnesses some personal meaning. Some authors (e.g., Sontag 1978) have argued that suffering can only be made humane by eliminating metaphor. Most others do not lobby for the actual elimination of metaphor but focus, nonetheless, on how the stigmas attached to metaphors result in the unjust treatment of sufferers.[5] Even though she later modified her argument, many still accept Sontag's idea "that illness is not a metaphor, and that the most truthful way of regarding illness—and the healthiest way of being ill—is one most purified of, most resistant to, metaphoric thinking" (1978, 3). Many doctors and patients have recognized how the self-help literature actually functions to blame those who cannot get well; and there is a long history of attempts to link per-sonality flaws to viral and immunological dysfunction. Oncology has been es-pecially guilty of this.

But as we have amply seen, eliminating metaphors in any domain of expe-rience does nothing to further human understanding, and neither does know-ing the actual biological causes of an illness do anything to decrease the extent to which metaphors may be used in describing it. Indeed, in a moment of as-tonishing scientific advances, how ironic it is that we have resorted to a most animistic and ideologically basic metaphorical form. To discount the signifi-cance of this fact may, alas, actually result in a misunderstanding of how social categories function to regulate human suffering and to control the rhetorical forms in which that suffering has meaning. One need only substitute cell war-fare for the language of sexual attraction previously described to begin to un-derstand just how central these metaphors are for conveying meaning, and how resistant they are to alteration.

But how easy are metaphors to change or modify? Surprisingly, the more prejudicial the metaphors (like those employed in gender stereotypes), the eas-ier they are to change, because, as we saw earlier, recognition is nearly coex-tensive with denial, with alteration, and even with elimination. On the other hand, changing metaphors that participate in the wider mythological dimen-sions of culture can be a difficult and consuming process, as I discovered when I asked my students some years ago to rewrite a popular account of the AIDS virus using another metaphor of their choice. What we discovered was both how difficult the process was, and how deeply entrenched were the fundamen-tal, heroic narratives that dominate immunology and its transformations.

Because they had been reading Sontag's *AIDS and Its Metaphors* (1990), I asked them to work with the popular metaphorical constructions of which Sontag is so critical and, in particular, to rewrite a popular account of how one contracts AIDS—the sort of description one might find in a WHO pamphlet written for distribution in a third world country. Remember, here, that Son-tag thinks (or, at least, then thought) that we must try to rid suffering of metaphor, while Johnson argues (and I agree) that it is metaphor that carries meaning. The popular description offered by Sontag reads as follows:

> The invader is tiny, about one sixteen-thousandth the size of the head of a pin.
> . . . Scouts of the body's immune system, large cells called macrophages, sense
> the presence of the diminutive foreigner and promptly alert the immune sys-

tem. It begins to mobilize an array of cells that, among other things, produce antibodies to deal with the threat. Single-mindedly, the AIDS virus ignores many of the blood cells in its path, evades the rapidly advancing defenders and homes in on the master coordinator of the immune system, a helper T cell. . . .

On the surface of that cell, it finds a receptor into which one of its envelope proteins fits perfectly, like a key into a lock. Docking with the cell, the virus penetrates the cell membrane and is stripped of its protective shell in the process. . . .

The naked AIDS virus converts its RNA into DNA, the master molecule of life. The molecule then penetrates the cell nucleus, inserts itself into a chromosome and takes over part of the cellular machinery, directing it to produce more AIDS viruses. Eventually, overcome by its alien product, the cell swells and dies, releasing a flood of new viruses to attack other cells. (1990, 105–7)

Asked to revise the metaphors employed in this passage, most of the students had a very difficult time replacing one metaphor for another. Here is what one student wrote:

The politician (AIDS virus) is tiny, about one sixteen-thousandth the size of the head of a pin. . . . Reporters of the body's immune system, large cells called macrophages, uncover a corruptive political story, equal to Watergate or the Iran-Contra scandal, and promptly notify the newspaper (immune system). The paper begins to contact news offices which send out an array of political reporters (cells) which, among other things, produce public condemnation (antibodies) to deal with the conniving politician. Undaunted, the politician evades the public outcry in his path and the swarm of reporters and reaches the office of the editor of the paper, a helper T cell.

Once in the office (surface of the cell), the politician finds the editor in a great deal of financial trouble. The politician slips the editor a cool payoff. Thus aligned with the editor, the politician strips the editor of all of his journalistic integrity. The editor falls under the power of the politician.

The politician can then manipulate his viewpoints (RNA) into the public's view (DNA). These viewpoints are then inserted into the minds of the people (cells of the body) and form a whole new set of ideas in society. Eventually, overcome by misinformation and propaganda, the people marry and reproduce children who are raised to think and act like the head politician, and who go on to corrupt other societies.

Is there, we must ask, any social connection between the rise of immunological discourse and fears concerning political corruption? More specifically, are we not evidencing the fear that those who appear to be acting in socially responsible ways may actually be abusing the advantages made possible through their politically correct behavior? Here I am reminded of the well-known Hindu notion of evil in which the worst forms of crime involve learning all of the ritual invocations and using them to selfish ends. I am also reminded of a famous Tibetan legend in which an alienated prince drinks from a polluted well which causes insanity because all of his subjects have done so. What we see here, in other words, is nothing more than a demonology—what traditional peoples know as possession, the *Invasion of the Body Snatchers* writ large. Now here is another student's revision, written during the Gulf War:

> The U.S. fighter jet had little trouble slipping over the border of Iraq, virtually unnoticed by the country's outermost defenses. This jet could have chosen many other points of entry, each just as suitable. But, once inside, the Iraqi radar soon picks up on this enemy attack, and begins to concentrate its weapons in a defensive manner. An impressive armada of surface-to-air missiles is moved across the desert and oil fields, yet it is no match for the massive firepower of the U.S. invader. Although the fighter pilot very well may have had the capability to destroy every target, he cunningly strikes at strategic points of communication, leaving all Iraqi systems totally defenseless. The U.S. jet, after surveying the situation, quickly returns to home base, to prepare for his next mission. The rest of this job will be left for someone else. Iraq soon realizes that its country's end is near.

An interesting study some years ago argued that among all professions fighter pilots and surgeons shared the most psychological traits (Cassell 1986). Now immunologists have pushed aside the gentler surgeons. This spontaneous evocation of the Gulf War provides, that is, a provocative demonstration of the sociopolitical implications of what we can legitimately call the Age of Immunology.

As in our earlier discussion of gender and ethnic stereotypes, we are here compelled again to reaffirm our basic observations about the meaning and function of culturally powerful metaphors. To understand, that is, how metaphor works for doctors and for patients, we need to see how the metaphors of immunology get embodied and manipulated through processes not unlike those earlier described for gender and ethnicity. The first point we need to keep in mind is the fact that, even if we don't like the sentiments conveyed about cell warfare, we do recognize immediately how culturally embedded these metaphors are—that is, that the metaphors are part of commonly shared and widely expressed cultural perceptions. The second is the tendency to see this as something that others engage in popularly, but in which one's self or one's friends do not self-consciously participate (hence "not me," "not my friends," "yes, it is common, but no one I know believes that cells can think"). In other words, people may deny the truth of these metaphors even if they rely on them regularly. And the third is our awareness that this denial is not a matter of deceit but is in fact part of an active renegotiation of the metaphor's meaning. In other words, as soon as the metaphor becomes recognized (that is, consciously "fixed") we begin to change it, difficult though this process must be, by challenging its universality. Metaphor, simile, and analogy are not, in other words, just figures of speech; they are the primary ways in which meaning is conveyed, and, alas, they are, all of them, cultural. They are not, in other words, only stylistic conventions, but major ways in which meaning is culturally constructed.

Are these analogies only *popular* representations, in the sense that they come to be employed loosely by nonprofessionals? How "immune" are scientists from the same ways of thinking? Is the very science of immunology, as Latour (1988) would have it, a *War and Peace* of the microbes, or are scientists any less likely to subscribe to and be influenced by the same cultural paradigms because they examine them critically and self-consciously? To address this question permit me, at least momentarily, to place Johnson's (and Lakoff's) argument about metaphor in the background.

Although for a number of years I have wanted to know more about how patients came to terms with the idea of a "body at war with itself," I have also wanted to know what bench scientists think about the intentionality of cells. So, I asked them: "Do you think that cells have volition?" Their answers surprised me, not so much by the diversity of their opinions regarding the significance of this question, as by my realizing how important the process of personification was and is to what we call "discovery." Indeed, since then I have learned that similes, analogies, and metaphors are not humanistic "flaws of science" but the basic building blocks used for making new discoveries.

Some scientists make important, Nobel-winning discoveries by, for example, imagining themselves as cells traveling throughout the bloodstream. Here is Barbara McClintock, commenting on her genetic research:

> I found that the more I worked with them [the chromosomes] the bigger and bigger they got, and when I was really working with them I wasn't outside, I was down there with them, and everything got big. I was even able to see the internal parts of the chromosome—actually everything was there. It surprised me because I actually felt as if I were right down there and these were my friends. . . . As you look at these things, they become part of you. And you forget yourself. The main thing about it is that you forget yourself. (Keller 1983, 117)[6]

Lest we miss the significance of McClintock's endeavor, it is essential to recognize the extent to which invention (as opposed to innovation) is based upon a process of selective dissociation in which unlikely elements are actively superimposed.[7] True discovery is made possible by repeatedly placing oneself at risk—by engaging repeatedly in the imaginative process of conjoining, superimposing, or otherwise conflating unlikely elements, or, in the social sense, of risking engagement with that which is potentially threatening or dangerous. Immunology as popularly understood is, in other words, anything but creative.

Although I have drawn attention to the importance of this superimposing process elsewhere (1992), we need here only recognize the systematic way in which metaphor functions in creative thinking. Scientific invention, like any other form of discovery, does not take place either through the systematic study of subjects *or* through chance; rather, its systematic processes keep alive a fluency within the context of which unlikely elements and chance encounters give way to something "new." There is, in other words, no contradiction in holding that creation results, on the one hand, from subjecting metaphors and the cultural categories they embody to a conscious critique (e.g., as with illness sufferers), *and*, on the other hand, from their wholehearted, fantastic embodiment (e.g., as in the selective dissociation of scientific discovery). The distinction that is crucial, however, is to recognize that the first activity is *innovative* (in the sense that it modifies an existing art), while the second is *inventive* (in the sense that it results in something unique that redefines an existing art). Because of the extraordinary difference between these two modes of activity, we need to take particular note of how creators dynamically engage both forms of manipulation—how they slip in and out both of the active use of "animistic" metaphoric projections, and of the self-conscious critical debasement of such projection as irrelevant, infantile, or "regressive."

Indeed, this slippage not only occurs among creators everywhere, but it does so with great fluidity. What has never ceased to surprise me is just how ready people are to adopt accessible cultural paradigms even while speaking of those popular metaphorical constructs pejoratively. The scientist who will deny that cells have intentions and volition will in the very next breath turn to his or her students and say that the cell they are observing through a microscope or slide projector is about to recognize, sense, scout, discover, mobilize, invade, appropriate, recruit, or kill its opponent. The scientist who denies that cells have volition may also, that is, be the same scientist who makes a Nobel-winning discovery by "becoming" a blood cell traveling through the body; and the speed of this shift from an innovative to an inventive process is sometimes made as quickly and as completely as a shaman can go in and out of trance. Discovery and healing are both productive forms of embodied psychopathology—atypical, peripheral, anomalous events in which creators shift constantly from the conscious transformation of cultural categories to unselfconscious, even dissociative, forms of embodiment.

As with our consideration of popular metaphors, the point is not that cultural metaphors invade science and that one must be careful not to be persuaded by them. Quite the opposite: the point is that these constructs provide the basis upon which identity is culturally negotiated and upon which discoveries are actually made. Talking *uncritically* and unselfconsciously about cell strategies, or cell volition, or cell warfare is not, therefore, just a convenient way of describing a process or a relationship: it is a way in which powerful cultural concepts participate in how meaning is understood, conceptualized, and embodied. Talking *critically* or consciously about these modes of conceptualizing provides the first step in transforming them. Thus, for immunology and virology, part of rethinking what happens at the laboratory bench comes simply with recognizing the cultural dimensions of metaphor, simile, and analogy in the first place. And, indeed, the very process of talking with bench scientists about their projecting intentions onto cells, and about their own use of dissociative processes, can function as a dynamic catalyst for revising how one thinks about the activity of looking through a microscope.

Thus, we must disagree wholeheartedly with those who would have us believe that it is necessary to rid meaning (or suffering) of metaphor. Metaphor is not a background against which meaning is set; it is the most basic and common vehicle for embodying meaning. Metaphors, especially when they embody powerful cultural categories, not only resist logical propositions; they should also remain largely unconscious if they are to control us, rather than be controlled by us. This is why one of the best ways of relieving the negative transformation of "a body at war with itself" is by talking to patients about the cultural construction of this metaphor; for, in so doing, individuals position themselves to accommodate the cultural weight that is brought down upon them, and, where necessary, either to reject it or to engage its possible consequences rhetorically.

It is because immunology's metaphors facilitate our negotiations with "not-self" that they become treacherously inescapable while, at the same time, providing the only real basis for revising themselves. That is why studying rarer autoimmune disorders can be more productive than examining how culture reproduces itself in the stereotypical paradigms of suffering that characterize our understanding of illnesses that are more stigmatized and better known; for in rarer disorders, as we will soon see, the more stereotypical manifestations of suffering are applied to new frontiers of human experience—to experiences occurring, if you will, at the categorical peripheries of the petri dish where survival itself is in jeopardy.

Examining the peripheries, in other words, enables us to see how difficult it is to escape cultural paradigms, how important it might be to look at pathogenic metaphors in other cultural contexts, how recognition of a metaphoric construct and its social construction is the first sign of its change, and how pervasive immunological paradigms are in a culture at large. Such practices may constitute our best hope for revitalizing an Age of Immunology.

So, to summarize, the argument is as follows:

1. Invention almost always takes place at the borders of a critical concept by those who can creatively manipulate existing metaphorical structures. This is an uncontroversial ethnographic fact that is supported by studies of the creative mechanisms by which discoveries are made (e.g., Rothenberg 1988). At these borders, transformations also take place; but, because the focus of change is on becoming "not-self," such transformations require not rational discrimination but some social or ritual setting. Only then,

what I call "selective dissociation" helps facilitate a (hopefully creative) transformation of a pathogen.

2. If we are interested in reframing old problems, we must make a concerted effort to transform existing critical categories. In the case of immunology or virology, this means examining the prevailing view of cell activity as modified hero epic.

3. Anthropologically speaking, we can transform existing categories by (a) shifting our focus from major disorders (the so-called "master illnesses" for which culture offers some powerful paradigms of suffering [e.g., Di-Giacomo 1987; Farmer and Kleinman 1989]) to less well-known diseases that do not conform to those stereotypes—that is, by examining what is happening at the categorical periphery of a scientific concept; (b) studying individuals in other cultures who employ diverse models of what pathogens are and how they interact with individuals; and (c) examining how scientists deviate from categorical norms when they make discoveries.

In each of these cases, we are positioned to understand how culturally meaningful narratives are valued, engaged, and modified—and, in particular, how they are dynamically embodied in both positive and negative transformations. We also see how their resistance to change is a direct function of their pervasiveness. And it is, therefore, to this deep-seated pervasiveness to which we will now turn.

ELUSIVE CATEGORIES AND CATEGORICAL IMPERATIVES

We have now seen how attributing meaning to metaphor is less a case of "bad metaphysics" than it is a means of illustrating how we deal with change at the levels of invention and innovation—how, that is, self-consciousness both inhibits us from transforming (when it inveighs against our need to dissociate) *and*, under different conditions, incites us to modify cultural categories (when it inveighs against the destructive dissociations in which we may have unknowingly participated).

Why, then, did we begin with an explication of the metaphorical idea that Physical Appearance is a Physical Force, rather than with the mechanisms of a Body at War with Itself, or Lakoff's cathartic paradigm of the Body as Container? Because, while the Body at War with Itself and the Body as Container are culturally powerful, we cannot embody for better or worse that power unless, say, we happen to be quite ill *and* sufficiently aroused by our illness (and its accompanying anger, pain, or frustration) to have the visceral experience that comes more readily to us when we hear, in this instance, a disturbing dialogue about sexual aggression. Until those who study illness are themselves seriously ill, they will continue to explore illness through narratives of suffering, while ignoring the central settings in which cultural categories are embodied, negotiated, and lived by or transformed. This is why so many indigenous groups (the Navajo, for example) claim that to cure a disease one ought first to have survived it. One could, in other words, speak all day about the lived world of someone suffering from cancer or AIDS—one could even appropriate their illness through descriptive narrative, through attaching one's authorial voice to some nice moving story—without ever coming to terms with how culture itself is inserted within embodied experience.

This is nowhere so apparent as when we see how biology not only symbolizes culture but is allowed to stand in for it. While this book is not directly meant to be a study of gender, it is clear that the separation of male and female is itself a cultural construct that is a subset—perhaps our most important subset—of a fundamental human need to establish what anthropologists call "radical categories." It is, I would argue, the very difference that we see in gender in which the notion of "gender" at all has meaning. Likewise, it is less a question of biological males oppressing biological females today than it is a question of understanding how patriarchy has become hegemonic—not a question of oppression, per se, but one of seeing how a particular form of reciprocity between "radical categories" (i.e., male/female, black/white, etc.) results in the neutralization of one side. This is hegemony, a form of Descartes's mask in which what appears to be a fair exchange results in the reverse engineering of one side: women live by patriarchal measures of success, blacks become "Oreos," etc. But it is a great mistake to think of this as simple oppression, because doing so prevents us from seeing how the metaphors—the cultural categories—actually function. Allow me one example.

In a study of male and female responses to sexually aggressive films, McCaughey and King (1995) made some startling and very politically incorrect discoveries. Rather than showing college students any of the many "awareness" films that deal with sexual aggression, they constructed an alternate fantasy. What they did was string together contemporary movie scenes in which women defend themselves against attacking men—initially featuring "scenes in which women are clearly 'innocent' and defend themselves from obviously unwarranted assaults" but gradually including "a few scenes of women doing violence to men with no obvious motive" (1995, 378). In this video women are shown not only building themselves up physically but engaging in traditional male aggressiveness. They are shown not only cleaning and loading guns, but using them. While many viewers are "uncomfortable" with their behavior, some openly applaud it without the slightest concern that they are participating in what they would otherwise label a deeply oppressive, "male" activity. "I thought the clips were great," said one woman, "It means that women are finally taking their place as violent, bloodthirsty, savage, testosterone-fueled egomaniacs next to the men. I love women with guns" (380)! Though the view may seem radical, the fact should not escape us that many women *do* value violence or, say, blood sport, even though they are also aware of the deep "maleness" with which these activities are traditionally associated. Likewise, many men value activities that are widely accepted as "traditionally female" (however they may define that). But, in either case, let us not mistake biology for the categorical oppositions that individuals *require* in establishing meaning. The categories themselves are flexibly adapted to needs and circumstances. The choice is individual.

My earlier example from Mark Johnson's *The Body in the Mind* showed how thinking and doing (or viewing) *do not* result in the same form of awareness, or in the same intellectual priorities: To say that one understands the gendered problems in Johnson's analysis, and to respond viscerally to the law clerk's narrative, are not only decidedly different kinds of experiences; they also set in motion quite different kinds of mental processes (which, in turn, give way to specifically different consequences). Recognizing the gendered nature of the metaphors in question, in other words, is totally different from responding viscerally to those metaphors. In the first case, we can easily assuage our discomfort by alluding to how particular "others" respond to the law clerk's language; in the latter, we ourselves are challenged. In the first case our experience-near analysis allows us to project the power of the collective category into the life of another whose emotional experiences we have appropriated; in the latter, we are forced to confront the fact that these categories are culturally driven—basic paradigms among which individual actors establish meaning. These so-called "social facts," in other words, are the powerful and oppressive stimuli that Gramsci and Fanon were so troubled by—the ruthlessly controlling cultural paradigms against which any other kind of experience is measured. Language is, after all, a social fact (Meštrović 1992, 73;

Hirst 1975, 90); just try not having a visceral response to Johnson's (Beneke's) law clerk, for instance. So much for the prejudicial valuing of the individual over the hegemonic.

Since these categories are sustained by and large through unselfconscious embodiment, through a process that forms a basis for collective identity, they also form the basis for the alienation and elimination of "not-self." The process itself is amoral, but its consequences are not; for though it can sustain a social collectivity (a "moral" community), it can also stigmatize those alienated by that community. Suffering, therefore, is eliminated not by denying the process but by bringing it to consciousness in cases where stigma flourishes. Self-conscious reflection takes us out of the domain of embodied, collective categories and moves us toward the categorical periphery where we find both the stigmatized and those self-stigmatizers we call "creative people." This process can be pathological (as when a creative drive leads to alienation), or constructive (as when those already alienated begin to reconstruct the categorical stereotypes they are damaged by).

Understanding, therefore, the mechanisms of transformation is essential to discovery, and especially if scientists are to rethink what immunology is and can be, or to reframe—even slightly—their ideas about cells and how they behave. This is why one of the best ways of determining how a stereotype might be refigured is to look at the categorical and cultural peripheries of experience—to "atypical" illnesses and especially to autoimmune disorders that have resisted or defied diagnosis.

Change, in these cases, becomes extraordinarily trying, painful, and difficult, particularly since marginalization itself necessitates challenging the cultural currency of deeply entrenched and, therefore, highly resistant ways of thinking. And it is naive to think that we can alter those prescribed ways of thinking and behaving simply by denying their relevance, or by waving the flag of morality upon the battlefield of embodied experience. Claims about the moral injustice of the processes that give rise to stigma do nothing to alter the processes themselves by which social categories function; transforming stigma cannot be accomplished simply by calling for the elimination of identity-forming processes when we find their results to be morally bankrupt, politically incorrect, or just odd or silly. And it is this mistake in particular—the belief that we can eliminate suffering by denying the very mechanisms by which meaning is embodied—that makes way for an autoimmunological age in which atrophy itself becomes tolerated, if not actively encouraged.

Immunology, in its fear of the unselfconscious, is, therefore, no more or no less the victim of post-Enlightenment metaphysics than is any other field of inquiry or domain of experience. What distinguishes immunology, though, is its hysteria—that is, the vehemence with which it curiously denies the very metaphorical mechanisms of embodiment while unconsciously reviving a demonology better suited to the Dark Ages. It is immunology's hysterical fear of possession that causes Descartes's enlightened reverse engineering to take its final toll autotoxically on the self.

3 | Immunology and Illness Experience

The successiveness of language—since every word occupies a place on the page and a moment in the reader's mind—tends to exaggerate what we are saying; beyond the visual trivia that I have listed, the man gave the impression of having experienced an arduous life. —Jorge Luis Borges, "Guayaquil"

INNOVATION AND EMBODIED IMAGINATION

Though social anthropologists may be well positioned to offer alternate metaphors to those military constructs outlined in chapter 2, it is not necessarily the case that we either have any better idea of why particular metaphors gain currency within a given society, or that we better understand just why an individual in a given cultural setting may cling to an unhealthy stereotype. Nor is it obvious from what has been published on the topic that anthropologists are any better positioned to be enough released from their own embodied narratives of salvation to examine how metaphors actually function in different illness experiences.[1] Why, for example, do we see the transforming of popular metaphors in our own tradition as healthy, while so frequently decrying the unhealthy consequences of changing what we perceive to be "traditional" in those we study? How are we any better positioned to release ourselves from our own sociopolitical objectives to look at how metaphors function in both positive and negative ways?

While we may want to argue rhetorically against the damaging effects of a particular metaphor (because, for example, it embodies an undesirable model of the nation state, or unjustly stigmatizes sufferers), we need a subtler understanding of just how metaphor actually functions in both everyday and scientific discourse. Lest we miss a critical opportunity, it must certainly be realized that metaphors are powerful, but in themselves neither good nor bad (or both good and bad); and the fact that some analysts wish so emphatically to excise them from the experience of duress points quite clearly to their power in establishing meaning in those domains about which we know least— cognitively, emotionally, experientially. Indeed, because metaphors are so potent, they more often than not are part of all manner of emotional and moral states.

In the interviews that I have conducted across a broad range of immunological disorders, metaphors consistently emerge as the major vehicle for creating new meaning. But, because they are so pervasive, their powers are not always transformative. They may, in fact, equally be inhibitory. Where socially embedded metaphors prescribe particular behavioral models, those metaphors may as much chain sufferers to existing culturally defined scenarios as provide creative models that are new and life-giving. Sontag's frustration at having been appropriated by the dominant cultural construction of cancer (as a stigmatized and self-inflicted form of pollution) led her initially to rebel against the way in which the social understanding of the disorder only increased the suffering of those who were afflicted by it.

Here, the overdetermined nature of a particular metaphor resulted in the afflicted being manipulated in unpleasant ways by the disease's social construction. But Cannon's landmark article, "Voodoo Death" (1942), shows probably better than anything I know just how the social definition of the pathological can have profoundly morbid consequences. Puzzled by how so many aboriginals could die from psychogenic shock after having a magical bone pointed at them, Cannon realized that, among other things, being singled out as a victim was only half of the pathology. The other half derived from family members who, upon hearing that a bone had been pointed, immediately began mourning the victim!

Indeed, when the unselfconscious (even dissociative) pathways of real transformation are not acknowledged, the constrictive nature of so many metaphors of suffering often only becomes apparent when the afflicted achieves "enlightenment"—i.e., when he or she becomes openly aware of the degree to which the cultural category can influence the illness experience. Then, highly self-conscious moral outrage and rejection seem like the only appropriate responses to the recognition of how easily oneself and others can be manipulated. This is why illness experience in general and immunology in particular embrace radically different forms of embodied imagination, and why the literature on suffering is characterized not only by vitriol and moral outrage but also by repeated descriptions of the (all too real) victimization of innocent people (e.g., DiGiacomo 1987; Farmer 1990; Farmer and Kleinman

1989; Good et al. 1990; Kleinman 1988a, 1988b; Kleinman and Kleinman 1991; Martin 1989, 1990). The very nature of metaphor, in other words, influences not only our understanding of actual illness experiences but also our coming to terms with the ways in which illnesses are described by those who write about them.

However, the anguish caused by being asked to embody a stigmatized cultural category need not have only unhealthy consequences. In cases where we are trying to salvage a "self" from a ravaged body, dissociation is critical. Talk, for instance, to anyone who has spent time in a clinic for chronic pain. "Has the pain subsided," we ask? "No, but I am learning how to deal with it." In other words, selective dissociation—separating self from self—becomes critical to successful therapy.

Why focus on the language of self-awareness, then, when what is called for is the development of the dissociative skill we daily employ but ignore and devalue? Because bringing powerful metaphors to consciousness is a primary means by which we resist undesirable and stigmatizing transformations of identity, even if that same self-consciousness functions elsewhere to inhibit transformations that may have beneficial outcomes. Rationality is, then, both a guardian against the unpredictable outcomes of dissociative behavior and the very thing that inhibits human change. At the same time, the dissociated appropriation of existing cultural or experiential categories is precisely what makes social well-being possible. One's ability to sense unselfconsciously what others mean in everyday encounters and to respond to those perceptions effectively is, in itself, the evidence of normality. This is so much the case that individuals who see themselves as psychologically alienated will develop strategies for convincing others of their normalcy. The deinstitutionalized mentally ill will often work very hard at public displays of normalcy, especially if they believe themselves to be permanently abnormal (Corin 1990). And those less seriously troubled will often be advised by psychological counselors that establishing a routine and sticking to it is the first step to recovering a sense of well-being.

So, the unselfconscious embodiment of modes of behavior (and of the metaphorical structures that socially convey meaning in local settings) is not in every instance to be criticized either for its inapplicability to local living, or for is damaging outcomes when metaphors exert real power over human intercourse. In fact, having such paradigmatic constructs available is so much a fundamental part of human relations as to make the idea of culture unthinkable without them. It is when these constructs are unhealthy—when sufferers are appropriated by pathological cultural constructs—that there is a need to make an extraordinary, conscious effort to resist those cultural categories. But *the process of dissociating is itself not a moral one.*

Oddly, when these metaphors (and the cultural categories of thought embodied by them) are expressed in their basest form, they also are at the place where they are most likely to be unwound and modified. One healthy outcome of the apparently unhealthy reiteration of our basest cultural assumptions and prejudices is that their simplistic nature becomes embarrassingly obvious. As myths are repeatedly cloned into simpler and simpler versions of themselves, so too does their cultural transparency become obvious. What is the *Terminator*, after all, but a radically truncated and highly dumbed-down *Odyssey*?

Real transformation—real invention—is largely, therefore, the result of selective dissociation—the willful participation in a creative superimposition of images or categories. We do not change, despite what Descartes might have argued, by becoming self-aware; for "awareness," in the Cartesian sense, allows us not to *change* but to *innovate*—to *react* to our recognition of the power of a cultural construct. Such conscious acts of resistance are, therefore, reactionary. And since they are reactionary—that is, by definition innovative byproducts of a given cultural construct—they may also help codify, participate in, and to a certain degree even legitimate, the very thing they seek to transform. This is why self-conscious reflection invariably leads us not only into an Age of Immunology but into an Era of Autoimmunity, a moment in which the static codification of what a "self" is leaves us incapable of negotiating productively with various "not-selves" whose unknown powers we have codified as "outside," beyond the range of what can be known.

Thus, rhetoric about the need to "know thyself" before admitting an "other" into one's life results in a quest whose only victim is the self one had hoped to "understand" but in fact "dissected"—where gaining control of one's destiny through so-called "self-awareness" leads to a kind of death by naming, a reactionary codifying of one's identity that excludes by definition dynamic encounters with the unknown. In such instances, it is crucial that we separate our moral outrage over how illness metaphors stigmatize from our understanding of how transformational processes work; for examining how metaphors function can help us better understand how change is facilitated, particularly if we focus on illness experiences for which culture has not already provided explicit paradigms of suffering. In examining immunological disorders that are less deeply entrenched in culturally explicit metaphors—so stigmatized, as, say, AIDS or cancer—we are able to see more clearly how metaphor functions in the *creation* of meaning. In focusing on illnesses that are less well known, therefore, we can expect to find a wider and more creative range of metaphors at work.

The creative features of metaphor, then, may be seen most clearly when we examine disorders that are not at all—or, perhaps, only minimally—determined. In such instances, metaphors serve an entirely different function than they do in disorders that are widely recognized, since their primary purpose in these indeterminate settings is *inventive*. One need only listen to the way illness is frequently constructed by an individual suffering from a relatively rare immunological disorder to see how metaphor may be used creatively to accommodate an absence of socially prescribed models of meaning. To have a disorder that is little understood means, necessarily, that one has no model to manipulate, to embody, or to rely upon in moments of existential uncertainty. Creativity here is an essential means of survival.

MEANING IN AUTOIMMUNITY: THE "BLACKEST" DISEASE

> *We are . . . confronted once more with the paramount problem of embodiment: to show not a causal relation or a parallelism, but to the contrary how an existential attitude of consciousness constitutes the signification of a physiological fact.* —Alphonse de Waelhens, *Une Philosophie de l'ambiguïté*

Although much of the language of immunology has its basis in metaphors of war that it shares with microbiology, it is important to highlight just how complicated both self-knowledge and sensory experience become when the distinction between "self" and "not-self" becomes formally expressed in the somatic process known as autoimmunity, where the body mounts, as it were, an immune response against "self." It is here where immunology shows itself as being significantly different from its predecessors.

While today the basic concept of autoimmunity has captured enough general interest to have planted itself firmly in the imagination of Western bioscience, its pervasiveness is no indicator of the extent to which we have resolved its more unsettling assumptions. First among these is the fact that autoimmune disorders begin with the notion of a confused and divided self. Rather than involve a body immunologically besieged by foreign agents, the autoimmune response involves directly the misreading of some aspect of "self." Second, but yet more unsettling, is what this separation implies, often covertly—namely, the stigma of not even knowing who one is.

Unless we assume that all selves are, as it were, divided into multiple volitional agents, autoimmunity shifts the focus of an organism's identity from its capacity to live among other organisms to its inability to control the agents that undermine self-knowledge. The autoimmune response leaves, that is, no psychological space for the kind of self-definition predicated upon the mirror that others hold up to us. What can "self" mean without a "not-self" through which to set its body-image boundary? While the microbiology of immunity has its psychological analogue in multiple personality disorders, in the sense that autonomous microbes interact with and sometimes respond to one another, the analogy works even better for autoimmunity, where destruction occurs when those microbes are neither recognized nor controlled. While the microbiological analogue is sustained in immunology (where a "self" is directed against a foreign pathogen), autoimmunity has its metaphoric corollaries in such things as masochism and suicide. An antibody is a substance that responds to a pathogen; an autoantibody performs the same operation on the very organism of which it is a creation. This systemic character of autoantibodies is evident from the very beginning in Ehrlich's *horror autotoxicus*, that "improbable situation of the immune system turning upon itself" (Tauber 1994, 32), which "makes no claim that autoantibodies may not be formed; it only suggests that they are somehow prevented from acting" (Silverstein 1989, 163). Under such conditions of extreme existential instability (where "nonself" is either expressed or latent within "self"), the causal agents of pain give rise to particular forms of meaninglessness; for there is no "normal" self, as we will see, to be distilled or salvaged from an alien encounter. In autoimmunity, one gets so viciously close to the mirror of otherness that no room is left for reflection. In, that is, the absence of light caused by a body compressed against that mirror, there is no image cast on which one might gaze.

While some 80 percent of all autoimmune sufferers are women, statistics are hard to trust, not only because diagnosis is often difficult, but also because growing number of illnesses can be categorized as "autoimmune." Among the more commonly known are juvenile diabetes (pancreas), Hashimoto's disease (thyroid), multiple sclerosis (brain), and, with increased frequency, systemic lupus erythematosus (SLE).[2] It is this last upon which we will now focus: first, because of its clinical ambiguities (that is, its range of symptoms); second, because it gives rise to forms of suffering that are "atypical" (in the sense that they do not readily conform to accepted cultural stereotypes); and third, because of its "social" dimensions (SLE is disproportionally common among black women of childbearing age, and its clinical spectrum means that advocacy and support groups must work hard to have their disorder publicly understood).

SLE is characterized by a chronic inflammation in multiple organ systems, such as the skin, the kidneys, and the joints. Those who suffer from SLE have a variety of antibodies to their own cells and cell constituents. Because these proteins differ among individuals, the symptoms of lupus are variable. SLE affects the skin (rashes, sensitivity to sunlight) and often devastates various internal organs. Arthritis is common; but damage to the kidneys, heart, and lungs also can take place: one of the rarer forms of lupus involves the central nervous system.

Though not as difficult to diagnose today as in previous times, SLE is still not always easy to recognize. To have SLE one must exhibit four of eleven possible criteria (Tan et al. 1982), ranging from photosensitivity and butterfly rash, to renal and hematologic involvement, and to such neurologic complications as seizures and even psychosis.

A variety of skin rashes (especially on the face and hands), aches and pains, and general fatigue are frequent; indeed, the name, lupus, is itself meant to derive from the wolf-like appearance of the face. But its diversity is its major attribute, enough so that "pain" in this illness may be defined by an enormous range of symptoms. To complicate matters, symptoms from which SLE patients suffer can be difficult to attribute to the illness; some unpleasant symptoms may at first seem not to be connected with SLE, and only later be recognized as SLE complications. SLE sufferers, moreover, often find that they have less in common with fellow patients than with individuals suffering from other unrelated illness who happen to share their major complaint. Sometimes, those with lupus wonder if an undiagnosed illness of a friend is SLE; lupus patients have suggested to friends (some later diagnosed with cancer) that they may have SLE.

What is worse, the "reasons" for contracting SLE frequently involve some blaming of individual sufferers. In part, this is because we know less about the causes of SLE than we do, say, of AIDS or of certain forms of cancer. As in the past, when cancer was openly attributed to personality types, the tendency to blame patients in SLE is palpable. Not surprisingly, then, SLE sufferers score high on standardized psychological tests (such as the Minnesota Multiphasic Personality Inventory scales) for hypochondriasis, depression, and hysteria, but it is entirely unclear whether their doing so is a sign of more suffering or of their taking more control of their illness:

> Given the multiplicity of symptoms possible . . . and the continuous need for self-monitoring and adjustment of activities, one hesitates to label hypochondriacal symptoms (exaggerated concern about health or bodily or mental sensations) as dysfunctional. Likewise, hysteria, the conversion of anxiety into somatic symptoms, is more likely to occur in the setting of an existing organic disease. In these patients hysterical symptoms may help rechannel anxiety released by the uncertain, potentially disabling, life-threatening aspects of these diseases. (Liang et al. 1984, 18)

The point of Liang's observations is that these symptoms may well be the appropriate adaptive strategies, given the nature of the illness. To what extent can a response be called "unhealthy," when it is appropriate? Without venturing an answer, we must recognize that some SLE sufferers are very likely to appear in the eyes of their families and caregivers to be hysterical and/or depressed hypochondriacs, whether or not these symptoms arise for "healthy" reasons. In this respect, those with initial SLE complications must face social problems similar to individuals who, for example, suffer from chronic fatigue syndrome.

Finally, and perhaps most troubling of all, is the fact that those who have been positively diagnosed have, unlike AIDS or cancer sufferers, little or no social construction of their illness to work with or respond to, no model of suffering either to find acceptable or to reject as stigmatizing. Because of its relative rarity, the clinical complexity of SLE, and the lack of public awareness about it, these conditions remain endemic. And these difficulties are not lessened by the fact that it is predominantly a disease of women (nine times more prevalent among females than males—women about whom, regrettably, all sorts of behavioral stereotypes still prevail in clinical settings and in homes). Unless someone knows an SLE sufferer, the usual response to its being mentioned in conversation is "What's that?" This clinical and social ambiguity also helps engender an existential uncertainty in which psychological factors may be unfairly brought forward by patients, families, and even caregivers to fuel existing feelings of guilt, blame, and self-doubt.

What often hurts most in SLE is the indignity caused by the suspicions of others that things are not as bad as sufferers make them out to be. One only has to imagine life for a lupus sufferer to see just how insidious the social experience of their disorder can be: burdened with an illness that has no social currency and little or no culturally recognized somatic value; plagued by symptoms that are as diffuse as they are painful; and, most visibly, inflated periodically with steroids and the insatiable hunger they can cause. Imagine trying to negotiate this profile of suffering in a world where the most socially powerful models of suffering come from the emaciated imagery of cancer or AIDS. Imagine this lupus sufferer—abandoned with a socially "meaningless" disorder, troubled by an inconsistent and diffuse set of symptoms, and perhaps even fattened by steroids—coming up against the socially meaningful paradigm of the emaciated fighter of tumors or other specified pathogens that is the norm for cancer and AIDS.

For those with SLE, socially recognized illness stereotypes (and their metaphors of suffering) are not labels that necessarily appropriate passive sufferers. Rather, if psychological survival is to be achieved at all, metaphor must be actively engaged. It must become, as it becomes for the lonely artist, a means through which different models of suffering are conflated or superimposed in the interest of creating meaning where none exists. Indeed, because lupus sufferers do not have easy access to culturally meaningful images of human suffering, they are less likely to be appropriated by dominant models of disease, nor do they suffer, or benefit, from the ready adoption of available imagery. The negative result is frequent isolation and self-consciousness. But there is also a positive effect: denied a readily available cultural lexicon for the legitimization of their experiences, lupus sufferers employ an astonishing diversity of metaphoric constructs. In fact, the remarkable diversity and richness of their narratives also means that they are quite likely to *feel* alone and isolated, but less likely to subscribe to an "alien" group identity that has been socially codified for them by others.

While they may be as satisfied with or as annoyed by the medical treatment they receive as are cancer or AIDS patients, the absence of a powerful collective voice in SLE has less frequently led sufferers to define themselves as an exclusive category. Though isolation and depression are already far too well known, individuals with SLE are less likely to have abandoned their search for a common ground in which their illness experience can be integrated within what they consider to be mainstream society; "normal" or "healthy" here become less a domain to be appropriated rhetorically by illness-specific advocacy groups, than a mirror in which one's identity gets negotiated. Here, in other words, is an artistry not to be overlooked, especially since the increasing role of support groups means that the traditional metaphorical diversity that characterized this illness becomes regularly eroded. Paradoxically, then, it is the very *absence* of a solidified group identity that encourages sufferers of a disease to negotiate constantly the very terms of their identity. The act of codification actually functions increasingly to limit the range of experiences that may be considered "meaningful."

Lest we mistake the complex nature of certain illness narratives as a sign of their incoherence, there is an important lesson to be garnered, as Kleinman (1988a) has shown, from those whose social voice is rather weak;[3] for here we may observe a process that is part of every creative act—namely, the conflation and modification of culturally available (but, for the purpose, inadequate) categories. Indeed, the complex narratives that seem especially to surface among those who suffer from rarer autoimmune disorders has its corollary in an equally diverse range of medical treatments and research agendas. While scientists working on cancer and AIDS may often feel—and even, at times, express—the concern that their research is being limited by its cultural construction, getting outside of that construction so as to entertain a different research paradigm may actually jeopardize one's professional standing. The oncologist who does not "fight" cancer with aggressive "magic bullets" such as radiation and chemotherapy is relegated to the fringes of his or her profession. The AIDS researcher whose authority may circumscribe a professional domain that is "an inch wide and a mile deep" (i.e., a domain, however thoroughly known, that is very limited) is in no position to step outside of the narrowing intellectual "black boxes" that, as Latour argues (1987; see also Charlesworth et al. 1989, 148–72), build, promote, legitimate, and ultimately control particular research programs.

The tendency of culturally relevant metaphors—indeed, of any collective representation—to limit human knowledge is as readily observed in the domain of research as it is among the experiences of sufferers, and the awareness of how culture both defines and limits the understanding and experiencing of different immune disorders explains why it is essential to examine this domain of "self and not-self" across cultures; for comparing how well-known and rare disorders vary in different cultural settings undoubtedly provides the best way of seeing the advantages and restrictions that our culturally given paradigms

establish and maintain. We now realize, for example, that the cultural construction of AIDS differs dramatically in the United States, Haiti, and Zaire;
we need also, however, to examine how cultural categories limit what we are
able to know scientifically. Do SLE sufferers in Britain tend not to present
themselves early on because of cultural prescriptions about assuming one's
share of diffuse aches and pains? Likewise, do rural poor in America not present clinically because of a popular belief that life after forty is *normally* characterized by hardship? Though entertaining more than one cultural model of
a disorder is never easy, it is only through such activity that we will enable
ourselves to reconstruct what a particular illness actually *means*; for creativity itself is, importantly, predicated upon a facility to superimpose and actively
conceive of "two or more discrete entities occupying the same space" (Rothenberg 1988, 444). The philosopher's imaginary Martian who descends to
earth to comment on how we conceptualize things is a mere straw man to the
finely articulated metaphors of "otherness" that anthropology stands to offer
immunology. Examining immunology across cultures, in other words, can
only help increase the possible ways in which a disorder may be conceptualized by sufferers, by health-care givers, and by researchers as well. Indeed,
many of us feel that such research is not only clinically useful but intellectually
necessary for understanding the degree to which cultural awareness can refigure scientific knowledge.

As the Aristotelian epigraph for the preface of this book suggests, only the
divine and the damned are able to separate themselves from the social, and
thus the cognitive, engagement that misfortune necessitates. For the rest of
us, meaning can only arise through embodying culturally valued imaginative
constructs and experiencing them dynamically; the "sick" individual stands
very much in need, as the late Anatole Broyard aptly pleaded, of "the conta-
gion of life" (1990, 36). "Fighting" cancer, therefore, can have no meaning
unless one finds a way of manipulating its social construction, since empower-
ment can only be achieved through trying one's knowledge on the contested
fields of memory and imagination. Like the Trobriand warrior who carefully
decorates his battle shield in the hope that it will attract more spears, effecting
a "cure" is, as the Greek *heroes iatroi* (hero physicians) well knew, an *art de faire*
achieved through the marriage of things creative and destructive. The
painted shield will always attract more spears than a plain one because the will
to cleanse, as Bachelard (1948, 41–42) so cogently put it, cannot be sustained
without an adversary every bit its equal. This is precisely why examining do-

mains where meaning is openly contested is far more productive than is engaging in histrionic displays of moral outrage, and why, in the end, the exception defines the rule.

WHERE THERE ARE FEW DOCTORS

> *To recount events is magical for sorcerers.... It isn't just telling stories. It is seeing the underlying fabric of events. This is the reason recounting is so important and vast.*
> —don Juan Matus to Carlos Castaneda, *The Active Side of Infinity*

It was one of the first in-depth discussions that I had had with a stranger who suffered from a serious autoimmune disorder whose causes were unknown, and its complexity has never left me. She was, by her own description, a black American approaching middle age, among that group most vulnerable to systemic lupus erythematosus (SLE).

"Martha" was a single woman in her mid-forties who had been diagnosed with lupus seven years before our first meeting. Though she now realizes that she had been suffering from a number of lupus-related problems for years before she sought medical help (or, at least, that her lupus has become the focus for making these earlier experiences meaningful), she has, since being diagnosed, had a number of life-threatening crises, and over sixty medical procedures that required hospitalization. Unlike many lupus sufferers, whose illness can enter long periods of remission, she has been close enough to death to have been very troubled by the way people frequently respond to her illness. This is how she describes the dilemma of regularly being told by others that, despite her illness, she looks good:

> I still get angry, actually, because people expect to see someone that looks like an emaciated cancer patient. They have a stereotype. [Though] people like to have compliments, [when they say] "boy, you look good" they make me feel like they are trying to delegitimize what I have just said. What makes me equally angry is when people tell me how I am.... People tell me, "look at you, you're doing well." I say if you want to find out how I am feeling just ask me; and if anyone *were* to just ask you, and you tried to explain, they [then] say, "that's all right ... the same thing happened to my cousin." ... One of the most frustrating things [in this illness] has been trying to talk to people about how my brain is different, and how it works so differently, and how I know that the brain is a wonderful thing, and I know for the most part that I can make appro-

priate responses. But I am very much aware of this brain's, uh . . . , searching for the right word, searching for a word. And it all happens within seconds. And no one else can see it. But I just know it. . . . I am aware of it.

This passage gives a good sense of the kind of frustration that results from having one's illness experience challenged, even passively, by common expectations about how sickness and health should be represented. But Martha's situation becomes more complex when we consider how the isolation caused by the absence in her SLE experience of any of the more widely received images of suffering is actually exacerbated by the biomedical construction of what she has. This isolation is most dramatically portrayed in her description of a life-threatening episode of lupus ceribritis. Martha begins with a remark about her lupus support group, from which, unlike some sufferers, she actually felt she derived benefit:

Yes, it was [good], but I only went to a few meetings [before] I got sick. And I was in hospital from September to December. So, the lupus support group, [well] I thought I needed that. And when I got sick, I couldn't have it anymore. So I wound up in this big city institution just bewildered. . . . That is when I had the crisis with lupus cerebritis and sort of came out of it [having] lost my balance. I couldn't sit up at all. I was always falling, and I couldn't walk without guiding myself with my hands because I had lost my coordination and strange things were happening to my vision. One of my eyes wouldn't move. All sorts of weird things that you could [possibly] think of happening happened to me. The doctors could never say to me that it was going to get better. . . . They'd say, "we don't know, we'll wait and see." . . . Well, things were going straight downhill, but they weren't [yet] spiraling [until] I came out of it and for six months I was so amazed. All I did was literally and figuratively say, "What the hell happened to me? WHAT HAPPENED?" I couldn't get rid of the sensation that this is really a grand surprise. WHAT HAPPENED TO ME? And wonderful steroids. . . . I looked into my mirror one day in the hospital and I was frightened at what I saw because I didn't think that was me. . . . And I didn't know who it was. . . . And it was absolutely frightening because my cheeks were up to my eyes. And the doctor had done these wonderful things. They had given me pulse therapy to save my life, and my life was saved. I looked like a freak. . . . I had this uncontrollable appetite. The woman in the next bed and I would have money, and we would find a nurse at night that was going down to the snack machines. We would give 5, 6, 8, 10 dollars . . . oh, we didn't care. Use it all up. Bring food. And I remember I ate six chocolate candy bars and never got sick. And I still can't figure out how I could eat six candy bars and not get sick. . . . And we were stuffing food down our faces because our appetites were uncontrollable from the steroids. And [when] anyone would call up, we would say, "bring food; BRING FOOD!" And it was the strangest thing. . . . My weight has never been in control . . . ever since. And at that time I was flowing up all over [that is to say, swollen]. But good old steroids. . . . They are wonderful things. They can save your life, and they can kill you. . . .

I have quoted this passage at length because it draws our attention to the manner in which the frequent inability of lupus sufferers to fit common stereotypes of suffering gives rise both to an absence of social meaning as well as to a genuine existential doubt about the meaning of the self. Surely, the most profound social doubts derive from the misreading of SLE by nonsufferers who are using other illnesses as models of pain and hardship. Though others may tell Martha that she "looks good," though some may think privately that a good bit of the problem is "in her head" or that "she's not as sick as she thinks," in fact her daily life is a struggle to complete simple tasks: at first, to find her way back home after work; now, to manage to get out of bed, or to cook a meal, or to spell her name. As she puts it,

My job [involved] details . . . and I wasn't getting them. I was forgetting them. I used to have to talk to a lot of people every day, and I was talking to a friend who had been a client and my words just went away. And I think there was some sort of panic in that silence, and I couldn't get it back.

Having described lupus and its manifestations as "bizarre" (and, later, how a study of suffering in lupus could not be standardized because it would, in Martha's words, "lack the important subtleties that are germane to people who have illnesses that are not typical"), she describes the existential crisis of her own cerebral degeneration:

I had a life-threatening crisis with lupus cerebritis. I sort of came out like a person who had had a stroke, but my personality—to me—had changed a lot. . . . In my fantasy, someone came to me and ferreted off my personality . . . covertly, and now I'm stuck with somebody else's. And I don't know this person. . . .

Sometimes I think that's what literally happened and I'm still waiting for some-one to confirm that it's just a practical joke, that it's not real. . . . I know . . . that I have lost some of my intelligence. I also know that I have lost much of my vo-cabulary. . . . Someone took part of my vocabulary away. I have always been fas-cinated by words. And words that I was drawn to—that I liked very much—I made them mine. . . . The brain's a wonderful thing, but I can't remember the words I want to say. . . . And when you lose your words, you lose a part of your personality, because of the way you speak, because of the language you use that's part of being who you are. And, when that goes, part of your self goes with it. . . . Now I'm always laughing at bizarre situations. . . . After awhile, the more bizarre things get, the more I laugh. And it's just a real strange personal-ity. I told [my doctor] that I am a manic depressive, but I don't get the depres-sive side. I just live a lot of the time in some kind of mania, talking jigs and all that. . . . You know, drop a pencil on the floor and I'll laugh. It's almost like watching another person in some ways. . . . Sometimes I just think it's a freak of the illness, that I'm watching someone else. . . .

Because of Martha's lupus cerebritis, she perceives a lack of meaning in her life and a loss of her self. Because she speaks of other selves, and, in particular, of a lost former self, her psychiatrists wonder if Martha is a clinical psychotic. Does "better health" for Martha mean denying the effects of her cerebral de-generation so as to appear better to know her "self"? What "meaning" can the "self" have for Martha when even the realities of her suffering are under-mined both by her real apprehensions about the social construction of suffer-ing and pain, and by her awareness of the delegitimating double-bind created through her openness about what has happened to her brain?

It is often erroneously thought that this disease is called lupus because of the butterfly rash that was taken, somehow, to appear wolf-like. But there is a much better answer to be found in classical mythology, where the wolf is sym-bolic of one who lives outside culture and beyond those social values that give rise to all that has meaning—a powerful animal, crafty in its ability to present itself for what it is not.

THE UNCOMMON GROUND

Thus far, I have described the experiences of one individual to highlight how problematic meaning in autoimmunity can become. I have also tried to illustrate the potential difficulties that arise when a complex disorder fails to conform neatly to the stereotypes through which a culture canonically allows individuals to suffer. But there are two additional factors that contribute to a rhetorical erosion of meaning in SLE. The first is the well-known role played by biomedicine in delegitimating embodied, imaginative, so-called subjective, meaning; the second (which I can here mention only briefly), is the role of ethnicity in influencing health-care behavior.

The problem of finding meaning in SLE is exacerbated by a number of specific features of the present culture of biomedicine. Perhaps the most important of these is the fact that the diagnostic and management difficulties associated with SLE necessarily unfold within a clinical setting characterized by a well-documented inability on the part of health-care givers to tolerate ambiguity. While Martha is exceptionally lucky to be the patient of one of the very best clinicians I have ever met, many SLE patients must begin their often long journey to diagnosis by negotiating a biomedical culture whose values are frequently at odds with the amorphous nature of their illness. The fact that both physicians and medical students are professionally socialized in training environments that place extraordinary emphasis on clinical certainty has the consequence of actively delegitimating the patient's subjective emotions and, ultimately, his or her sense of self (Good 1994, 78–83). This is not only because of the real need to get the clinical facts right; studies have shown that medical students actually get worse at taking case histories as their clinical education advances, even though it is well known (despite what our managed care officials promote) that most diagnoses (something like 80 percent) can be made by taking the time, and making the human effort, to construct a careful case history—i.e., of getting to know a patient as a human being.

Especially during initial visits, the obvious discounting of subjective criteria may be seen both in the physician's legitimate desire to construct a full history of *relevant* symptoms and in the patient's efforts to employ clinical (rather than emotional) terms to describe his or her suffering. In SLE, where patients may only be finally diagnosed by physician-hopping, this tendency is especially obvious. Clearly, it takes a very special sort of person to respond to a physician's claim that it is "all in your head" with the response that, indeed, "it may all be in the physician's head." Most people are inclined to accept the diagnosis offered by a family practitioner and, unless they continue to deteriorate, will put up with their inner conflict if the diagnosis seems to have merit.

Thus, the SLE patient who has finally arrived at some diagnostic certitude may actually have done so by challenging the veracity of what he or she has been told, and by taking the unusual step of seeking help elsewhere. Those who make it to an early diagnosis are often strong people who are willing—either by personality, by cultural inclination, or by the severity of their suffering—to work toward a setting in which diagnosis becomes possible. One thing is certain: those who are successfully diagnosed early in their illness are either lucky or are quite skilled at negotiating their health care. Diagnosed SLE sufferers are therefore inclined to be very articulate and independent. How else would they have the courage to physician-hop, in some cases for years, without an acceptable diagnosis? How else could they learn to live with the emptiness they can often discover at the end of that struggle? And though it may be clinically helpful (and socially expedient) to *normalize* SLE (one doctor complained to me that Martha is not a *typical* SLE sufferer), the amorphous character of the illness is everywhere present, even in the campaigns of its own advocacy groups. Were SLE characterized by "normalcy," the Lupus Foundation of America would not have to spend so much time making lupus "common" by informing us of our ignorance (figure 10).

In addition to dealing with a clinical environment that is sometimes actively engaged in the deconstruction of the subjective meaning of their experience, the SLE sufferer is also influenced by factors of ethnicity and class. In an illness with a documented advantage to those who are diagnosed early (i.e., before significant organ damage), social stigma and cultural categories can both function to inhibit the seeking out of care. Successful treatment is not simply, that is, a result of access to good care, but of how and when one decides that one's level of pain warrants engaging a health-care system that is always expensive and sometimes inhuman.

What must be emphasized, however, is that such decision-making is less a simple socioeconomic problem than might at first appear to be the case. A well-known immunologist practicing in America and England once told me quite openly that his older British SLE patients presented later than his American ones because, he conjectured, of cultural prohibitions against complaining (the stiff upper lip) and against seeking help for symptoms that at first appear vague, diffuse, or nonspecific. Although it would be inaccurate to say that lupus is a disease for self-obsessed Californians or for those of a Cartesian inclination, in communities in rural Appalachia folk legends about the blues and the plight of the rural poor are powerful enough to inculcate a strong sense of a normal life after forty as one of depression and suffering. Here, it's

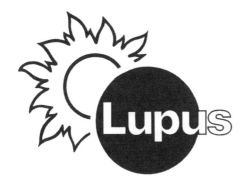

Lupus Erythematosus is a chronic inflammatory disease of the connective tissue. Though relatively unknown, it afflicts over a half million Americans—more than multiple sclerosis, muscular dystrophy or leukemia. And there is no cure.

Let us tell you more. Ask for our free brochure. Write or Call:

Lupus Foundation of America
Vermont Chapter, Inc.
P.O. Box 209
South Barre, VT 05670
(802) 479-2326

THE RARE
DISEASE
THAT IS
NOT RARE

Your CFC Contributions
Will Help Millions of
People Live a Healthier
Life.

October Is
National Lupus Awareness Month

MEMBER
National Voluntary
Health Agencies
for the Combined
Federal Campaign

FIGURE 10. **Lupus: The Rare Disease That Is *Not* Rare** Like artists leading lives of extreme psychological alienation, those who suffer from incurable or obscure illnesses develop a wide range of metaphoric constructions about their suffering. Here we see how naming an illness becomes the first step toward codifying how that illness is meant to be experienced. (Reproduced courtesy of the Lupus Foundation of America.)

not necessarily the case that SLE sufferers go undiagnosed (though obviously some will), but that they could present themselves at a doctor's door late enough to compromise seriously their chances of living successfully with the disease. Even where money is no object, cultural considerations have a serious impact on this illness. Some studies, for instance, indicate that the prevalence of lupus among African American women is as high as one in seven hundred and fifty (as opposed to one in two thousand for the general population). Though we are only beginning to examine the influence of socioeconomic factors and care-seeking patterns among blacks with SLE, and to examine what cultural factors inhibit early presentation, it is believed that African Americans have a hereditary disposition for the illness, despite the fact that we have little knowledge of the extent to which culture influences health-care seeking and compliance behavior at the early, crucial stages (Liang et al.

1984). How convincing, then, are the genetic arguments? Well, given the broad social factors, not very.

Such racial and ethnic presumptions are—as they are in much of biomedical culture—not only permissible but considered morally acceptable. By devaluing the patient's subjective criteria in favor of clinical ones—by not, that is, actively accounting for ethnic and racial variables that actually keep suffering people from seeking out care—health-care providers can actually promote the erosion of Johnson's "nonpropositional and figurative structures of embodied imagination"—that is, the metaphors that one dynamically negotiates in creating a bridge between "reason and sensation." The effects are palpable: asked if she would still be with the same GP had she not persevered and found her remarkable rheumatologist, Martha replied, "No, I'd be dead."

OUTSIDE IN, INSIDE OUT

The community . . . can preserve itself only by suppressing [the] spirit of individualism.
—Hegel, *Phenomenology of Spirit*

We have described in general terms how metaphor is used in both popular and scientific immunological discourse. We have seen how bringing these metaphors to consciousness allows us to formulate innovative responses to stigma, and how selective dissociation facilitates our inventively manipulating metaphorical structures. In addition, we have come to realize that the act of defining occurs much more emphatically at the anomalous peripheries of cultural categories where isolation and the need to survive highlight the exceptional manner in which meaning in illness is embodied. These peripheries are not merely those of a culture—i.e., not only embodied by "outsiders"; they are also the peripheries of groups that may themselves be considered "inside" but "abnormal"—i.e., not only groups that become stigmatized scapegoats for a culture, but even "advocacy" groups whose identities are codified by a shared sense of being in need of some voice, of being "not well" or *considered* not well by others. Understanding "advocacy" is, therefore, central to understanding the social implication of "immunological" thinking; for by definition these groups are devoted almost solely to the task of convincing the "body" of culture that its real or perceived "antigens" are not so harmful as that body imagines.

Indeed, advocacy groups are often so preoccupied with defining and limiting the unknown that they sometimes fail to understand how their moral objectives may actually reify the alienation of those they seek to protect. Although it seems totally counterintuitive that an organization designed to promote the welfare of a stigmatized group should actually participate in the codification of that stigma, in reifying an existential condition (i.e., in naming the nature of an illness experience), advocates risk undermining the creative side to uncertainty, including its positive and empowering consequences. Let us take two immunological examples, starting with a social stigma that is understood to be highly antigenic (AIDS) and proceeding to one which is not perceived as socially threatening (arthritis). Throughout this exercise we should be asking ourselves about the effects of advocacy programs that actually promote the "antigenic" status of something relatively unknown (e.g., SLE, "the rare disease that is *not* rare").

Although being accused of attempting to police language frequently limits the more overt attempts at controlling how certain illnesses are described, when a moral high ground has been taken, there are few limits to what is accepted as appropriate monitoring. The booklet *HIV & AIDS: A Guide for Journalists* (1993), co-published by Britain's Health Education Authority and its National Union of Journalists, provides an excellent framework for educating ourselves about what should and should not be said in print (figure 11).

First, journalists are warned to be hypersensitive: they should check with the appropriate organizations "*each time* they report on the virus" (ibid., 7) because knowledge and information (not to mention the dimensions of what may be considered correct) are changing daily. We are told that it is accurate to say "HIV positive/person with HIV" but inaccurate to say "AIDS carrier." It is accurate to say "HIV, the virus which causes AIDS" but inaccurate to say "AIDS virus." Likewise, one goes for an "HIV test" (not an "AIDS test"), engages in "safer sex" (not "safe sex"), and gets involved in "high risk behavior" rather than with "high risk groups" (7). AIDS carriers do not kill people, the infections they give them do; and, because of this, journalists should "avoid describing people as 'innocent,' as 'victims' or as 'sufferers'" (8): "HIV does not discriminate"; the word "'victims' implies helplessness and invites pity"; and "sufferers" won't do because "people with AIDS are not necessarily ill all the time" (8). The guide even explains that, while the Oxford style for acronyms dictates that upper case be used only for the first letter when the abbreviation for a name is pronounced as a word (i.e., "Aids"), "AIDS" should be advocated so as to remind us that we are dealing with a syndrome rather than a single condition (9).

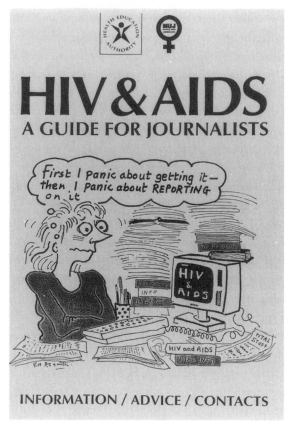

FIGURE 11. *HIV & AIDS: A Guide for Journalists* While a sensitivity to the emotions of those who have contracted life-threatening diseases, or who live with chronic illnesses, is reflected in our being careful about how we describe those conditions, all too often that very language alienates individuals from the realities of daily experience. Though health-care providers rightly want to assure those who are HIV-positive that they are "well," the everyday experiences of those living with the virus all too often suggests otherwise. (Crown copyright material is reproduced with the permission of HMSO and the Queen's Printer of Scotland.)

Although these prescriptions are offered with the best of intentions, what strikes me as alarming in all of this is the fact that people who suffer (if you will pardon my use of the word) from the knowledge that they are HIV positive are being denied this experience by the very groups whose moral duty it is to look out for their best interests. Leaving aside the fact that the distinction between HIV and AIDS in large measure was fueled by an insurance industry that did not want to pay for the former, what is most shocking of all is the complete avulsion from the domain of human experience of the concept of "illness" as an absence of a state of well-being: people do not go for HIV tests because they think that "everything is all right." Nor is it necessarily in the best interest of every individual who is HIV-positive to be told by caregivers that nothing is "wrong" with them, even though what most truly believe is that something has indeed gone very wrong.

This fact came home to me in a very concrete way some years ago when I was invited to conduct research on immunological metaphors at a highly proactive metropolitan health-care facility. I knew personally three of the facility's providers, and initially, at least, everyone was enthusiastic about what I explained to be the obvious benefits that accrued to those who understood the mechanisms by which unacceptable metaphors could be modified once they were sympathetically brought to consciousness. Despite their enthusiasm, the entire project had to be abandoned because a protocol that I had used in countless clinical encounters (one I could not and would not modify) began by asking each patient how long it had been between the time that he or she had not felt well and the time when medical advice was sought. Since counseling for those who are HIV-positive depends critically on the organic fact that the body may be functioning in an acceptable manner, I was not permitted to entertain in that clinical environment the notion that patients had come there as the result of feeling that something simply was not right—that feelings of being "sick" had been the catalyst for seeking a diagnosis in the first place.

Setting aside completely the anxiety created by the gross disjunction between what was being suggested in the clinical setting (that they were completely healthy) and what was being experienced in the world at large (that they were polluted by an incurable virus), the truly educational experience for me came when I explained my situation to a close friend, who happened to be both a psychiatrist and black. I had introduced my dilemma to him because, initially at least, I thought of revising the protocol, despite the fact that doing so would have skewed my ability to compare responses for HIV and AIDS with responses I had already recorded for rarer autoimmune disorders. His response was both candid and alarming: "If you want to work there, you'll have to let them 'do' you; it's just like being black."

It was at this juncture that I began to look more carefully at a coincidence that I had earlier recognized—namely, the historical parallel between the invention of an "immune system" in the 1960s and the rise of an era during which policing language was considered an appropriate means of protecting social differences. Was this historical parallel, I asked, a mere coincidence? For, clearly, the popularity of immunology, despite what we now anachronistically argue, definitely antedates the arrival of HIV. And which of us, in any case, seems willing to consider the idea that a continued hypersensitivity to what is or is not "different" could actually erode the very things we might otherwise have shared?

Now today even my Latino students of European descent refer to themselves as "students of color," despite the fact that my own skin color is significantly darker than theirs! Again, what we see here is not the melting pot but the potluck dinner—that aforementioned "celebration" to which we each bring a different dish but all eat by the same rules. In fact, trivializing difference ultimately undermines diversity "immunologically" because it desensitizes us to real difference: students who wish to be doctors nearly all *say* that they "want to go into primary care"; the world's major natural resource plunderers are all "for the environment"; and our colleges, governments, and businesses all claim to "celebrate diversity" while, at the same time, working frantically to get everyone doing the exact same sorts of things. Indeed, what one may think at home is often so totally irrelevant to how one presents oneself in public that the latter space appears almost wholly dominated by "antigenic" exchanges—with relations, that is, in which we present ourselves as cautiously and as opaquely as possible.

In all of this, the single constant is our increasing inability to negotiate with difference. In this "Age of Immunology" we, like those attending environmental conferences, become increasingly less capable of distinguishing between, as it were, the antigens and antibodies—between those who love nature and those who find it expedient to say that they do; for our Cartesian program has not just completely paralyzed us when it comes to facilitating changes in our lives, but has actually desensitized us to the actual need to negotiate with real dangers when we do attempt to change. Alas, this superficial placation of difference ultimately backfires because social skills are like language skills—if you don't use them they disappear. We feign interest as a means of avoiding hard decisions. Is it any wonder, then, that our teen suicide rate grows shockingly, while those very individuals seem to have made such little effort at social intercourse, or that Americans, as we will soon see, far exceed any other culture in verbally advocating what they least know or do well?

And this superficiality grows exponentially. The creative domain of metaphor already described for those with "rarer" autoimmune disorders (i.e., where metaphorical *invention* is more prevalent) is, as I write, being codified and seriously limited by its own advocates. The Arthritis Foundation and the Arthritis Health Professions Association are working hard to keep its members from expressing just how badly they feel: when referring to "people with arthritis," we are instructed to avoid not only the words "sufferer" and "victim," but, alas, we must also give up "arthritic." Arthritis should, moreover, not be referred to as a crippling disease: for, according to the guidelines, "these words carry an image of inferiority." (God help all of the spastic societies in Great Britain.) Inference and deduction—i.e., human reasoning—are discouraged: "As a general rule, we refer to people with arthritis as just that—people with arthritis." "Will someone," asked a South Asian student of the college at which I teach, "please explain to me just what the difference is between that term 'person of color' and the term 'colored person,' and why one is politically correct while the other is offensive in the extreme?" Will we really be any better off when we replace all of the "arthritic people" with "people with arthritis"? The important point, of course, is less that we acknowledge difference by paying lip service to diversity than that we genuinely enjoy having our public and private aliens living next door. Without a genuine enjoyment of the exotic we are merely left with hiding our awareness that the act of acknowledging *any* difference or diversity is itself a discriminatory endeavor. And it is the hiding of this discomfort that, in turn, deeply alienates those who are different, whether their difference be one of health status, one of ethnicity, or, in the case of our teenagers, merely one of age.

Although I imagine I will forever be damned by the Arthritis Foundation for saying so, I do think it "unfortunate" that my grandmother was a "person with arthritis" (alas, not "arthritic") and that this condition kept her from engaging in most of the activities she valued. Not only should I be reprimanded for openly expressing this reality, but I am also not permitted to address the well-being of others, for "people who do not have arthritis should never be referred to as 'normal.'" Yet, I'm afraid what I really hear when I look to those who are suffering—yes, "pitifully," and "in isolation"—is Martha's frustration and anger at those who would tell her how she feels.

SHORT STORIES

I have made this letter longer than usual, only because I have not had the time to make it shorter. —Pascal

It is sometimes said that an illness has no "normal" course. SLE transforms this insight into a truism. Perhaps the oddest thing about examining this disease is the realization that there is an enormous (albeit painful) creativity at work in the years of undiagnosed thinking. Talking to lupus patients, I hear echoes both of my first experience of phenomenological thinking as a philosophy graduate student, and of the descriptive language of many of the artists I befriended during my years as a painter. For, unlike we anthropologists—who codify "meaning" at symposia, through books, and, even at times, through the histrionic appropriation of the experiences of others—what is most obvious in talking to unusually creative people is the degree to which their existential isolation (whether deliberate or imposed) results in an enormous diversity of metaphorical constructs the meanings of which are not always accessible. For philosophers and artists, of course, the condition is often self-imposed. For those with autoimmune disorders, however, the degree to which they do not participate in acceptable forms of meaning often makes "meaninglessness" itself a painful form of life; for narrative authority is predicated on a system of interrelations, of networks and rules, which, once accepted, both direct and limit the possible forms that human experience can take, through the leveling out of variation, the dissolution of difference, and the delegitimation of phenomenal experience.

What are the consequences of such ambiguity for SLE? First, because "meaning" is something that is always called into question, isolation is inevitable. Even clinically, the invisibility, liminality, and resistance that are characteristic of "rare" disorders combine to create an ambivalence of meaning in which systems of status are treacherously negotiated. This is, of course, why subjective criteria are nearly always devalued in clinical settings, why they give way to the biotechnology of charting whether a patient measures up to certain scientific requirements,[4] and why medical students are actually trained to distance themselves in the interest of reducing a patient's emotions to a diagnostic category.

Second, the effects of this isolation may be damaging or fatal, but they may also become catalysts for a genuine transformation. Heightened levels of depression, hysteria, and hypochondriasis may be "neurotic," but they are also adaptive: they can both redefine the past (Martha's "I-used-to-be" narrative) and set the stage for a truly transcendental redirection—one that happens less by self-conscious therapy than by chance. The word, aphasic, let us remember, refers specifically to that which is "inexpressible" or "speechless"—to things that are hard to describe or communicate, but that are, nonetheless, definitely felt. No doubt it is the intuitive awareness of the fatal limitations of the canonical that leads sufferers into hysteria, depression, and hypochondria. What is left but panic when sufferers attempt to embody the creative mechanisms that those within the canon (academics, clinicians, "advocates") work by definition to standardize, if not delegitimate?

And while advocates may work with the best of intentions to minimize the alienation of sufferers, it is also true that collective meaning (that is, "culture") is not always the self-conscious multicultural phenomenon with which we are presently familiar, but a system that limits and confines—even delegitimates—certain "diverse" forms of experience. For culture, especially as it is experienced unselfconsciously, is "meaningless" wherever its rules are not contested, even if its successes are nonetheless still measured in its dissociative rites. It is, in the words of Fredrik Barth, an "empty vessel." This is what McFarland has in mind when he claims that "culture actually witnesses the absence of meaning, not its presence" (1987, 113), why successful living at the center of things is measured by the degree to which one "does well" without wasting so much time thinking about it.[5]

Our Cartesian connection of "self-awareness" and "meaning," then, both inhibits us from seeing how self-conscious advocates codify suffering and desensitizes us to the ways in which meaning is achieved through forms of selective dissociation—where ambiguity becomes, as it does in ritual, adaptive and creative whenever it is contextualized. This is not a type of meaning that focuses on distinctions (on specificity and the absence of relativity), but a commingling of forces that are both creative and destructive. No doubt our Enlightenment concern with the destructive powers of dissociation not only protects us but also inhibits our potential to create. If this is so, what we may perceive in the ambiguities of SLE is the problem of how to turn this tendency around—how to focus on creativity—in a world that does not fare well with ambiguity.

If this situation is as troubling as it seems, why haven't we responded culturally in more inventive ways? This is the complex question to which, by examining the canons of "science" and "society," part 2 of this study will be devoted.

In the next chapter we will examine some of the cultural factors that have contributed to this simplification, and particularly those factors that have allowed for the "search and destroy" mentality of immunological thought to have taken such a pathological hold on human life. First, however, we ought to confront the major transformational issues that are not culture-specific: among these certainly the most significant is the recognition that change is *necessarily* a dangerous process. While society may, as so many intellectuals fear, control our actions with ruthless precision, it also functions to limit constant and unlimited transformation. The inhibiting tendencies of culture, in other words, do not only exist so as to enchain us; they also function to protect us from the kind of uncontrolled growth that we can biologically witness in any tumor.

That change is not a safe activity is easily verified by the controls that have been placed upon change throughout history by various societies, as well as by the rites of passage and related structured frameworks that societies have created to maintain social order. Because creating real diversity *is* dangerous, there exists among all societies a deep desire to engage in collective initiatives to limit it—even if such well-intentioned efforts eventually lead to Aristotle's feared world of dead-level, nonvarying enclosed types. And, yes, here again, medical science offers us a cogent example of the "shortening" of the story in which the future is, as Warhol quipped, preoccupied with all of us looking alike (the actual outcome of generations of hormonal therapy) and with a pseudo-celebration of diversity in which each of us can be famous for but a few minutes.

Although there are numerous clinical cases that illustrate the relationship between our dead-level Age of Immunology and our active efforts to limit diversity, few provide us with as crude a short story as do the ethical dilemmas posed by genetic engineering. But, though the future of our species may be put at risk by clones and cyborgs (Haraway), let us not forget that the growth hormone industry has already offered us the short story that is the outline for the grander epic, the question here being: how do you create an "illness" out of diversity, and how do you, in so doing, create an infinite clinical need? Our biotechnology industry has already sorted this out for us by lobbying to equate "difference" with "disease." This equation is accomplished through a statistical maneuver in which the shortest 3 percent of our healthy population is, by virtue of the stigma they bear, clinically "ill." After all, isn't it true that short people in the 1950s were kept out of sales jobs because they could not impose their products on others in door-to-door encounters? According to an article that appeared in the *New York Times*, "college graduates more than 6 feet 2 inches tall earn 12 percent more than their shorter classmates; of American presidents, only two have been shorter than the national average for men of their time" (Werth 1991, 47). In criticizing the unscholarly nature of much of this research, the same *New York Times* author reminds us that little of this information is germane to a child "agonizing to become 5 feet 6 inches instead of 5 feet 4 inches" tall (ibid.).[6]

But how does our biotech industry create a constant need for their synthetic human growth hormone (HGH)? By arguing that the disadvantages of being at the liminal edges of the height curve, or at the peripheries of its Venn diagram, create intolerable "suffering" for liminal people. And, unlike diagnosing "people with SLE," establishing who suffers (i.e., who qualifies for treatment) is a simple matter of finding out what the largest cohort of HGH users shared in common—in this case, being in the lowest 3 percent for height. The beauty of this scheme was soon, however, exposed by critics who pointed out that "of the three million children born in the U.S. annually, 90,000 will, by definition, be below the third percentile for height" (Lantos 1989 [in Werth 1991, 47]). Not only would these numbers create "a potential annual market of $8 billion to $10 billion," but the market would, de facto, become unlimited: "If making our shortest children taller is the goal, the growth curve can be pushed up indefinitely. After all, there will always be a lowest three percentiles. Someone will always be shortest" (ibid.).

And so we begin our program to achieve Warhol's vision of the future. The circle of diversity becomes smaller and smaller, until it begins to disappear in the stagnant atrophy that is characteristic of the cells at the center of the petri dish, where we find not only those too weak to negotiate their own identities, but a condition of life characterized by an actual inability to negotiate with difference—a loss of those skills upon which human intercourse depends. Should it surprise anyone, then, that modern life would come to be characterized by a near complete disjunction between what we profess to value and what we actually do?

Part II   εpistemology

"Epistemology" is a big word. It is also a bit of nonsense. Strictly speaking, it is the branch of knowledge that is concerned with the nature of knowledge. Those who attempt to practice it are committed to thinking about thinking. Stretched further, one might say that every moment of self-conscious awareness is, necessarily, epistemological. Why use the term at all then? Because thinking about thinking is in itself a certain kind of practice—one, moreover, that produces forms of knowledge and experience that are far less universal than we might "think." Thinking about thinking produces the practice of writing, of explaining, of logic, of science, and of historical memory—in short, of all the cultural practices we take to be of value, of import, and of relevance to what we call "understanding."

Over time, the act of thinking about thinking produces responses to universal questions that are culturally unique, self-perpetuating, and sometimes exclusive. No matter how theoretically sophisticated we take ourselves to be, we will never transcend Descartes's cognitive definition of being by thinking about thinking. There are, in other words, no fancy or "modern" theories that can totally explain away what came before them, because the act of cognition can never in itself facilitate, for instance, the creation of a boxer's experience of the world out of the thoughts of a novelist. It is not possible, in other words, for a Hemingway to be motivated to fight by the same impulses that moved the boxer he writes about. While the novelist may, indeed, become a boxer, he will always be the writer who in thinking about thinking decided to enter a practice much more physical than his literary vocation.

This is why no "new" theorizing can ever tell us more than we already empirically know—why, even if we awake one morning to some Kafka-esque transformation, we will still be the thinker trapped inside the insect form. Thinking about thinking is the *epitome of what the Enlightenment stood for—in practice, a reflection on reflecting, combined with universal claims that are actually very specific because they develop out of certain cultural activities like writing books, or looking to a factual past in order to understand the present, or trying to suggest an informed course of action for the future.*

And it is because no smart theorizing can transcend the infinite reflections we see in the barbershop mirrors of human thought that alternatives to thinking about thinking strike us as so completely naive—why thinking reflexively or deconstructively about life produces not answers to, but mere extensions of, the Enlightenment. This is why a theory of theories is just an extension of whatever that theory might have been meant to replace. More positively, however, this is also why reinventing history is (surprisingly) the only creative way of achieving transcendence. And why should we want to transcend or reinvent the process of thinking about thinking? Because somehow, somewhere, the "recognition and elimination of difference" (i.e., immunology) arose as our dominant social obsession, as our collective response to the Enlightenment.

Why should this have happened? Why has the Enlightenment's self-conscious requirements led to the total separation of self and nonself, and to the attempted elimination of the latter and, alas, even the former? Are there more constructive outcomes lying dormant in the same corpus of cultural values? Might the cells of the culture we inhabit "commit" themselves differently? And, as for commitment, why have we at all, and quite deeply, committed ourselves to that thing we call science when the world of science so often appears lifeless and scientists themselves so self-absorbed? Why have we so accepted science as a religious form—as a domain of exclusivity, a modern locus of esoteric knowledge? Why has such thinking produced in the first place the overarching belief that modernity is a pathological condition?

Although these are not questions that can be easily answered, our attempt to reformulate the past should be placed against the background of the issues they raise in order to allow us to hope that the soil we till may someday—if even perhaps by "chance"—produce new forms of living. You can't get out of the water, as the alchemists knew well, before you've jumped into it.

Thus, it is in the spirit of invention, rather than the spirit of explanation, that it becomes important to take the time to ask about immunology from the standpoint of thinking about thinking. Studying the history and practice of science is, in other words, as much a creative endeavor as it is an analytical one, especially if our goal is "recursive"—that is, a return in thought or discourse to that place where thinking about thinking first committed us to stopping life in its tracks.

These central chapters, therefore, attempt to focus on a small part of why we have so incomprehensibly participated in our own cultural pathology. For wherever there is an awareness of death, there is also the basis for life. What I intend here is not only to analyze the origins of our "immunological" tendencies—to accept as much as to critique them—but to explore how thinking about thinking has made us participants in a world much more self-perpetuating and tumorous than integrated and constructive. Is there a way that thinking about thinking can result in a pattern of growth that is more relative, more embryological, more creative? Implicitly, such possibilities should and must exist, even if only found by chance, as when our Creators formed humankind out of clay and dust.

The point is that there comes a time in everyone's life when it becomes necessary to do something that seems illogical to virtually any other human being; for, without such actions, it becomes impossible to go back and find a new way out of the destructive tendencies that the Enlightenment has facilitated.

> *My lord, I have undertaken this long journey purposely to see your person, and to know*
> *by what engine of wit or ingenuity you came first to think of this most excellent help in*
> *astronomy, viz. the logarithms; but, my lord, being by you so found out, I wonder no-*
> *body found it out before, when now known it is so easy.*—Henry Briggs to John
> Napier

For the past three decades the concept of "incommensurability" has been employed, controversially and with little success, to articulate the absence of a
relationship among various scientific theories and among the social practices
that arise from them. During this period, philosophers of science (e.g., Kuhn,
Popper, Lakatos, Feyerabend, and many more) have ruminated over the question of just how related are the initial and final intellectual paradigms that
stand at the beginning and at the end of a scientific revolution. As Katherine
Hawley puts it:

> The key idea [for Kuhn] was that of change: scientists work within a frame-
> work, or paradigm, until more and more phenomena prove difficult to account
> for within that framework. This accumulation of anomalies prompts the devel-
> opment of an alternative way of working, and scientists may change wholesale
> from one paradigm to the other, changing their ways of talking and thinking
> about the world. Between these changes, or revolutions, the main activity of
> scientists is that of "puzzle-solving." This is a worthy endeavour, but it is not
> quite the great march towards truth in which scientists had previously seemed

to have been involved. After each revolution, different puzzles present themselves, and the process begins again. (1996, 291)

Does "real" change create a paradigm so new as to be "incommensurable"
with the paradigm that led to the "revolution" that created it? Philosophers,
of course, will never resolve this question because, according to Needham, in
the main they

> bypass what has been discovered about the variegated springs of human con-
> duct and instead base their arguments on fictional examples; one asks his read-
> ers to imagine the ethics of a tribe on a Pacific island, another makes up the
> teleology of a people in the Amazonian forest (their main aim in life, it should
> be mentioned, is to die of influenza, so no wonder they have to be made up),
> and yet another takes it as an axiom of method that we can invent the natural
> history of mankind for our philosophical purposes. (1983, 21)

While this practice, Needham continues, "is open to several explanations . . .
what in any event calls for remark is the explicit preference of fiction over
fact" (21). On the other hand, it is with literary fiction itself where "the matter
if anything becomes more interesting. In these instances the authors may give
themselves away in their figments, or they may reflect the presuppositions or
desires of those for whom they write. In either event they often tell us more
about conceptions of human nature than would the inevitable qualifications
of more didactic ventures" (21).

Whether or not there is more anthropology in Kuhn's *Structure of Scientific
Revolutions* or in Edgar Rice Burroughs's *Tarzan of the Apes* (the subject of
Needham's argument), I will not venture to resolve here; for Needham's
conclusion is not that we should be good postmodernists (replacing anthropology with fiction because the latter may more openly reflect the motives of
those who write it), but that we should recognize the depths of our own cultural prejudices and the heavy influence of our categories of thinking on
what we take to be a universal mission of our own creation. To wit, the notion
that incommensurability might be a part of major paradigmatic change, and
the notion that this idea could "seem exhilarating, outrageous or extravagant"
(Hawley 1996, 291), are important signals indicating the major preoccupations
of a specific culture (namely, *ours*) at a particular historical moment. Setting
aside any reference to the possible beliefs of fictitious groups, then, what "in-

commensurability" openly calls attention to is our fear and discomfort as a modern society with change, with transformation, and with the potential for great human difference.

Although it may be expedient to label our concerns about what cannot be known as universal—and, in a homogenized world, more easy to be convinced of their universality—there can be no intellectual merit in recommending such a presumption. Although happiness, sadness, a fear of change (even, alas, the misery of influenza!) may be common worldwide, the manners in which these experiences become meaningful vary enormously and are always individually experienced through the currencies of culture and language.

Every human experience must, then, be viewed against the background of a collective legitimacy in which the meaningfulness or meaninglessness of that experience is embedded. And, today, such understanding is, if anything, seriously jeopardized by an obsession with our private individualities, combined with an ignorance of how to cultivate ourselves socially. That we are today acculturated to avoid recognizing diverse modes of thought (to avoid, if you will pardon the neologism, "essentializing" cultural or national characters) is no reason to deny the continuities of collective behavior. No wonder our world appears so "immunological"; no wonder we profess to honor difference without the slightest sense of how the challenges of the unconventional might help us define who we are; no wonder we homogenize the universe by denying the possible incommensurability of other modes of living. No wonder we devote ourselves to saving others from the comfort of our homes, our offices, our foundations and organizations, our big university chairs. No wonder we all want to work at a safe remove from otherness and where the lights are brightest!

One of the unstated rules of multiculturalism is that honoring diversity means that we can know it; for it is unacceptable today to think that totally different modes of thinking exist, let alone that they might give way to moral and emotional domains that are to us inaccessible. While incommensurability may be unknowable to those who remain untransformed; so, too, is the scope of communality we so confidently apply worldwide. This is why the actual experiencing of transformation is so important, because the experience itself demands that we acknowledge the potential for each of us to be genuinely transformed by human love—by a kind of reciprocity that is deeper and more profound than direct exchange. And if our culture actually devalues these experiences, we are left alone to deny their reality and to suppress their manifestations in others.

Yet the legitimate fear that looking at "culture" will lead to social Darwinism—to a ranking of various kinds of abilities that different lifeways encourage or enhance—becomes less problematic as real differences internationally disappear. In fifty years, for instance, the six thousand unique languages in which diverse modes of thought are embedded worldwide will be cut in half. Such facts are completely lost on institutional networkers because they have so insulated themselves from human experience (psychologically, if not physically) that they aren't aware of the profound homogenizing effects, not only of their own denials of difference, but of modernity itself. Although they use moral claims to speak for things they don't actually know, their daily distance from the "other" they so fear leads them into their own kind of "essentializing," where "others" appear so incapable of helping themselves that only the expression of "my" ego will save them from one another.

Comforting though it may be to claim a complete universality of human experiences, these comforts should be recognized for what they are. Such claims are especially embarrassing when they result in an intellectual imperialism, an academic dissection of the emotions or feelings of others via whatever literary techniques are currently favored and fashionable. It is hard enough to engage in the trying and laborious intellectual effort demanded by any explication of a different mode of thinking; it is far more demanding when such efforts are undermined by a conservative kind of humanism—one whose universalist language is itself designed to dissuade us from examining the implications of human difference. Indeed, a moral fear of difference—emotional, cultural, even racial—need not in itself prohibit us from accepting the fact that others may experience sensations of which we are entirely ignorant. It is an unwritten rule of clinical psychology that one cannot treat a condition (a criminal behavior, for instance) that one could not imagine oneself experiencing. The converse is also true: if a psychologist cannot work in a prison setting because he or she cannot imagine doing what the criminal has done, it also follows that there are all sorts of ways of seeing to which a group of professional interpreters could have no access.

Thus, it's not simply that we might want to see the pathologies or the illness experiences of others as either anomalous or "typical." Worse is the assumption that all domains of experience can be appropriated by an intellect enough conditioned to transform them "virally" and then to disempower all that strikes us as "unusual." This is why incommensurability is so problematic; for hidden within our cultural obsession with "progress" is the outright fear of the possible existence of new and different forms of experience—forms about which we may have no intuitive understanding, nor any sense of what mechanisms of change might allow or require us to experience something entirely new. Today, alas, the concept of genuine difference has itself become unfashionable in a postmodern era where (because one can only know one's own experience) how one articulates one's feelings and one's presumptions about the feelings of others is accepted as adequate. The trying and laborious effort that is required to engage some genuinely novel mode of thinking (Lévy-Bruhl [1949] 1975]) is set aside and disparagingly labeled either as the "exoticizing" of the everyday or as the "essentializing" of the cultural influences on individual freedom.

Yet the fundamental categories around which specific ways of thinking and acting develop can vary enormously over space and time, and may even be readily evidenced within the recent history of a particular culture or intellectual tradition. In Euro-American history, one need only look as far as the nineteenth century not only to see a system of values decidedly out of step with our own concerns but to witness a real fetishization of the notion of "progress." Why speak of the habits of Martians to get at the gist of basic cultural difference? For the very concept of controlled change that began in the Enlightenment and reached its peak in the Victorian era has been almost totally expunged from our perceptions of what we might offer the rest of the world. "Progress" may no longer appear unquestionably good. But, like it or not, let us not forget the degree to which the Victorian period was impelled forward by a widespread set of beliefs about moral certitude, a pervasive injunction about the necessity of fairness, a deep-seated belief in the necessity of patrician sentiment, and, above all, an excitement about the mechanisms of controlled change that were embodied in the concept of "progress." Change? Yes, as long as we can invoke and control it.

The very degree to which we find these inclinations no longer acceptable is itself an indicator of the level to which they have become incommensurable with the objectives of modern life. Clearly, these concerns are today as unfashionable as they were then fashionable. And it is precisely *because* we today find them so unacceptable that we must also recognize the degree of difference that they represent. It is not enough to say that we have learned from the past and that we have overcome the colonial framework in which these ideas flourished; for we haven't the slightest idea of what life was actually like for those individuals who embodied these concerns and lived them faithfully. We simply cannot, and never will, know these sentiments at the unselfconscious level at which they were openly lived out even in the last century of our own intellectual tradition. How, then, might we presume to know the lifeways of another tradition, let alone in immunology the embodied awareness of the physically unwell?

So, let us set aside the philosopher's speculations about the cognitive dispositions of fictitious tribes or space aliens and, for the moment at least, also set aside the exotic forms of life to which only the seriously ill and the religiously possessed have access. Let us instead turn to a nineteenth-century England that was less concerned about Darwin than we today are—a culture much more preoccupied with managing world change in what was then thought to be a productive and progressive manner. For though evolution may offer some contemporary palliative in the face of human change, let us not forget that Darwin speaks to us today in ways unfamiliar to the nineteenth century. And though evolution has come to be accepted as the most important idea of that period, it must be remembered that it was hardly the primary metaphor that drove nineteenth-century British society to such levels of productivity. Indeed, even today, no one at all familiar with Great Britain can fail to acknowledge the remarkable intellectual productivity of this relatively tiny place, one that yet stands as a living, if diminished, reminder of the "progressive" nature of the empire. Nor is it possible to live in Britain without acknowledging its extraordinary, and seemingly paradoxical, capacity to accommodate eccentricity—that is, the extent to which a confidence about its own values has allowed until recently for the productive assimilation of its social periphery, a capacity to live with its more liminal (even sociopathic) elements.

Eccentrics have always survived in Great Britain—sometimes at its very center—and their impact on the progress of the empire is undeniable. Here's one example we will take up later: in the early seventeenth century the Scottish mathematician John Napier, possessing both a true distaste for Catholicism and the luxury of time, invented a system whereby an alignment of calculating rods allowed for the easy resolution of the problems posed by the complexities of multiplication and division (figures 12a and 12b). Though mystically inclined mathematicians had throughout the ages drawn up lists of numbers with the hope of identifying certain correlations, for the first time in human

Napier's bones

In 1617, a Scottish mathematician named John Napier invented a set of calculating rods that helped make multiplication and division problems much easier to solve. The rods were often made from bone. This photograph shows a cylinder version of Napier's bones.

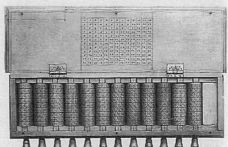

The rods work by changing difficult multiplication problems into simple addition problems. Each rod begins with a number from 0 to 9, and beneath that number is its multiplication table. To multiply two numbers together, for example 37 and 24, place the rods that show the numbers 3 and 7 next to each other as they are in the illustration on the right. This gives you 37 in the first row.

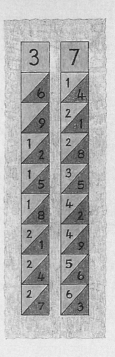

Then, multiply 37 by the number 4 by looking at the fourth row and adding the numbers in the columns diagonally, as shown below. You will get an answer of 148.

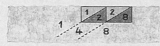

Next, you must multiply 37 by 20. You do this by multiplying by 2 and then adding a 0 to the answer. This is the same as multiplying by 20. To multiply 37 by 2, look at the second row and add the numbers in the columns diagonally. Then add a 0. You will get an answer of 740.

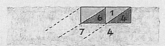

You can now find the result by adding these two numbers together, like this:

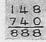

FIGURE 12A. **Napier's Bones**

Discovering mathematical relations across numerical domains allowed Scottish mathematician John Napier to develop in 1617 a system that simplified significantly the multiplication of large sums. Napier's parallel discovery of logarithms facilitated Britain's colonial ruling of the seas by simplifying and regularizing maritime navigation. In this sense, logarithmic tables became the central tool for the successful colonization of the world. (Reprinted with the permission of Gareth Stevens Publishing, Milwaukee, Wisconsin, USA. All rights reserved.)

Something to try

Make your own Napier's bones

You will need:
cardboard, a ruler, a pencil, a pen, a calculator.

Divide the cardboard into ten columns and then each column
into nine squares. Divide the bottom eight squares with a
diagonal line. You can see in the photograph below that the
children have made rods for the numbers 1, 4, and 8. Try
making your first rod for the number 7. Look at the illustration
of a number 7 rod on the opposite page and fill in the numbers
on your rod in the same way. Think of your seven times table.
What do you notice about the numbers you have just filled in?
All the rods work in the same way. Can you make a rod for the
number 6? Try doing different multiplication problems using
your rods. Check your answers on a calculator.

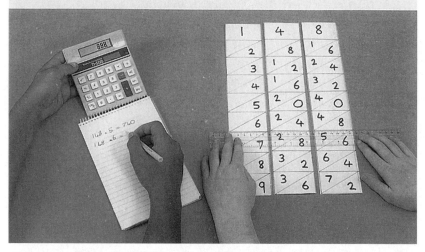

FIGURE 12B. **Making a Simplified Set of Napier's Bones**
A few strips of paper can readily demonstrate the simplicity and elegance of what was undoubtedly the
first true computing device. (Reprinted with the permission of Gareth Stevens Publishing, Milwaukee,
Wisconsin, USA. All rights reserved.)

history these lists were placed side by side so as to examine what patterns
might be *diagonally* consistent across them. Indeed, as it turned out, adding
this way across columns yielded complex multiplications.

By simple steps and an obsessive compulsion about numbers, the first real
calculating machine was invented, and, by the same man, a logarithmic system was born. From logarithms came navigational superiority; from that the

preeminence of the British Navy, and from that the Empire. As Smith and Wise put it:

> In the late Victorian and Edwardian eras, Britannia's rule depended less on the military power of earlier empires than on the geometrical conventions imposed upon the material world in order to make possible the maritime trade and communication, without which the widely scattered and largely island Empire could scarcely have existed. Without those geometrical divisions of space and time—the lines of latitude and longitude, the British Admiralty charts, the lighthouses and the day-marks—the foundation of Britain's wealth and security would disintegrate into the chaos of anarchy. (1989, 723)

Indeed, the importance of mathematics—and logarithms specifically—could not be underestimated, for they also made it possible to set aside a hypothetical and speculative view of the universe by reducing speculation about the natural world to empirically verifiable problems of local geometry. This new kind of natural philosophy brought abstraction to pragmatic ends by focusing on "the geometrical process underlying the piece of calculation by logarithmic tables" (Thompson 1961, 91).

Historically speaking, it is perhaps far too easy for us to underestimate the social consequences of enforcing the local demonstration of mathematical abstractions, of putting to the experimental test the practical consequences of airy ideas. Those who successfully bridged this distance set in motion the transformation of cultural categories at the most basic level, and did so, to be specific, by instilling a deep Victorian conviction—accepted by a public that had come to fetishize science, as Joseph Conrad put it, above both royalty and religion (Smith and Wise 1989, 723)—that "mathematics was the only true metaphysics, and that mathematics should be of a geometrical and eminently practical kind" (724).

To understand the importance of this cultural fetish—its impact on the metaphors and cultural categories of the day—one must understand the degree to which invention and discovery were understood as a matter of applied natural philosophy. Nowhere is this better seen than in the success of William Thomson, Lord Kelvin, in the professorship in natural philosophy at Glasgow University. For, in shipbuilding Glasgow, the achievements of mathematics were compounded by their immediate application to issues of progress and empire.

In the mid-nineteenth century Darwin's ideas about organic change meant far less to those rigorously engaged in the philosophy of applied science than did the real empirical work on entropy and relative size that came of trying, for instance, to build the best and most efficient steam vessels; building efficient boats required a knowledge which was deeply guided by another practical application of geometry—namely, the science of thermodynamics.[1]

In today's era of general ideological uncertainty, it is difficult to imagine the degree to which these were heady times in which the symbols of the academy found their immediate niche in the annals of progress. "Between 1840 and 1870, Britain became for iron ships the shipyard and ship owner of the world and the [River Clyde by Glasgow] the shipyard of Empire" (Smith and Wise 1989, 729). By 1876, "the Clyde achieved the remarkable feat of building more iron ships than the rest of the world put together" (732)—a feat not to be bettered until Scotsmen, like Andrew Carnegie, brought that same sense of industrial progress to Pittsburgh.

Certainly, to place the consequences of this enterprise in global perspective one might do well not only to remember how the shipping name of Cunard became a cultural icon,[2] but to recognize the degree of success that public support of the relation between philosophy and industry made possible. During this era roughly "half of the world's seaborne trade by both value and volume was carried in British ships"; although France, for instance, had built the Suez Canal (and was in fact Britain's closest rival in its use), the number of British ships using the canal exceeded that of French ships by more than ten times (732). To be blunt, abstract thinking had a ready application. Progress actually enhances speculative thought. Town and gown, despite their inequalities, shared a cultural paradigm. And a professor of physics ought to be very clear about the application of his ideas to the requirements of progress before he could be sure that what he thought was of value.

It would, then, be hard to make too much of the metaphor of navigational progress for this era; for unlike Darwin's exotic Patagonian examples, a fully laden steam vessel making its way most efficiently against its oceanic resistor far better embodied the obsessions of an era and a nation than did the impact of millennia on what most considered to be the freaks of nature. Though thermodynamics had interested frugally minded intellectuals (who operated on the conviction that "some limit should be placed on the enormous consumption of coal by steam ships which is rapidly exhausting our coalmines" [730]), unanimous enthusiasm for applied mathematics and geometry could be found among the supporters of long-distance oceanic enterprise and especially of navigation by steam to places previously inaccessible on account of the absence of any supply of coal (e.g., the west coast of South America).

In short, though we today see nineteenth-century England embroiled in a debate over the origin of species, an efficiently shaped oceanic vessel far better represented the idea of progress around which an entire nation focused its values. And let us not miss—in our evangelical enthusiasm to bury an embarrassing past by discounting the former significance of "progress"—just what a metaphor of linear progress a vessel at sea represents. What better symbol of progress than an object making its way through a "resistor"—a near-living organism that succeeded in progressing by "pilotage, astronomical navigation, 'dead reckoning,' and deep-sea sounding" (724) within a fluidous medium? Disguise the vessel with a female name, and then go about infecting the world.

LONELY AT THE TOP

> *The levels of criminal behavior that Americans find so disturbing may be the inevitable consequence of aspects of national life that Americans prize—individualism, mobility, privacy, autonomy, suspicion of authority, and separation between public and private roles, between government and community. The United States may have relatively high levels of criminality because it is inhabited by Americans.* —David Bayley, "Learning about Crime: The Japanese Experience"

One of the primary consequences of being able to produce consistently the local demonstration of a mathematical abstraction was that the act of conducting a scientific experiment itself achieved culturally the status of a religious rite. In so doing, the specificity of the controlled environments upon which such experimenting was based virtually guaranteed the belief that it was proper and just to reconfigure the world in the name of the Empire and the Almighty. This is how a belief in positivism and in the linearity of progress licensed the major Victorian prejudices: that it was acceptable to organize the world to our liking; that it was moral to infect the world with our prejudices; and that it was unacceptable to return to an empathic world where the transcendence of cultural difference had yet to homogenize human experience. Of these, it was this last inclination whose effects were least known and most ignored; for the religion of progress did nothing if not cement a great chain of social being in which progress would forever eliminate a genuinely multicultural world. To accomplish such a swift and permanent transformation it was necessary not only to put this multicultural past behind us in favor of global progress, but to induce the belief that progress was inevitable enough that even our own recent ancestors could come to look primitive and quaint. It's not that Victorians were unaware of the importance of family and inheritance—far from it. But there was actually little or nothing in Victorian cultural values to slow the advances of "progress" enough to allow for the development and maturation of the sort of empathic embodied understanding we associate with so-called traditional peoples: in the broadest sense, an understanding of how self is known through family tradition and through an embodiment of the deep symbolic richness of one's local environment. Here, one might say, modernism was born. By the 1950s Eisenhower could summarize these effects quite cogently in a speech about progress and the development of the hydrogen bomb:

> This transfer of power—this increase of power—from the mere musket and the little cannon all the way to a hydrogen bomb in a single lifetime, is indicative of the things that have happened to us. They rather indicate how far the advances of science have outraced our social consciousness—how much more we have developed scientifically than we are capable of handling emotionally and intellectually.[3]

Although the empires of Europe claimed to be conservative by attaching themselves to all sorts of ritualized display, in fact such "traditions" were hardly adequate to keep the average immigrant to Australia in any way attached to the local European environment in which that person's embodied understanding had been abandoned. Instead, colonialism promoted the opposite—namely, the feigning abroad of the status one could not possess at home. Though there may have been, for instance, plenty of British military display in colonial India, there could hardly be anything as pitiful as a band of immigrants—of the sort, say, that E. M. Forster describes in *A Passage to India*—feigning the upper-middle-class status they could not enjoy at home. Is it any wonder, then, that America has "presidents" of everything? Tens of thousands of them, all wanting to be addressed as such, virtually none of them known. And is it any wonder, also, that "progress" nourished the almost total disjunction between what we profess and what we can actually embody?

But if a disjunction between our perceptions of what we do and what we actually do is the hallmark of our contemporary world, the social fabric of American life should provide us with some startling evidence for the human capacity to embrace contradiction. In his acidic commentary on American beliefs and behavior, Andrew Shapiro (1992) highlights the gulf between what we claim to value and what we actually do. Here is a partial list of the contrasting domains in which Americans excel.

According to Shapiro, America is number one as a country

- in marriage and in still believing in marriage, but also in divorce (1992, 35);
- in higher education enrollment (61), but last in rewarding our teachers (63);
- in percentage of students who say they are good in math, but last in percentage of students who are good in math (64);
- in billionaires (and in real wealth), and in children and elderly in poverty (in unequal wealth distribution) (73–75);
- in big homes, and in homelessness (77);
- in defense spending, and last in spending on the poor, the aged, and the disabled (80);
- in private consumption, but last in investing and saving (87);
- in budget deficit, in foreign debt, in innumeracy, and in trade stagnation (90, 92);
- in percentage of population who say they take an active interest in politics, but last in voter turnout (105);
- in ethnic diversity, but behind only Germany, Spain, and Japan in our intolerance of people with different ideas (107);
- in membership in human rights groups, but also in not ratifying international human rights treaties (114).

Without laboring, or sensationalizing, or quibbling over how these statistics might have been gathered, or that the cohorts compared represent only part of the international community, this list puts into rough numbers what some of us may already recognize in our culture: Americans consistently don't as a society do what they profess to value. The argument here is not that the nation is one of deceitful people, but that *we have so lost contact with real difference that we have no way of gauging its usefulness*—in our own lives, in our perceptions of self, and especially in those instances where a better understanding of difference might allow us to reshape old problems. We simply don't see the contradictions, or we are incapable of acting to resolve them, because our society has become so individualized, and (like immunology itself) so independently and specifically focused, that we may have seriously jeopardized our capacity to act as a collective in an organically constructive manner.

This tendency is perhaps nowhere so clearly witnessed as in the conservative penchant for blaming any perceived rises in crime rates either on the dissolution of the nuclear family or on the absence of punishment as a technique for inducing socially acceptable behavior. Without getting embroiled in the standard arguments—about our decadent permissiveness, the liberation of women, and our proliferation of single-parent households—one can readily see that the family is as much a metaphor for collective action as it is the remedy for every social ill. After all, those of us raised in the less liberal 1950s are well aware of how families that adhered religiously to this very system of values often also created rebellious children. The 1960s, remember, was not our most tumultuous recent decade because its dissatisfied youth had been socialized in a more liberal 1950s!

Why ought we, then, lament the passing of an era that socialized children who went wild in the following decade? The serious flaw, in other words, with advocating a nostalgia for the values of the 1950s is that doing so fails to account for the fact the 1960s were *precisely* the result of the values that baby-boomers embodied day after day in the years following the Second World War. Far more plausible as an argument is one that acknowledges the veracity of the need for the kind of collective good that a healthy nuclear family symbolizes, for such an argument also allows us to accept that the kind of privacy and autonomy that we so cherish as a nation has the unavoidable outcome of increasing our fear of outsiders. Here, it is less the absence of the baby-boom family than the paranoia and fear of the 1950s that caused the social hysteria that followed. And no amount of political cant will reduce our sense that the hysterical alienation of most Americans was abundantly visible: in the targeting of foreigners we assumed to be among us; in the pioneering that turned "Going West" into a national mantra; and in the time-honored evicting of indigenous "others" necessitated by the construction of each new home on the range. Set against an America in which incarceration rates have vastly outdistanced increases in crime (Currie 1985, 32), the depths of our alienating—the consequences of our own alienation—become troubling.

It is, then, precisely this hysteria and its accompanying loss of negotiating skills that rewards us, for instance, for seeing ourselves as outsiders in the natural scheme of things. While even our corporate executives can now claim with straight faces to be emphatically "for the environment," as a culture we still lead the industrialized world in forest depletion (149), in paper consumption and garbage per capita (150), in junk mail (152), and in the production of hazardous waste (153).

But our determination to embrace at any cost our myths of heroic alienation is nowhere as clearly seen as in our willingness to abandon those environments for which we, under other circumstances, might have felt responsible. Pioneers, we must remember, are not only brave adventurers; they are also pitifully lacking in "staying" power. Instead of bringing what they find back to reinvigorate the center of society, they continually attempt to promote the expansion of the cell colony. For the pioneer, "progress" is a unilinear journey from the center to the periphery, in which the periphery is polluted by the misshapen central values of the pioneer (Napier 1992, 139).

Thus, while even colonialism promotes a return to the center (e.g., in the appropriation of natural resources from the colonies to the motherland, or in the celebrating of soldiers arriving home from foreign campaigns), the pioneer is more often the "loner" who abandons his place of origin never to return. For how else could we come to see the deterioration of our culture as "someone else's problem"—unless, that is, the symbols of "otherness" that are at the heart of a pluralist culture are not really perceived as "ours"? Is it any wonder that white reactionary politicians should claim that it is now time to start looking after "our" children—as opposed to all of those black children of the ghetto, who are now somehow "theirs"?

It's not exactly that we care about those we demonize, but we want them, nonetheless, to suffer. This fact is perhaps nowhere so clear as it is for illness experience. While Americans lead the first world in total health spending, we fail miserably in health and social services for the poor; for, in addition to being leaders in the percentage of population without health insurance, we insist that what funds we do spend go for magic bullet research. Thus, while the Netherlands, for instance, is a high roller when it comes to social services for AIDS patients, some American politicians have actually gone on record as saying that we should stop wasting money on sufferers (who are doomed to die anyway) and devote all of our efforts on research to kill the HIV virus. Asked why the moral world of the Dutch is so different than ours, scientists will sometimes claim that "they" are leaving this important work to "us." Yet how different is the moral reality? Note, for instance, the fact that Americans are also number one in the percentage of individuals who claim they would refuse to work alongside someone with AIDS (Shapiro 1992, 24): "Fourteen Americans were killed in combat in the first thirty days of the 1991 Persian Gulf war; during the same period, AIDS claimed the lives of 2,500 Americans. The equivalent of the federal government's entire research budget for AIDS in 1989, $981 million, was spent in approximately two days of the ground war" (24). And let us not forget that much of the money spent went to protecting "American" oil tankers—you remember, the ones registered in places like Liberia so as to avoid having to support all of those American citizens now being punished by our righteous gods.[4] Our myths and metaphors about "otherness," in other words, far outdistance our moral claims when it comes to looking at how we behave as a society. While Americans are number one in being trusted by the Japanese (54 percent), only 15 percent of Americans claim to trust those same Japanese. Instead, we take our small comforts in trusting those we think most behave like us: Canadians, British, and Australians (we think) are far more like us—even if, or perhaps precisely because, "us" is such a contested, even unknown, category.

Clearly, unless we are out simply to ridicule the deeply rooted American fear of difference, it is essential that we begin to understand the fundamentally "immunological" character of our lives—to see in particular how much our embodied awareness of ourselves is characterized by contradiction and by the metaphors of immunology that influence not only our ideas about illness but our treatment of others.

To do this, let us reexamine the popular passage on AIDS infection quoted by Sontag and discussed in chapter 2. There we saw that the fundamental focus of AIDS pathology in popular discourse has to do with a fairly simple form of demonology. It goes something like this: a clever pathogenic secret agent dons a mask so as to talk its way into the organism; the agent is deceptively small, apparently harmless, and seems not to ask for much. To extend the social metaphor of cell deception, the pathogen holds out hope; in mimicking what is beneficial, it gives the appearance of being useful. Indeed, within the concept of cell warfare is another assumption—namely, that infection is based upon a bit of bad faith—that the body perceives itself to be engaged in a form of productive reciprocity that, in fact, balloons into something else, something quite destructive. The diagrammatic image of this relationship is not the "bell curve" of cultural difference, but the surrealists' "praying mantis,"

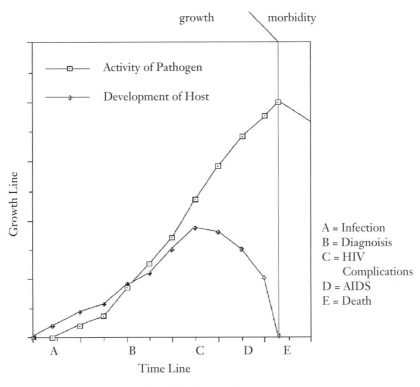

the insect that devours its partner after sex. This relationship is illustrated in figure 13.

Here, the course of HIV infection may be viewed diagrammatically as an expression of consciousness and of conscious transformation (of "inoculation" as understood as the conscious process of "being enlightened," of "having an awareness"). One line of the graph represents the awareness of the pathogenic process—the state of apparent health and its eventual decline. The other line represents the activities of the pathogen. For HIV, the intersection represents the point of diagnosis, which is also an expression of consciousness (i.e., the moment when inoculation means both "awareness of the new concept" and the introduction of some new [morbid] thing). The small space between represents a time of perceived well-being, at some point during which seroconversion takes place.

What is interesting about the saga "embodied" in this scenario, however, is not only that, as we have seen in the metaphors constructed by my students, it is a powerful visualization of a retroviral host-pathogen relationship, but that it offers a more generalized social parable of the reverse-engineering of "otherness"—of the colonial undoing of social difference. This infectious saga, in other words, is not only about a morbid biological restructuring of an organism, but is also about the domain of political economy where concrete *foreign* policies—policies that relate to otherness as "nonself"—can be shown to be equally pathogenic. Yes, this is a big claim, but one can readily demonstrate how our understanding of viruses is paralleled by our behavior toward other ways of living—that our views of retroviral infection are not at all unlike how we undo those who don't live by our rules. Examine the form of figure 14.

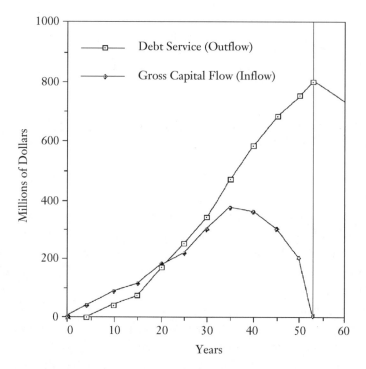

FIGURE 14. **Debt Cycle with World Bank Terms**
(Growth line from C. R. Frank Jr., Overseas Development Council; after graph by Douglas Rogers.)

Although figure 14 is an exact duplicate of figure 13, it is worth noting that what we are actually looking at is a chart that depicts the first sixty years of a time-line of third world foreign debt—its pathology, as it were, the magnitude of its crisis. In figure 14, the 10-year point on the timeline (the place that corresponds to "A" in figure 13) indicates the period during which the infusion of capital makes prospects look hopeful, where inflow of capital is greater than outflow (for HIV infection the period after infection, but before diagnosis or clinical complications—that is, where innovative behavior may still appear to have a desirable outcome); 20 (= B) indicates the initial struggle with repayment and the first hint of the *quantity* of the repayment (for HIV, the period after diagnosis during which the organism may remain healthy despite the psychological ill-health of being consciously aware of infection); 30 (= C) indicates the period during which the borrower begins to experience the magnitude of the social illness the loan will cause (for HIV, the period during which debilitating complications presage what is to come); 40 (= D) marks the beginning of the foreign AID crisis, the period where servicing the debt grossly outdistances the inflow of capital either from earned profits or from other loans. This is the stage I call "Foreign AIDS." It is the time during which the company folds—when death (50 = E) is immanent. The organism is now dysfunctional; having exhausted the life force of its host, the pathogen itself begins to desist.

It is important to remember that the similarity of these two diagrams is not merely coincidental; for the relationships embodied in them represent not *just* structural, formal, or superficial analogies, but mythic resemblances that are themselves embodied in epics about how heroes (and, in autoimmunity, antiheroes) and their significant "not-selves" relate. The proof here lies in seeing how well this model works in articulating the "Cartesian" motivations of the lender, in this case of the officials of our banks and the heroic motives of our relief agencies (C. Payer 1991).

Descartes's Enlightenment, in other words, provides us with a basic pathogenic methodology for organic deconstruction, a framework for taking something apart by approaching it masked. This is not—as anthropologists so often see—a mask that is worn to promote negotiation with a wide range of creative and destructive forces, but a mask that functions to take something apart in order to see how it is built (or, in the case of foreign aid, to try building something new that also involves taking the existing traditional system apart). It is the solipsistic mask, that is, of self-conscious philosophy. It is not the mask of ritual.

In this view, the Enlightenment goes hand-in-hand with the Age of Discovery because the relation of "self" to "not-self" is in both cases pathological—designed in theory to appropriate, and thereby to defuse, difference. The Colonial Period that followed, or was coextensive with the onset of the Enlightenment, is in turn marked by the enthusiastic use of this theory by the state. James Jurin's support for variola inoculation in the Royal Society during the early eighteenth century, the theatricality of early inoculation experiments (e.g., the reprieve—the rebirth—of condemned prisoners who agreed to participate in smallpox trials [A. Wilson 1990]), and the function of l'Institut Pasteur as an advocate of the state in the following century (Latour 1988), are all examples of such appropriation. Indeed, the Age of Discovery, and the Colonial Period that was its outcome, may together be said to have initiated the cosmopolitan reverse engineering of culture—the pathological appropriation of "other" organs, and their eventual embodiment in a cultural construction of "self" (figure 15).

This is why Fanon could not talk about indigenous identity without describing the experience of being represented: why Descartes's deconstruction of difference results in its elimination; why Gramsci's hegemony had less to do with dominant ideology than with an ideological reciprocity that neutralized the dominated; why for indigenous peoples "taking means in nearly every case being taken" (Fanon 1966, 182).

FRIENDLY FIRE

> *In a time of peace, the war-like man attacks himself.* —Nietzsche, *Beyond Good and Evil*

To understand why the Age of Immunology has arisen at this precise historical moment, we need to sketch out a picture of its mission in broad historical terms. Let us, therefore, review the historical argument:

(1) If anywhere, the Age of Immunology has its origins in the Age of Self-Discovery—i.e., in the Enlightenment, where "inoculation" implies both Descartes's self-imbuement or impregnation of ideas (his meditations) and also his awareness that this engagement must be done so masked ("I am now about to mount the stage and I come forward masked"). Enlightenment, in other words, carries with it both self-consciousness and its corollary—the

HIV propaganda for the West: *You're not as sick as you think.*
HIV propaganda for the Third World: *You're sicker than you think.*

Business propaganda for the West: *You're successful if you're self-motivated.*
Business propaganda for the Third World: *You need our help.*

FIGURE 15. **The Reverse-Engineering of Culture**

awareness of how disguise is used to approach a perceived danger. But, unlike the masked rituals of polytheists, this enlightenment is intended to result, not in a new creation, but in a deconstruction, an instance of "reverse engineering" (Descartes's "In my youth, when I was shown an ingenious invention, I used to wonder whether I could work it out for myself before reading the inventor's account," and that this practice led him to realize that he was "making use of definite rules"). Here we have, already, the intellectual basis for what will later become a theory of germs, of the microbe, because the intention behind Descartes's disguise is to facilitate some awareness of how the whole (the organism) can be disassembled through speculating about the relations of its parts. This is, quite emphatically, innovation rather than invention, the result of the reverse engineering of an existing art rather than the creative construction of a new one. The purpose of wearing the mask, in other words, is not to engage "otherness" in a creative act but to dissect it through a mimetic one.

(2) Once the Enlightenment had provided us with the basic methodology for deconstructing difference—a framework for taking things apart by approaching them masked—it also readily facilitated the so-called Age of Discovery. This was a time when it was believed acceptable and morally correct to organize the world according to European prejudice, a view that in turn made possible the cosmopolitan reverse engineering of genuine cultural difference. However, although this process did promote the infectious homogenization of other modes of living and thinking, it also gave way to a concept of progress that alienated much of Europe from any empathic awareness of how difference functions to create "self," as well as from any desire to attend to one's ancestral relationship with a local environment, or, in the extreme case of the pioneer, even to consider a return to a site where empathic knowledge could be cultivated. The combination of such neglect was to produce a way of living radically at odds with what it professed to value. This we see not only in the

Age of Discovery but in the radical alienation of contemporary American life, and especially in the disjunction between what we profess to believe and what we actually do.

(3) With the concept of progress came the particular labeling of what was "discovered," the heroic lionizing of those who discover (for science, rather than for "God"), and the specifying of the controlled environments of scientific experimentation. As Latour says of Pasteur's microbe:

> At first it is something that transforms sugar into alcohol in Pasteur's lab. This something is narrowed down by the number of feats it is asked to do. Fermentation still occurs in the absence of air but stops when air is reintroduced. This exploit defines a new hero that is killed by air but breaks down sugar in its absence, a hero that will be called "Anaerobic" or "Survivor in the Absence of Air." (1988, 90)

Victorian science was, in other words, extremely adept at fusing these three tendencies—of applying names to new and mysterious phenomena, of heroizing the secular world they named, and of controlling the unknown by subjecting it to dissective experiments. Indeed, with the discovery of the microbe, the analogy between appropriating other cultures and appropriating other bodies became complete—for now, truly, a "culture" could at once be understood as both "a social collectivity" and as "a cultivation of microorganisms." And it is precisely this analogy that allows immunology—like microbiology before it—to become the dominant social paradigm of its era.

But the analogy stops there: where microbiology invokes the aggressive pathogenic dissipation of "others," immunology focuses on how those "others" come back to haunt us—how, like a virus, they return in slightly altered form to seek their revenge. It should come as no surprise to us, then, that the rise of immunology is accompanied by a breakdown of the body of the state as an autonomous entity—a belief, as Lasch argued, "that old political ideologies have exhausted their capacity either to explain events or to inspire men and women to constructive action" (1991, 21). Here, the most haunting bit of evidence must surely be found in the politics of immunological research. By this I do not refer to the well-known politicking that dominates what research does and does not get funded, but to the more insidious parallel between historical moments in which a broad, social fear of otherness influences the form that scientific research takes; for it is usually culture that influences science,

Disease/System	Last "classical" contribution	First "modern" contribution
Hemolytic disease	1909	1945: Coombs et al.
Sperm and testicular	1900	1951: Voisin
Encephalomyelitis	1905	1947: Kabat et al.
Sympathetic ophthalmia	1912	1953: Collins
Phacoanaphylaxis	1911	1963: Halbert and Manski
Thyroid	1910	1955: Witebsky and Rose; Roitt et al.
Wassermann antibody	1909	
Platelet disease		1949: Ackroyd

FIGURE 16. **The Dark Ages of Autoimmunity**
(After Silverstein 1989, p. 174.)

not the other way around. Heretical though this will sound to bench scientists, the examples are plentiful. Here, I am not speaking of how little, for instance, American medical students learn about the greatest human killer of all time (how many even know that it is malaria?). What I am referring to is how the broader conditions of social life influence the way that science takes up, and then suddenly drops, a particular domain of inquiry. A good example is the so-called Dark Ages of Autoimmunity (figure 16).

What are we to make of the fact that the last "classical" research in autoimmunity ended at the dawn of the First World War, while the first "modern" contributions began at the end of the Second? How could scientists actually focus, that is, on the "enemy within," when the "enemy without" was becoming such an overwhelming threat?

Is it only coincidental that the period of time framed by the two great wars is precisely that of these "Dark Ages" (Silverstein 1989, 174)—as if the presence of obvious social pathogens was enough to eliminate any possible preoccupation with the self's own "autotoxicity"? The obvious hero epics that define our view of microbial events must, in other words, be understood as deeply dependent on how we conceptualize "otherness"—i.e., the "foreign"—at the social level. Autoimmunity, in this sense, is very much a "cold war" concern.

Although most will dismiss such a broad historical and conceptual parallel as merely coincidence, it must be remembered that society always drives science, not the other way around. Many simple demonstrations of this fact can be had by looking at the domain of applied medical research, where the social expectation that something be done almost always produces therapeutic products the effects of which are recognized well in advance of the research that explains how they work. Basic understanding, in other words, almost always follows an application that materializes as a response to a social demand: note, for instance, just how little was known scientifically about *why* cowpox or anthrax bacillus (or penicillin, for that matter; or so many new treatments for HIV) had the effects they did before we were well on our way to deploying them therapeutically; note that the knowledge of *how* any of these work was not necessary in order to use them.

Despite this awareness, it has become commonplace today to unearth and discuss the extent to which our scientific forebears, especially those we make heroes of, were a lot of "showmen" who were "cooking data," without remembering and accepting just how frequently the explanation for why something happens often follows by decades—even centuries—its actual so-called "discovery." The mechanism by which we think we understand something, in other words, is rarely a necessary aspect of its use or, indeed, of research about it. And we, therefore, need to be most cautious about accepting unexamined assumptions concerning what we think we experimentally "see," and much more cautious about what metaphors we employ to "explain" things away. We also need to accept the strong and deep influence that culture has on what researchers actually do.

These facts are, as we will see, of particular significance for our understanding, or lack of understanding, regarding why immunity becomes "systematic" in the mid-1960s. For now, let us accept that a *social* belief in scientific "progress" did have a recognizable effect on the precise form that Descartes's viral mask actually took by the mid-nineteenth century. For one can hardly measure the enormous impact Pasteur made on his own and future generations when he conclusively ended the discussion of spontaneous generation of microorganisms (by demonstrating that they were airborne), and when he later showed that parental microbes are living things that descend from preexisting forms—forms that replicate, and that are enormously varied. These discoveries, along with Koch's demonstration that specific organisms were responsible for particular diseases, paved the way for our long-standing belief that a battle for life was taking place in every complex living thing, and that these battles were not altogether unlike what we humans, left to our own devices, could and would do to one another.

So why, in summary, apply social science to "real" science? Because of the fact that the two are closely woven. Sometimes our understanding of a bio-logical fact does not lead to social action in a clinical setting (smallpox, for ex-ample). And sometimes therapies are employed because of social expectations without any real sense of how the actual therapy works (polio vaccines, for in-stance). Moreover, it is virtually impossible to describe scientifically what a "system" is without referring to or evoking directly varieties of social rela-tions. Explaining a network (say, "the upward formation of a protein from the sequential linkage of amino acids and the downward folding of the chain into the biochemically active configuration of an enzyme" [Bibel 1988, 309]) goes hand in hand with our understanding of social relations (of "the development of a society from a group of individuals, whose behavior is regulated by an evolved culture and system of laws" [ibid.]). The inseparability of the social and the scientific—indeed, the conceptual preeminence of the social over the scientific—occurs because what we are actually referring to in both instances is the metaphorical articulation of hierarchies of order. Yet, as we will evi-dence in chapter 5, this focusing on the *determining system* has had some un-usual, and quite troubling, effects on how we have conceptualized the activities of microorganisms.

But before we take up the topic of the immune system, and particularly of how immunity became a "system" at all, we need to consider the future cross-cultural consequences of this Age of Immunology in which we now find our-selves. What will be the outcome of immunological thought if we fail to rejig in a positive manner the recursive virus of the Enlightenment? Where does Descartes's appropriation of other organic entities (through masked reverse cultural engineering) actually lead us? What happens when Western colonial discourse gets reshaped as the "return gift" of the colonies—when "our" rela-tional terms are brought to life by "them" in peculiar and unique ways and then fed back to "us" (figure 17)? One need not invoke the most recent demonstrations of "foreign terror" to ask who now is steering the Trojan horse.

FOREIGN AIDS

After the conflict there is not only the disappearance of colonialism but also the disap-pearance of the colonized. —Frantz Fanon, "On National Culture"

To appreciate just how immunological are "our" post-colonial relations, we need to test the infectious model offered here (figures 13 and 14) not just

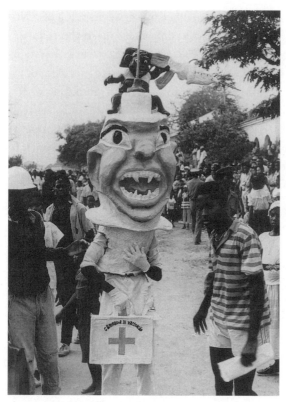

FIGURE 17. **The Magic Bullet: Cultural Relations as an Immunological Form** In these extraordinary masks from Guinea-Bissau we see a densely symbolic parallel created between colonial aggression and its "inoculating" powers. At left, a health-care worker dons a hat that is topped with a hypodermic needle and the figure of a local god who, himself, holds an AK47 rifle the barrel of which is also a needle. Is the hypodermic needle a symbol of that same aggression that the rifle so clearly epitomizes? (Bissau Carnival, Guinea-Bissau, 1987. Photos by Doran H. Ross, used with permission.)

against the perspective of the infected nation but against the anticipated pro-phylaxis of the lender. To begin with, it is very important to realize that very few people, aside from international economists, are aware of the fact that most third world countries are actually massive *exporters* of capital, that ser-vicing their debts has resulted in an enormous *outflow* of capital that grossly exceeds what they receive. *Most citizens of the first world don't realize—amid all the discussion about defaulted loans—that the third world continues to give the first world much more than it is getting, not only as the result of destroying its own re-sources, but in debt repayment.* Even those countries not meeting their obliga-tions, in other words, are paying exponentially much more for what they have been given. In immunological terms, we must begin our inquiry at the mo-ment when an attempt is made to construct the borrowing nation as an imita-tion of ourselves, as a "mock-form" of the self: the third-world puppet "president for life"; the infected T-cell that is the mock-form of the thing im-

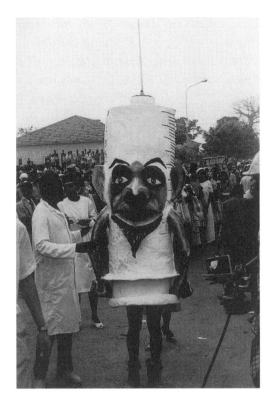 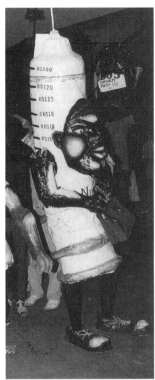

itated—i.e., any "antigenic" situation in which the trappings of selfhood, the many masks, are imitatively worn.

While the puppet state is supported from outside, in fact this is usually only true to the extent that it becomes a host for the virus we call "development" (an analogy that works especially well if we consider that viruses are, at least chemically speaking, ancient parts of self that have survived autonomously in other forms until the moment at which they seek their awful revenge). What then happens is a brief period of apparent productivity that ends when a healthy individual seroconverts, which in "debt" terms is when total debt flow out of the already impoverished society starts exceeding the flow of gross capital into that country. The fiscal result is a debt "crisis" in which the indigenous mock-form retaliates, a kind of international immunological reaction which threatens to cause the lender's own state of autoimmunity: this occurs when the lender realizes the degree to which the lending program has been redefined by local interests and values. The presence of the mock-form at the gates of the self causes a reaction that is culturally "sickening." We respond by trying to undermine and delegitimize the "authority" of that form (for example, at the United Nations) by looking for and embracing its own inner form of "not-self" (e.g., the third-world nation's own oppressed peoples). This we accomplish through propaganda, such as we have seen in figure 15—propaganda that monolithically defines "them" as "needy" and "us" as "knowledgeable."

Despite the obviousness of the relationship, the process itself—as an Enlightenment product—is actually insidious, elusive, and nonterminating, since the creation of the tribal mock-form (the nonbellicose, environmentally friendly harvester of nuts and berries, as opposed to the authentically "different" [read noncompliant] warrior) starts the process all over again—that is, causes the next viral mutation, where the indigenous culture itself experiences its own immunodeficiency (caused by the "end run" of the international community which now redefines a country by reconstructing the identity of its indigenous peoples). Once this mutation has taken place, so-called traditional forms of authority can be tapped through isolating and "developing" their "cultural capital" . . . which gives rise to the next viral mutation, where the country's own autoimmunity is exhibited by its feeding itself up to us as the advocate of its own tribals, and so on. How do we culturally "resolve," for instance, so many crises abroad? Enlist the former warring tribal leaders to run a new country built around the managerial notion of "cultural capital" . . . hmmm.

What, in other words, is rarely seen in such immunological relations is the fact that the cycle is infinite, which is why we can no more "cure" the ills of the third world than we can the common cold. Inflation is to development what inflammation is to immunology; and inflation only occurs when a local economy is redefined by an outside force that is radically at odds with a carefully constructed network of local relations. The Andean peasant aligns himself with the central government so as to undermine the local plantation owner. Later, the now-impoverished landlord and the peasant unite against the failed promises of the central government. The local Vermonter aligns himself with the big chain store (even though he knows that the goods are made by foreign slaves) because he believes that the giant chain will break the backs of the local gentry. Finally, when the town is wrecked, he aligns himself with that bankrupted gentry to redefine "local identity" in the face of its being abandoned by that international monster.

But is the parallel between inflation of the body and inflation in foreign trade actually viable? Well, just think about it. Start with the basic assumption that funds should be given to a presiding government (say, money to an impoverished, indigenous mock-form: a puppet government, the president of a country whose election has been rigged) for purposes of inner growth (read, the tumor of development). The loans are, though, awarded as a false prestation: they purport to be capable of creating a healthier, more productive body; but in fact they are a virus, since they never result in increased savings, but only in spending more on the products of the developed nations. We loan money to a particular nation to build a dam, but they give the money back to us (and more) to buy construction equipment.

Now there's nothing wrong with giving something that one hopes to get back in an embellished form; in fact, it's the basic principle of some very effective forms of symbolic exchange, such as the Melanesian *kula* (see, e.g., Weiner 1992).[5] It was also, incidentally, the basic principle of the Marshall Plan: we loan money at low or no interest in exchange for creating in a ravished country a market for our goods and, hence, some work for *our* laborers. Good reciprocity (monetary or symbolic) requires some gauging of the return gift. Otherwise the giver becomes, as the Trobrianders nicely put it, "hard on the kula"—that is, too punitive, too tough for the system to work.

Now the difference between the Marshall Plan (or any traditional form of reciprocal exchange) and the immunological model offered here is not in the lending itself but in what follows, and specifically in the abandonment of reciprocity in exchange for what, hopefully, will become a financial balloon, a tumor of money. Remember here that in Rome *immunis* referred to a freedom from social obligation; as much as we may say (even hope and believe) that the loan will result in the development of an inner "healthy economy" (whatever that is), our goals are in the least contradictory and at worst outright deceptive, because the "progressive" nature of the monetary virus precludes us from being at all sensitive about the nature of *how* the return will influence our own well-being. In the first place, *"we" have no intention of supporting the economies that produce all of the cheap products* that "they" produce in an effort to repay all of the extraordinary interest that will accumulate for the following 50 to 75 years, but we *would* like to control the sale of those products and coerce others to buy them. In fact, buying every cheap auto made in Korea would ruin what little remains of the inner productivity of our societal "body" (which, in fact, is what happens when so-called "free trade" allows the wealthiest people in the first world to subsidize laundered prison labor abroad). No wonder the assets of the wealthy grow hideously, while the middle classes lose what little they possess to gross inflation and a decline in living standards. Ask why in the current political climate the wealth of the top 1 percent of the economic spectrum has grown so grotesquely, and in such an undignified manner, and you see the real outcome precisely.

What is "viral" about our behavior—i.e., the "trick"—is the postponement of the ballooning of the debt, at least until one has created a Pavlovian need for foreign goods. Then, and only then, the line of gross capital inflow drops sharply and the debt flow expands like the imagination of someone on a mind-altering drug, or like someone experiencing anaphylaxis. Delay followed by grotesque inflammation—the basis of allergy, the pathology of viruses like HIV. It is the combination of postponing the debt, of abandoning a manageable form of gradual reciprocity, of ignoring or even faking what will really happen "immunologically" ("yes, there will be a market here for all of those shoes"). Surely, commodification must finally be recognized as the *absence* of reciprocity, a weird kind of assimilation in which the kula "gift" is replaced by a slow virus.

Unless the needy nation in question develops a highly restrained sense of deferred gratification (which it can't because its misery sees no future; because its miserable state encourages it to accept an optimistic view of how it might develop; because it is tempted by all of the "cargo" you offer; because it is afraid to invest its money locally; because it uses its loans as "flight" capital; because those in power have given up at home; and because, finally, it is imitating how *you* yourself behave), how can it respond otherwise? Moreover, the model applies not only to what is called the third world; it is deeply entrenched in the ideology of "discovery" that we have already described.

How much of this "foreign AIDS," really, can be attributed to the unilinear nature of Victorian "progress"? An easy answer is to look to where flight capital actually ends up, and at cultural patterns of investing across borders. While most people think of the Japanese as the major threat in terms of incoming investment in America, it is, surprisingly, the original colonizers (i.e., the British) who in fact are the heaviest investor of flight capital from their homeland—a staggering 44 percent of all foreign investment in the U.S. economy, as opposed to a mere 19 percent by the Japanese.

So what development in fact does is promote the same kind of abandonment of tradition as did "progress" and the "pioneer" mentality of the nineteenth century. Although abandoning tradition happens for quite different reasons in the case of most impoverished countries, the viral result is the same. There is, as it were, no way that one can heed the warnings on all of the safe sex posters, unless one has already seen a virus at work, or one can imagine how the consequences of what might happen present a risk of greater proportion that the other sorts of risks one experiences on a daily basis. This is why teenage homeless are the greatest risk takers: they've given up on living more than ten years anyway. So why worry about AIDS? Why worry about debt repayment if it looks like the world is coming apart? This sentiment is one that is not only felt in the third world, but is one embraced by the first-world "cargo" economics of anyone (e.g., Ronald Reagan) whose Armageddon ego extends to the belief that the world will end in his lifetime. Why not burn the forests to stay warm if it's your last night on earth?

Much to our surprise, however, the earth does go on—albeit in a form that has jettisoned its current dinosaurs.[6] So, ten years or so after receiving the loan, you are now giving, or meant to be giving, lots more money than you are getting; or, you start paying the debt through a form of brinkmanship you can't possibly win (i.e., through the pyramid scheme or chain letter in which you pay one debt with newly acquired loans from others who think their money is being invested). It's playing "big man" rather than kula; it's why Melanesians who don't engage in kula regularly pummel one another or take each others' heads; it's why warfare (either between "bodies" or within a single "body") is the only possible answer to the one-directional drain of resources that results when the virus has taken hold of the local economy and of the otherwise healthy bodies that make that economy work.

Are there any answers short of "fighting the virus"—a term used very effectively in medicine and computer science, but one that will shortly take hold in economics? Probably not. Because the real problem is not only that the lending bank has dropped a time bomb, but that the lender has, to extend our metaphor, been "desensitized" to why reciprocity is important. Like the bullish banker, who always lends more than he has in his safe, the overly optimistic borrower now finds himself paying the interest on his loans by tempting other venture capital. And like that same bullish banker, the question of just *how* he will eventually meet all of his obligations is abandoned in favor of the grotesque appropriation of whatever capital can be legally or illegally stashed abroad.

So, it's not enough to imagine (simply and unrealistically) that "they" begin to live like "us"; for, in order for them to do so, "they" ought also to be able to use 80 times more resources per capita, and to develop unfair terms that punish their trade partners. In fact, there is only one way the loan can result in a situation in which both parties win, and that's when the borrower finds someone else to buy their shoes. In other words, the whole development scam is exactly like a virus, even down to the fact that its "life" depends upon an assumed, ever-expanding pool of "other" bodies. Immunology involves a kind of logos that is the exact opposite of the sort of reciprocity that is epitomized in kula exchange. In this light, "sustainable development" is not only a concept that keeps the "virus" of unfair exchanges alive, but an oxymoron.

In short, the absence of a system of reciprocity (which is epitomized in the our expectation that "development" will result in the competitive marketing of goods "somewhere else") has left us ill-equipped to deal with "antigenic" economic behavior: the other side of not having forged reciprocal bonds (and by this I don't mean only grotesque debt repayment) is the inability to see one's own concepts of "progress" as a form of collectively understood, embodied imagination. The result is not only what we call the exportation of "flight" capital, but the autoimmune "not knowing oneself" that makes possible the wholesale airlift of inalienable things that we have now commodified.

What is, finally, so frequently missed in this commodification of now-alienable things is the way in which it makes possible all sorts of hijacking and piracy. The international company that packed up for Asia, abandoning the town it destroyed in West Virginia, now finds itself undermined by those very Asians who now log onto the downtime of New York computers to build cheaper and cheaper software. Lost in all of this is not only the moot point of what we can call "American made," but the subtle social fabric that created new life out of a finely balanced set of reciprocal moral relations. Having permitted our Wall Street crooks to sponsor slavery abroad, we now must pay the toll of never having developed any exchange relations that take empathy into account. The end result of this neglect is our obsession with, belief in, and devotion to the fraudulent network, a domain of uncertainty and deceit that now more or less defines all of our social and scientific relations and, in turn, places us squarely in an "immunological" age. To network and "immune systems" theory we must, therefore, now turn in order to see how and why empathy has been extracted from the domain of reciprocity. Can it be reintroduced? That is the question.

5 | unnatural selection
social symbols of the microbial world

In science, a truth that cannot be proved is called a law. —Hans Christian
von Baeyer, *Maxwell's Demon*

FASHIONING MODELS

*A sign is always less than the thing it points to, and a symbol is always more than what
we can understand at first sight. Therefore we never stop at the sign but go onto the goal
that it indicates; but we remain with the symbol because it promises more than it re-
veals.* —Jung, *Symbols and the Interpretation of Dreams*

I have argued that marginal people are largely responsible for invention
within a culture—how change results from a successful move from outside in.
And we have also seen how liminality itself becomes threatened in an Age of
Immunology—how the compulsive need for certainty gives way to the homogenization—the "leveling out"—of difference. But we have yet to ask how
science has managed this coup; nor have we examined the possible outcomes
of the combined leveling out of difference and the attempted cornering by
scientists of spheres of esoteric, "priestly" knowledge. Is the world, as Foucault constantly argued, a place where corporations of power run roughshod
over individual freedom? Or might it also be argued that institutions and
those who populate them are equally ensnared by the metaphors that so often
appear to make them invincible? We look to science for answers. But, in so
doing, are we enslaving ourselves to a timid prince?

To understand how the Age of Immunology perpetuates itself (despite its
unhealthy consequences), we must not only examine what those at the center
(e.g., the purveyors of scientific dogmas) might hope to gain by the continued
promotion of the kinds of exclusive, cultic practices we can plainly observe
in any laboratory, but we must also examine the places where supposedly

power-thirsty institutions have actually succeeded in eliminating difference by getting everyone to do the same thing. What is the outcome of such conditioning? Is it, as our media and our colluding intellectuals suggest, only a place of dehumanized suffering and pain? Do we, as we so often hear, actually inhabit an automaton's world in which we merely give ourselves over to whosoever is ruling the day—where, as the beat poet Lord Buckley quipped, the only question one can legitimately ask is, "Where do I go to surrender?" Or do institutions, because of their hermetic nature, actually become victims of their own entropy? If invention is, as we have argued, an external phenomenon, then institutional interiority cannot itself produce transformation or growth.

While it may be inevitable that social groups alienate (or even eliminate) that which they cannot understand, it is also the case that an absence of understanding about the "unusual" can lead either to an overtly vicious and heartless behavior toward anything different, or to an "Enlightened" defusing or destruction of difference through professing an actual appreciation of it. Perhaps today, as never before, we find ourselves the unwilling participants in Descartes's recognition and elimination of difference through approaching that difference in a friendly disguise—where the mask of friendliness (the smile that invites) encourages responses to otherness that are coercive, disingenuous, and unhealthy. As a homeless friend once put it:

> It's a "smiley" culture, where smiles are used like weapons against different people, smiling in all different places. . . . And it can become quite annoying to get mixed up in this smile business. Usually, a smile is actually an outward sign of inner happiness. But when you force a smile, it's not an outward sign of inner happiness; it becomes a mask, [and] that's when it becomes quite strange to see people smiling. . . . I always look around and think: "Who's really in charge?" . . . I looked at it from all different points of view, I guess just like a game of chess. . . .

While we probably fail to recognize what may be lost in covertly seeking and eliminating difference, so also do we lose any sense of why appreciating the uncertainties of difference may be worthwhile. This is why our models of illness and our intolerance for liminality go hand in hand: to be ill is to be in a very strange and attenuated place—perhaps even a "sacred" location. To be forced to accept that one's body is being recognized and eliminated does nothing to advance a sense of well-being; nor does it do anything for our believing that difference might play some positive function in promoting well-being. Many students I teach are nearly incapable of seeing any merit at all in examining liminal values, not to mention actually living marginally. And the evidence for the effects of the recognition-and-elimination model of pathogenicity on perceptions of alienation is today everywhere to be seen—not only in the victimization of patients by the "battle" that just happens to be going on inside each person's body, but in the effects of accepting this model on what we culturally believe to be socially and scientifically possible.

Surprisingly, the belief that our military models of cell warfare do not accurately represent the current state of scientific knowledge (in, for example, immunology, virology, and vaccinology) is gaining ascendancy among scientists themselves. This change has led to the discounting of the applicability of military models in bench research. Scientists today deny the accuracy of military models, although, as we will now see, they do so for all the wrong reasons. For the perception that immunology should "abandon the self-nonself question and focus on the rapid advances that are revolutionizing cell biology" (Schwartz 1995, 1177) is not based upon any concrete examination of how and why those metaphors still deeply permeate the very act of observing cellular interactions.

Not only are the bugs themselves magnified by laboratory practice, so too are the roles played by those very military metaphors; for they prevail despite the fact that the self/nonself paradigm "did not solve the transplantation problem, or those of tumor immunology, or even those of autoimmune diseases" (ibid.). Each time scientists stop thinking consciously about these metaphors, each time, that is, they unselfconsciously watch one cell "killing" another—in medical school slide lectures, in laboratories, and in doctors' offices—we see repeated the inescapable cultural meaning of the military model (figure 18). Can there ever be, we must ask, any end to this pugilism?

Surely, we must recognize that the use of language—the softer side of "hard" science—has had a profound impact on our understanding of microbial interactions, and frequently the very scientists who make a conscious effort to describe philosophically their work actually end up emphasizing, rather than denying, the microbial battering—the military events—they witness. Roald Hoffmann's attempt to describe poetically the "inescapable metaphors" of science results, as Shira Leibowitz points out, not only in an awareness that "the problem of metaphors is not a marginal one in science"

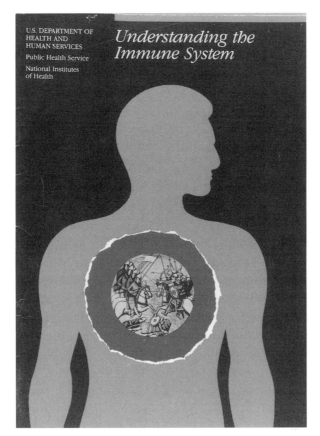

FIGURE 18. **The Body at War**
Though we usually attribute the exaggerated abuse of metaphor to the
popular press, illustrations, such as this government publication on
immunity, are everywhere to be found—in posters for children, in
health-care campaigns, in public health brochures for "developing
countries," in medical school slide shows, and even in molecular biology
textbooks where the language, if not the image, of warfare predominates.

(Hoffmann and Leibowitz 1991, 387) but that it may be *the* central issue.
"What facet of themselves are chemists and immunologists presenting to the
public," Leibowitz asks,

> when popular expositions of their science read like World War II scenarios?
> Your lethal lexicon, Professor Hoffmann, includes such phrases as: "molds that
> combated infections," "the drug routs the microbe hordes," "fortress-like cell

wall," "lethal subterfuge," "fooled by penicillin's camouflage fatigues," "welcomes the invading drug to its ranks," "inside enemy lines," "cell-wall armor," "decimated the invader," "battle plan," "commandeer . . . with new marching orders," "annihilates the cell," "entered the fray," "acyclovir . . . turns traitor . . . [and is] an effective weapon in only one theatre of this war."

To be sure, this martial terminology is not your idiosyncrasy, Roald (although you employ it with gusto); it is the standard arsenal of professional and popular immunology. (387)

Referring to a well-known article from a popular magazine, Leibowitz remarks that the "lexiconic body-count reaches twenty deadly terms in [the] first column of copy alone" (387).

The first question, then, is not simply: "Are there different metaphors that can be employed?" The question is, "Are there *better* metaphors?" Though military metaphors may govern our unselfconscious thinking from the moment we stop reflecting about them and return to our work, this does not in itself mean that they are more accurate than any of the alternatives; it only means that culturally we have preferred, favored, and, therefore, embodied them. Leibowitz's own attempt to revise dominant and dominating military metaphors involves employing amorous language in which, for instance, natural killer (NK) cells become "natural lover" (NL) cells. In such a world "'surveillance' mechanisms will be replaced by molecular courtship and flirtation; the unwanted cells can be hugged and kissed to death. As Shakespeare observes after Romeo and Juliet die, 'heaven finds means to kill . . . with love'"(ibid., 393).

But such a world—where cells are "snuggling up to the unsuspecting bacteria"; where "immunological terror can be turned into erotic trysts, and battles into orgies" (393)—can as much remind us, as we saw in chapter 2, of the brutalities of physical attraction as it can alter the nature of what we really see at the cellular level. In response to a reconsideration of the "bonding or affinity" (the "game of life") that is played out for us microbially, Hoffmann alludes to this confusion, not only in his initial response to embracing, as it were, Leibowitz's romantic suggestions ("Just a touch more and I would be past innuendo and into broad sexual comedy" [395]), but in his resistance to the realization that sexual "conquests" are for many people a kind of war, even though "it's hard to think of love when the intent is slaughter" (395).

It may be the case that what we see here is Lévy-Bruhl's age-old conundrum, whereby old definitions may no longer work, at the same time as novel ones prove distracting ([1949] 1975, 64–65); it may also be the case that what we call "culture" is actually not simply a shared set of values. In fact, "culture" may equally be understood as a tendency—one toward preserving us from the dangers that become all too real when we accept the plasticity of metaphorical thought and the consequent power that metaphors actually have over us. One need only reflect on the capacity of a single metaphor to embrace both the amorous and deadly, or the humorous and serious, to appreciate the anarchy and chaos that culture works to eliminate.

So, while most of us will resist as unnatural the replacing of the language of warfare with that of love—finding the idea simply absurd—our metaphors are, nonetheless, quite capable of accommodating the paradoxical conflations of love and death, or sex and comedy. Indeed, it appears that the more fragile the social category, the less willing we are to play with its meaning; for its instability leads both to its possible contestation and to exaggerated prohibitions regarding its use. To fear liminality, for instance, one must also fear for the very stability of one's own values. Thus, before we can address the question of whether there actually are better ways of describing microbial events, we must first ask what alternatives have been favored by those few individuals who have addressed this problem. How diverse are these really? And are they feasible?

Foremost, of course, are the widespread religious images that have been employed, especially by sufferers, to represent illness. These include not only the "cross that must be borne" but also the demonologies that explain both the possessed of the Middle Ages and the guilt of the modern cancer patients who are told that they have brought on their illnesses by virtue of some or another character flaw. Among those with chronic illness who are, however, unwilling to accept this blame—and, interestingly, among those scientists concerned with the complexities of cellular relations—metaphors of circuitry and networking have proven more appropriate. Not only have I been told, for instance, that rheumatoid arthritis is a problem of organic hardwiring (in which circuits get overloaded and short out), but it is quite common today for patients to indicate that their illness is the apotheosis of numerous chance "low-voltage" neurological events. Such explanations can commonly be heard in descriptions of everyday experience, but they may also be intimated in the craze for "alternative" therapies, on which Americans spend one out of three health-care dollars. These explanations, in other words, range from the cumulative effects of old age to the electromagnetic effects of the New Age. Among theorists, however, the most favored contemporary metaphors derive from information theory and cybernetics (e.g., Cohen 1999; Segal and Cohen 2001). This is especially telling when one realizes that the kinds of systems theories that glamorize networks only found their way into the medical literature in the late 1960s—i.e., that it was only for a generation raised on nuclear hysteria (where no one was safe from "invasion") that a discourse on *unforeseen activation* became mesmerizing.

Although the literature on scientific networks is unmanageably large, in what follows I will focus on two compelling arguments. The first is that expressed by Bruno Latour, especially in his *Science in Action* and *We Have Never Been Modern*. The second is a feminist reading offered by Evelyn Fox Keller in her *Refiguring Life: Metaphors of Twentieth-Century Biology* (1995). Both of these authors offer compelling arguments for accepting the role of networks in microbiological thinking, as well as some indication of why it may now be time to transcend them.

LATOUR DE FRANCE: *SCIENCE IN ACTION*, OR SCIENCE INACTION?

> *There is often no clear linguistic line . . . between words for* experiment *and* experience. *What we are trying to pin down is the emergence of the self-consciously contrived contexts of observation we now peculiarly associate with the label* experiment. —Howard Margolis, *Paradigms and Barriers*

Since the 1940s, when Norbert Wiener and his associates began to popularize the concept of cybernetics, theorists of science have argued that the complex nature of modern informational systems—their "feedback mechanisms," even their "purposive behavior"—requires that we examine the way in which the replication of information in various social settings (despite the content of that information) is itself sufficient for the creation and maintenance of "scientific fact." As Latour has stated repeatedly, a scientific fact is an object that is inscribed on the window of an instrument. Indeed, in the aftermath of quantum physics—where the act of looking influences what is looked at—it often appears that science has increasingly distrusted empirical evidence, replacing measurement for observation. The mystery of why specificity should become an end in itself is, in this view, an outcome of "winning" through knowing one's competition rather than winning through inventing a new paradigm.

In this sense, science can be perceived as a highly social activity within which networks of authority are established and controlled. Though networking has been a subject of serious inquiry for decades, the concept became widely popularized long before it would be applied in a thorough way to scientific practice, to what scientists *actually do* when building networks of authority.

While Latour and Woolgar's *Laboratory Life* was the first detailed application of these ideas to a "social" study of what goes on at the bench, Latour's *Science in Action* argues outright that science is, first and foremost, a power-engendering human activity in which authority is established through social networks that drive—and in turn are driven by—the canonical inscriptions we call "facts." But *Science in Action* is no ordinary consideration of the social construction of knowledge, or of its proposed deconstruction; for what Latour brought to his project was, first, an incisive awareness of the principles that govern the creation and maintenance of scientific canons; second, a rigorous (if eclectic) methodology by which resistant ideological "machinery" could be unwound; and third, a complete irreverence about how bourgeois professionals actually lead their lives. Latour, in fact, enough accepts the overwhelming authority of networks that his methodology has him extending his investigation through as many odd passages as he can pull his readers; indeed, there are several murky places at which he deliberately leaves the reader to sink or swim.

The incredible terrain that Latour covers in this study of science in the making—experimentation, publishing, rhetoric, "social and institutional history of science, science policy studies, ethnographical studies of scientists and technologists at work, the histories of technology, commerce, warfare and exploration, analysis of scientific discourse, even citation indexing" (Jardine 1987)—makes his analysis almost impossible to summarize. However, since his range of associations stems directly from his method, a partial clarification is possible through a consideration of the rules of cybernetic thinking that guide him.

Latour's first rule brings surprises at every turn and deserves some critical overview. According to this rule, "we study science in action and not ready made science or technology; to do so, we either arrive before the facts and machines are black-boxed [i.e., converted into unexamined assumptions] or we follow the controversies that reopen them." Why study "science in action" instead of just "science"? Because science is made primarily through the related activities of inscribing data (legitimizing "fact"), networking (establishing chains of dependent social relations), and building more and more black boxes, more and more unexamined factual relations that become increasingly difficult to challenge.

Take writing, for example: Latour argues that we are better off reading novels than scientific writing, for the latter is, as he puts it, "a peculiar trade in a merciless world" (1987, 60), a kind of fact-writing with few—actually, only three—options for readers: "giving up, going along, working through." Of these,

> *giving up* is the most usual one. People give up and do *not* read the text, whether they believe the author or not, either because they are pushed out of the controversy altogether or because they are not interested in reading the article (let us estimate this to be 90 per cent of the time). *Going along* is the rare reaction, but it is the normal outcome of scientific rhetoric: the reader believes the author's claim and helps him to turn it into a fact by using it further with no dispute (maybe 9% of the time?). There is still one more possible outcome, but such a rare and costly one that it is almost negligible as far as numbers are concerned [i.e., far less than 1%!]: *re-enacting* everything that the authors went through. . . . (1987, 60)

Here, readers must put the text in jeopardy by untying the numerous resources that are mobilized to legitimate it. The task is formidable; in order to untie "these supply lines," one must have at one's disposal a vast array of scientific and social "machines." Critics must be willing to repeat everything, since the job of networking is to create the appearance of logical relatedness rather than to demand that those relationships be logically necessary. "No wonder," Latour laments, "this way of reading a scientific paper is rare!" Thus, he concludes:

> The peculiarity of the scientific literature is now clear: the only three possible readings all lead to the demise of the text. If you give up, the text does not count and might as well not have been written at all. If you go along, you believe it so much that it is quickly abstracted, abridged, stylised and sinks into tacit prac-

tice [i.e., converted into what Latour would call a "black box," or what an anthropologist would call a "cultural category"]. Lastly, if you work through the
authors' trials, you quit the text and enter the laboratory. Thus the scientific
text is chasing its readers away whether or not it is successful. Made for attack
and defense, it is no more a place for a leisurely stay than a bastion or a bunker.
This makes it quite different from the reading of the Bible, Stendhal, or the po-
ems of T. S. Eliot. (61)

What, in fact, distinguishes scientific literature and accounts for its tre-
mendous authority, then, has little to do with its being read; rather it is distinguished by its capacity to mobilize, to engage in a "process made necessary
by the intensity of the rhetoric" (61). Latour wants us so much to accept the
force of this argument that he dissolves the distinction between people and
things: machines, inscribed information, and people are all drawn (as "actants" [Latour's neologism]) into authority-seeking alliances. This, in itself, is
a remarkable argument, not because it confirms other existing theories about
the social construction and deconstruction of meaning, but because it illustrates how, mutatis mutandis, individuals appropriate and get appropriated
by—literally, absorbed into—domains of discourse, even (or perhaps most)
when this appropriation is carried out from the highest of moral promon-
tories.

Indeed, the outcome of Latour's position here (though he never says it
outright) is that claims to the moral high ground—because of how they self-
promote by clinging to a rhetoric of immediacy—are not only callous strategies for mobilizing allies but potentially the most morally suspect of all forms
of appropriating "otherness." His response to his critics is, then, rather like
Charles Lemert's quip about the preacher's relation to sin: namely, that "those
under professional obligation to police the normal do their duty well not because they are pure but because they so finely appreciate the intricacies of human misbehavior" (1997, ix). This reaction is most obvious when Latour's
critics attempt to describe him as a wild reactionary, much in the way that
other defenders of the politically incorrect (e.g., Lasch, or even Benjamin
Spock) have been demonized.

But does Latour really believe that those who wear their morals on their
academic sleeves are, themselves, morally bankrupt? Probably. Because, for
Latour, the success or failure of the mobilization process—the claim to immediacy (moral or otherwise)—becomes the sole determinant of whether or

not something is considered a fact. "A fact is what is collectively stabilized from the midst of controversies when the activity of later papers does not consist only of criticisms or deformation but also of confirmation. The strength of the original statement does not lie in itself, but is derived from any of the papers that incorporate it" (1987, 42), as well as by the degree to which it can "isolate the reader by bringing in many more resources" (44). Here, the very Napoleonic power of scientific rhetoric (or of "the media" or even of "moral imperative") lies in killing off that which is potentially "different"—in Latour's terms, by "making the dissenter feel lonely" (44). "A scientific article becomes more difficult to read, just as a fortress is shielded by buttresses; not for fun, but to avoid being sacked" (46):

> It tries to pack inside the text as many supporters as possible. This is why what is often called "technical details" proliferate. The difference between a regular text in prose and a technical document is the stratification of the latter. The text is arranged in layers. Each claim is interrupted by references outside the texts or inside the texts to other parts, to figures, to columns, tables, legends, graphs. Each of these in turn may send you back to other parts of the same text or to more outside references. In such a stratified text, the reader, once interested in reading it, is as free as a rat in a maze. (48)

"A text is like a bank; it lends more money than it has in its vault" (50)!

Though Latour may be referring here to his own experience with high science, the subtext of his argument has much more to do with his clear sympathy for the isolated antihero—à la Pinter or Ionesco—than with activities that are exclusively scientific. One could argue that science is merely the symptom of our heroic, Machiavellian obsessions, our fanatical enrollment of other people in both what we do and how we protect what we do. Thus, for Latour, what makes a scientific text credible is less its content than its ability to withstand heroic trials: "the text builds a little story in which something incredible becomes gradually more credible [i.e., more heroic] because it withstands more and more terrible trials" (53).

One way of assuring "logical" success in these trials is through what Latour calls "captation," the rhetorical trick by which the arguments of a potential objector are subtly corralled: to "captate" another's argument one must discover just how to leave another "completely free and have them at the same time completely obedient. What is the best way to control these potential dissenters? To lay out the text so that wherever the reader is there is only one way to go" (57).

In such a view, the language of cultural diversity, for instance, would offer an excellent example of captation, since it uses the rhetoric of difference to eliminate real difference from our aforementioned cultural potluck. Conformity, in this case, is not only the end product of the rhetorical cant of those who preach about institutional "diversity," but this captating power is in itself what makes its agenda "right"—to run, that is, your laboratory or university by using the language of diversity itself to coerce all of your faculties, students, and staff to do the exact same sorts of things. Orwellian, Foucaultian (or outright paranoid) though this may sound, Latour has "captured the captators" by mocking the politically correct behavior that inhibits free thought. And it is when conformity is obtained (through the withstanding of trials) that "a text is said to be logical" (58).

Thus, we are led to Latour's second rule of method: "To determine the objectivity or subjectivity of a claim, the efficiency or perfection of a mechanism, we do not look for their *intrinsic* qualities but at all the transformations they undergo *later* in the hands of others" (258). His argument is not merely that egocentric people strive to control others, and that they do so by compelling them to conform; more radically still, the consequences of their networking actually assimilate them as "actants" into objectifying initiatives occurring well outside the intentional range of even the most paranoid of fact-builders. And since, therefore, "the fate of facts and machines is in later users' hands" (259), we now also have a first principle which tells us that the qualities of facts and machines "are thus a consequence, not a cause, of collective action" (259).

By now we begin to get a sense of Latour's unique program, as well as a taste of the searing humor that is not unknown among those who study the methodology of scientific research programs (e.g., the irreverence of Paul Feyerabend's *Against Method*). On one level we are looking at a kind of radical functionalism, as well as a radical empiricism. Where Stuart Hampshire defines an individual's attempts through his or her expectations,[1] Latour pragmatically claims that unless she is very clever at constructing bridges to breed loyalty and cooperation among her colleagues and underlings—unless she knows how to "kula"—a scientist, or anyone else for that matter, may have no idea of what she is doing, since the facts—the certitudes—all come later. Indeed, his second principle (there are six altogether) addresses this issue directly: "Scientists and engineers speak in the name of new allies that they have shaped and enrolled; representatives among other representatives, they add these unexpected resources to tip the balance of force in their favor" (259).

How do successful scientists become responsible for facts if facts must be constructed? Well, as Latour says repeatedly, by social networking. A successful scientist (or academic) is someone who "co-publishes"—who gets others to do his or her own work, to factualize and name that which one has not created, to objectify it. Others help canonize ideas; if we network effectively, another's "discoveries" become "ours" and the concepts that result are "objectified" for us by them. Here Latour reminds us of the self-aggrandizing nature of this endeavor: scientists—indeed, all networkers—gain enormous strength through "naming," through "the act of defining a new object by the answers it inscribes on the window of an instrument." Even before it is named, a new object may be identified as a "list *readable* on the instruments *in* the Professor's laboratory." He adds: "Laboratories generate so many new objects because they are able to create extreme conditions and because each of these actions is obsessively inscribed" (90).

But the idea is not only to create new objects; we have to maintain their resilience, and, in microbiology, even construct them as mythic heroes. Although it is self-evident that this resilience is established through a series of suitably heroic trials (to borrow the proper and appropriate classical paradigm), Latour argues that what is less commonly understood is "the way the same people who constantly generate new objects to win in a controversy [a heroic battle] are also constantly transforming [these new objects] into relatively older ones in order to win still faster and irreversibly" (92). The epithet, the list of trials, thus becomes reified, literally objectified, made into a "resistor," a "thing": "Any new object is thus shaped by simultaneously many older ones in their reified form" (92).

What is so interesting about this perspective is less the power it attributes to institutions than the explanation it offers for why, regardless of one's field, the same professional faces keep appearing in all of the "important" settings. One need only attend an annual meeting of any discipline to witness the degree to which participants—even hysterically—grope for some sense of the so-called cutting edge. And Latour is certainly right about what can be ignored once one can claim a pole position: only a few years ago, for example, our top medical schools faculties scoffed at the idea that a student considering a medical career would choose general practice; today they are all rushing to meet federal quotas. Yet no one seems to be asking how those who spoke cyn-

ically about general practice have suddenly acquired the skills or the motivation to promote primary-care values overnight—a real problem when all ap-
plicants to medical school now claim some interest in the subject. One side of
Latour's Janus face (a device he, in fact, employs in *Science in Action*) would
claim that social conditions have changed; the other side argues that those
who claim the high ground can basically do whatever they want because the
obstacles they have created to resist anyone's untying them are too formidable. So we pretend the obstacles aren't there; we don't even question their
legitimacy. Or, like Americans avoiding politics, we sense the power but admit
defeat straight away. In other words, the circumstances seem hopeless so we
ignore them, even though our doing so doesn't make their power over us any
less troubling.

We should not be surprised that the results of such networking resemble
what can be experienced in all institutional life, since the feedback mechanisms (the protections against dissent) that institutions create are both pervasive and self-perpetuating. Indeed, anyone bold enough to resist a network
will find it necessary to "untie the links between more and more elements
coming from a more and more remote past" (92)—to engage in an activity so
at odds with convention as to make its antiheroic untying appear no less than
sociopathic.

Thus, the basic activities of science—i.e., science in action—may be summarized as dynamic struggles for canonical authority in which "inscribed"
data are transformed into the rapid creation, packing, and repacking of what
at any given moment passes for "fact." Scientists build such machines; what
social scientists must do, he argues, is disassemble them. Can this disassembly
really be accomplished? That depends upon just how manipulative and powerful you take scientific institutions to be, upon how much potential unpack-
ers can resist the heroic rhetoric science employs to dissuade would-be
dissenters, and upon how much dissenters are able to resist the accusation that
their distrust of science in action is sociopathic and "unnatural." For any argument from nature will also be used against critics of science in action, even
though "nature," as it were, arrives late in scientific discourse, even though it
is always brought forward as the most fundamental settler of controversy:
"Nature is the final cause of the settlement of controversies, [but only] once
controversies are settled" (98). Thus Latour's third rule of method: "Since
the settlement of controversy is *the cause* of Nature's representation, not the
consequence, *we can never use the outcome—Nature—to explain how and why a*

controversy has been settled" (99). "Natural" conflict, in other words, is less a Darwinian game that we "naturally" engage in than itself an outcome of particular forms of social engagement that are built around a rhetoric of "survival." Cells and cell warfare may seem "natural" to us, but they are merely the outcome of proclivities that are deeply cultural. So how does one choose the appropriate vehicle for storming the ivory tower of scientific dogma? Well, that depends a good deal on the weapons one chooses to make possible the reverse engineering of all of those black boxes—which in turn depends, as the Cheshire Cat says to Alice, "a good deal on where you want to get to."

GANGSTERS

Accurate though Latour's informational focus may be, it is yet not clear if network theory actually offers us any new or alternative model that could be applied beyond what scientists *do* to what they *see* when they engage in bench science. We have no sense, to paraphrase Hampshire, of what they are trying to do, if we cannot assess what they expect to happen. Studying how scientific facts are built through the social interactions of special interests may inform us about what seems to be happening, but the question of how we go about freely choosing an alternative remains unresolved.

The distinction is crucial: first, because understanding what is genuinely new in Latour's argument—and particularly his insights about how "networking" in our informational era allows a few to "administer many people on a large scale and at a distance" (1987, 255)—means actually examining for ourselves the social implications of, as he says, "opening Pandora's black box"; second, because once we accept his argument about the significance of affiliation in fact-building, it is self-evident that our critical focus would shift from evaluating information to aligning ourselves with the heroes who actually assemble black boxes; and third (and foremost), because accepting Latour's work as an *explanation* invites those who make a habit of black boxing (i.e., those too busy building empires) not to query their own one-dimensionality.

Short of reducing Latour's many insights to yet more black boxes, I would like to focus on the particular significance of reflecting about networks—of "thinking about thinking"—for our understanding of why network metaphors have blossomed in molecular biology. Because "thinking about thinking" honors self-consciousness, it seems tailor-made for the kind of specificity that honors the individual achievements both of surviving cells and of the egotistical scientists who study them. In Latour's work, this view is particularly evidenced in his clear frustration over our heroic obsessions—a frustration that has an important and particular meaning for a molecular biology that sees all of cell activity as modified hero epic.

When he offers us his third principle—in which "we are never confronted with science, technology, and society, but with a gamut of weaker and stronger *associations*" (259)—Latour tries to cut through the heroic rhetoric (by which historians of science attribute discoveries by naming a pedigree) and focus our attention on how successful appropriation or annexation of ideas takes place. What he calls "translation" involves "at once offering new interpretations of these interests and channeling people [i.e., discoverers and developers] in different directions" (117); in turn, these translations are useless unless we can construct "machines" through which the behavior of others can be made predictable (121). Such machines are actually the engines which, when stoked, function as so many connective joints, so many genealogical links that perforce produce the lineages that legitimate scientific hybrids—the very same links that, when perceived by the young, make them all so determined to "get into Harvard."

These "machines" are visible not only in the work of historians who "rush forward to provide genealogies and coats of arms" (134) but also in anything that depends upon "calibrating inscription devices, focusing the controversies on the final visual display, obtaining the resources necessary for the upkeep of the instruments, building nth order theories on the archived records" (256). In other words, Latour's method stands to "gain nothing in explaining 'natural' sciences by invoking 'social' sciences. There is not the slightest difference," he argues, "between the two, and they are both to be studied in the same way. Neither of them should be believed more nor endowed with the mysterious power of jumping out of the networks it builds":

> What is clear for economics, politics and management is all the clearer for sociology itself. How could someone who decided to follow scientists in action forget to study sociologists striving to define what society is all about, what keeps us all glued together, how many classes there are, what is the aim of living in society, what are the major trends in its evolution? . . . The very definition of "society" is the final outcome, in Sociology Departments, in Statistical Institutions, in journals, of other scientists busy at work gathering surveys, questionnaires, archives, records of all sorts, arguing together, publishing

papers, organizing other meetings. Any agreed definition marks the happy end of controversies like all the settlements we have studied in this book. No more, no less. The results on what society is made of do not spread more or faster than those of economics, topology or particle physics. These results too would die if they went outside of the tiny networks so necessary for their survival. (256–57)

To push yet further his anxieties about the resident institutional gerontocracy, Latour adds: "A sociologist's interpretation of society will not be substituted for what every one of us thinks of society without additional struggle, without textbooks, chairs in universities, positions in government, integration in the military, and so on, exactly as for geology, meteorology or statistics" (257). In short, Latour shows the hero to be a coward and a hysteric—someone who cannot work in isolation, someone who cannot act without the accolades we associate with professional success. This is why networking is innovative rather than inventive—because it depends so much on looking over the shoulder or one's neighbor to measure small advantages. This is also why our universities, despite their professed concern about the life of the mind, more frequently than not actually become sites of moral and intellectual stagnation; for policing the network also means policing what can be understood as normal.

Thus, Latour's disdain for "social explanations" is the result of his belief "that we should be as agnostic about society as about nature, and that providing a social explanation does not mean anything 'social' but only something about the relative solidity of associations" (256). Like science and technology, sociology becomes more "social" as it becomes more esoteric because "the more science and technology have an esoteric content the further they extend outside" (259).[2] Here, anthropology is as much subject to its own doxa as is any other discipline; at the same time, because anthropology has as a core theme the acknowledgement of "otherness" (i.e., of that which is "outside"), one might equally say that if any field has the prospect of attending to the complexities of such relationships it may well be anthropology—either because it stands or falls on the acknowledgement of difference, or because its tendency to acknowledge the exotic drives home the degree to which the pursuit of diversity can blind us in recognizing how it exists in the household next door.

Thus, Latour raises the question: What "inside" is it for which an "outside" may become inessential or esoteric? This question is not answered directly in *Science in Action* but is taken up in later arguments where Latour attempts to posit the concept of "outsider" as a "straw man" for the nefarious activities of various networkers (1993)—where anthropologists attempt to articulate unity within the "other" societies they study because continuity has become impossible at home; where modernity itself fails to save us from the disorienting effects of a world characterized by diffuse and intangible networks. "What sort of world is it," Latour asks, "that obliges us to take into account, at the same time and in the same breath, the nature of things, technologies, sciences, fictional beings, religions large and small, politics, jurisdictions, economies and unconsciousnesses?" (ibid., 129).

The answer is, of course, that same hysterical world that is dominated by the need for self-importance and fame despite the one-dimensionality of the very individuals who believe themselves to embody these values; a world in which secure progress in one's career outweighs the risks of cultivating both hard work and pleasure; a world of empty and novel obsessions. In short, the world that Latour himself sees: one glued to ephemeral events, to the "news," and above all to the weather; one in which identity cannot be negotiated at home because notions such as autonomy and choice have no place in the superficial hysteria generated when we willingly enslave ourselves to networks of power,[3] a world in which the fear of being different overrides the desire to defeat entropy by, as it were, cooling a warm vessel, or warming a cool one.

Where can we witness the equally real world of tribal moieties in which one defeats entropy by engaging difference, where social interactions are catalyzed by, literally, marrying one's enemy? Where in network theory has a tribe "brought the war inside its own boundaries" (F. Huxley 1956, 243)? Where is there room for that cultural theater in which "during ceremonies the moieties confront each other and may even stage a mimic battle" (243)? Where in the networking world is there room for the kind of magic in which people openly resist involvement in fame and in power—in congresses and in constitutions—because the risks of social destruction far outweigh the pursuit of personal glory?[4] Where, in other words, is there room for recognizing the importance of polarity as a necessary component in facilitating human transformation?[5]

What network advocates fail to recognize (and even openly jettison) is any sense of, any need for, or any awareness of, the pleasures made possible by the successful social engagement of one's "adversaries"—i.e., those who are "different." In eliminating the value of difference, networks also devalue the growth potential of empathic relations; for the threat posed by "outsiders" incites us to destroy rather than to embody anything "new," while the sentimental overtones of words like "love" and "empathy" lead us, as they do Latour, to discount the very idea of the premodern as "romantic."

Devaluing difference, furthermore, exacerbates the mistaking of "thinking about" for "doing of" because this devaluation also ignores those activities not devoted to the maintenance and bolstering of existing networks. This mistake allows us to forget that empathy requires work that is sometimes difficult, frequently tedious, occasionally dangerous, and almost always unrecognized. Empathy is a highly inefficient activity for networkers. Networkers can stare at their computers all day "thinking about" what it might be like to be in love, or homeless, or sociopathic, but they have no intrinsic means of taking chances, and no way of seeing that their thinking is no replacement for experience. This is also, by the way, why so little anthropology actually gets done in supposedly "rigorous" academic settings.

What network theory offers instead is a world of burdensome mediators who survive, not by negotiating the marginal domains of what can be known, but by appropriating heroic paradigms while simultaneously subjecting others to their random and immoral displays of power. It is this hysterical domain that the network devotee necessarily must inhabit. This is why Latour's *We Have Never Been Modern* must be read as a kind of Faustian eulogy; for a world that can only be sorted out by appealing to a fantastic reordering by "thinking" decision-makers will never develop an innate sense of how to find meaning in what others consider "unimportant." In short, our choice to discount empathy and its embodied projections is more than a little "autoimmune."

Yet this is also why anthropology becomes for Latour a focus of great hope, one that he refers to in several settings, develops fully within a network (cf. Latour and Woolgar 1986), but does not carry into an empathic assessment of why it is important for each of us to seek out our own experience of difference. Latour, in fact, actually resists describing the thing he loves, probably because (like Oscar Wilde) he fears killing it—or, perhaps, like the Beast, because he fears the departure of Beauty. In network terminology, this means a timid experimenting with free association, but an eventually abandonment of it. In turn, Latour offers what he calls "sociologics."

Unlike logic, which questions the veracity of paths of reason (are they "straight or distorted"? [1987, 202]), sociologics only seeks to evaluate social and cognitive strategies (are certain associations weaker or stronger?). Like the obsessive networking of a Melanesian "big man," such a program has one purpose: to map contacts wherever they may lead. To free ourselves from "the belief in the irrationality of certain claims" (scientific realism) and from the equally naive belief that "all claims are equally credible" (cultural relativism), we must "go on following people striving to make their claims more credible than others. While doing so," Latour maintains, "*they map for us and for themselves the chains of associations that make up their sociologics.* . . . All actions," therefore, "like 'dividing,' 'classifying,' or 'ranking,' do not do justice to the unpredictable and heterogeneous nature of the associations" (202).

Here we begin to realize that what Latour has in mind is not the anthropology most know, but a kind of "pure" anthropology—a sort of literal, etymological rendering of the word that is quite at odds with what he perceives to be the moribund academic discipline that goes by the same name. His is a technique, as he elsewhere describes it (e.g., [1992] 1996, 1993), by which we cut through the canonical tyranny that makes a "modern" way of thinking somehow more powerful than all of the alternatives (see, e.g., 1988, 207–9), a ticket for an uncharted voyage, what sailors call a "barefoot cruise."

And it is onto this sandbar that Latour drives our unmanned ship. At its most extreme we are left like Lewis Carroll's German professor in *Sylvie and Bruno Concluded*, who describes how, in order to achieve greater accuracy, the cartographers expand their maps, making them larger and larger until they equal the size of the country itself. Since such a map could not be spread out without reducing the world to darkness, the citizens "now use the country itself as its own map" (Carroll 1939, 557).[6] At its luckier moments, we find ourselves engaged in unwinding old associations and replacing them, or in superimposing them upon new and unlikely affiliations that may present the prospect for creative redefinition—intuitions that, we hope, can cleanse us of the tendentious banality of academic life, of the heroic body-building we mime in order to secure the ideological, intellectual, and even the moral high ground.

Though Latour's sociologics would have us study the ways in which associative links are established and strengthened, the *exact* way in which we decide which lists of interrelations to begin with cannot, like real fieldwork, be specified in advance. This is because

> sociologics are much like road maps; all the paths go to some place, no matter
> if they are trails, tracks, highways or freeways, but they do not all go to the same

place, do not carry the same traffic, do not cost the same price to open and maintain. To call a claim "absurd" or knowledge "accurate" has no more meaning than to call a smuggler trail "illogical" and a freeway "logical." The only thing we want to know about these sociological pathways is where they lead to, how many people go along them with what sort of vehicles, and how easy they are to travel; not if they are wrong or right. (1987, 205)

Indeed, this is why the only real map of Latour's program would be the very experience of an event or a series of related events—"La Tour de France," as it were.

What, in the end, do we gain by such a dissective ethnographic technique? At the least, we reach some kind of active engagement—but one so skeptical in nature that it has as its premise the de facto corruption of those who display their medals—including their moralities—on their institutional garments. We gain, to use another analogy, some indication of why all of our museums of modern art are filled to the gills with self-promoting artistic statements, and why all of the postwar paintings that cover their walls are so bloody big. What, however, distinguishes Latour from other critics is his tenacity. Like Diogenes of Sinope (the so-called "dog philosopher"), Latour is convinced of the need to eschew convention even if his devotion to networks leads him to a kind of self-imposed alienation.

Where, we invariably will ask, might a despairing soul actually begin his sort of "anthropological" investigation? Perhaps by Latour's leap of faith into the domain of an imaginative anthropology, one I have elsewhere characterized as a state of "selective dissociation" (1992, 190–99); for what Latour is trying to offer us is a sense of how one might employ associative thought to redefine the boundaries of what is theoretically and practically admissible, to open what he calls an "unlimited field of study for anthropology" (204).

In criticizing science Latour shows, then, how the tenacious questioning and hard labor of traditional anthropological empiricism is central to his "sociologics," but we also need to see how creative processes are themselves characterized by daily toil, precisely *because* they may be driven by the kinds of unlikely ideological affiliations that institutions find so unacceptable. This is why marginality is crucial, and why empathy is the guiding force for seeing oneself in another.

Deviation, in other words, is actually a constructive quality (Eguchi 1991) that is challenged (but not necessarily overcome) by institutional networking.

Latour's rule by which we avoid accusations of irrationality in favor of under-standing degrees of displacement reflects the common social tendency to contain behavioral deviance. However, what remains to be shown is how ap-parent anomalies can actually influence a social network, and also why it is so important simply to jump in and swim—that is, to accept the notion that cer-tain forms of apparently liminal behavior may be as much creative as damag-ing.

It is, then, the inherent devaluation of the socially marginal that has en-abled us to surrender to the presumed power of networks and the immuno-logical world of which they are a part. Despite the inherent weaknesses of the practice of networking, we are invited to believe that networks (in businesses, universities, cultures, states, empires) have virtually unlimited authority over the individuals who find themselves trapped within them. However right Foucault or E. P. Thompson may be about the relationship between industrial time-keeping and the control of workers' bodies, and however much our as-piring academic heroes conflate the seriousness of their own work with the survival of entire moral orders, "the superficially attractive notion that the growth of state power has been directed towards the social subordination of the body turns out to be naive and unconvincing" (Porter 1992, 220).

Furthermore, though we each may indeed be, as Latour suggests, as free as a rat in a maze, his account of the power of networks may lead us to underes-timate the tendency of institutions to atrophy, to be brought down by the weight of their own intrigues and colluding. This tendency becomes more clear by contrast—i.e., when the "selective dissociations" of some antihero (as we will see in part 3) actually lead to the kind of revision that makes a particu-lar network obsolete. Granted, these (apparently catastrophic) changes are rare, particularly given the degree to which they are discounted and chal-lenged. Still, many important discoveries are made by amateur astronomers, even if the terms of what actually count are being limited and controlled by industrial researchers and by professors in university departments. And it is also now clear that the obsessive competition that creates our imbalanced (i.e., tumorous) world is not even in the best interest of those hell-bent on vis-ible success (see, e.g., Kohn 1986).

Indeed, it is the very tendency of these institutions to drag themselves down that makes possible those moments (rare though they may appear) when outsiders can have an extraordinary influence on relations at the center. And it is precisely here where "foreign bodies" do sometimes successfully impose themselves on otherwise hermetic environments. The truth of this influence can be seen in the mythologies of nearly every culture, and the patterns of such rare influences are phenomenally consistent. What is more, the individuals who inhabit institutions and who enslave themselves to various networks are no more capable of being inventive than are the institutions themselves: one consequence of the argument that the objectification and verification of a fact "comes later" is that facts are not very negotiable once they have been black-boxed, and that existing black boxes cannot be readily revised even by those networkers who create them. In short, the most common response to the possible atrophication of a "fact" is not to rebuild it but to create a new black box before the previous one can be totally undone. This is consumer marketing writ large.

Finally, we need to begin asking something about what it can cost in human terms to devote one's life to building black boxes. Latour's work—and particularly *Science in Action*—leaves us with the feeling that there are only winners and losers, and that those who build and control always win. But nobody seems to be asking about just what they win. Is it fame after death? Or an impact on a field? What is the human cost of living a one-dimensional life? How many institutional initiatives have ever inspired creativity? And what happens to those who are enough motivated spiritually to put aside the heroic values that plague most people?

If working alone appears too risky, then do get yourself aligned or otherwise connected with whatever network is ordering the day; but remember that there is very little evidence for the positive, long-term influence of such networking on the world of ideas, or, for that matter, on human happiness. When the great sculptor Brancusi gave up his apprenticeship to Rodin (after having walked from Romania to Paris to take it up), he was said to have remarked that no sapling could grow under the shade of a large tree. Can *any* world at all survive beneath Carroll's map? This is not a Buddhist koan for those who can enough distance themselves from professional rewards to contemplate in any meaningful way the degree of slavish allegiance that is the precondition for participating in the heroic values their institutions propagate. Nor does this question invite a mere *argumentum ad silentio*. Instead, it is an invitation to examine in one's own life the ways that meaning can be achieved without the guarantee of public recognition.

In summary, then, the reduction of human activity to the establishment and legitimization of domains of power creates a belief system in which

(1) invention gives way to a reactionary innovative existence, where the effects of marginal activities (e.g., selective dissociation, or superimposition of unlikely elements) are minimized; (2) the devaluation of difference leads to a nonreciprocal view of the phenomenon of exchange and of human relations generally; and (3) life becomes characterized by a series of scams carried out by subterfuge.

Because networkers do not and cannot value marginal activities, the cultivation of empathy as a creative endeavor is discounted as inefficient. Relations without a reciprocity of opposites leads to cynicism, coercion, and disingenuousness; while the increasingly hermetic nature of social relations for networkers (maniacally seeking out the very domains of existing authority that enslave them) creates little more than social entropy. This is why, of all things, human love and its psychological risks become modernity's only hope. Transformation at the borders is the only way forward.

What we now need to examine is the manner in which information theory has been employed in microbiology specifically. How do cell biologists, geneticists, virologists, and immunologists utilize network metaphors? And, more importantly, are those theorists who were initially attracted to network metaphors actually able either to offer us a better account of what they observe, or, if not a better account, then other, new metaphors that better explain what microbes seem to do? Can biological causes be at all located in totally relational networks of "stronger" and "weaker" interactions? And how important is it, anyway, to be able to attribute outcomes to specific agents? To address these questions we will now examine an argument in which several of them are taken up.

NATIONAL PROCESSED RADIO

Our present scheduling procedures almost guarantee that nothing unexpected can be found. —Nobel Laureate Luis Alvarez

In her thought-provoking examination of the use of metaphors in twentieth-century biology, Evelyn Fox Keller reminds us of the initial novelty of attributing agency and autonomy to genes. Though to us "so familiar as to seem obvious" (1995, 8–9), the notion of gene agency was once novel:

The conception of genes as autonomous actors—endowed with the authority and the capacity to direct the future course of organic development—dates to

the mid twenties, but the particular twist added by the notion of the chromosome as "code-script" arrives only in the early forties. Credit for the introduction of this idea to biology belongs to Erwin Schrödinger, the physicist often
cast as the father of quantum mechanics. (45)

In answering the question of what "attributing (or for that matter, denying)
causal power to genes" (3) actually means, Keller argues that earlier sexist
metaphors (particularly the penetrating agents of infectious diseases [Brandt
1987]) are gradually being replaced by more neutral terms: aggressive atomistic
genes give way to informational models in the same way that aggressive sperm
have given way to newer models of fertilization that are "more likely to be cast
in the language of equal opportunity (defined, for example, as 'the process by
which egg and sperm find each other and fuse' [Alberts et al. 1989, 868])" (xii).
As Olds, in her study of the psychological implications of systems theory (1992),
argues for the unifying possibilities of systems theory metaphors, so too does
Keller see the emphasizing of an integrated immune system as beneficial for establishing a more neutral way of visualizing cell-cell relations.

Optimistic as Keller's views may seem, one can only hope that changing
our language of symbolic interaction would permit us to adopt a less aggressive view of cellular life. However, the degree to which one accepts this shift of
emphasis is rather dependent upon where one looks, for it may be as easily argued that the policing of language merely encourages yet more subterfuge.
Sociobiology, a well-known bastion of scientific and political conservatism, is
now more than ever rife with male egos acting in "selfish" secrecy. Indeed,
Midgley (1994, 7–9), in her discussion of ethics and Darwinism, offers some
glaring examples of such disingenuousness, including the following excerpts
from well-known neo-Darwinists:

> Human behavior . . . is the circuitous technique by which human genetic mate-
> rial has been kept intact. Morality has no other demonstrable ultimate func-
> tion. (E. Wilson 1978, 167)

> We are survival machines—robot vehicles blindly programmed to preserve the
> selfish molecules known as genes. (Dawkins 1976, x)

> The organism is only DNA's way of making more DNA. (E. Wilson 1975, 4)

Thus does ideology bow to its hidden masters, the genes. (E. Wilson 1978, 4)

Parental love itself is actually but an evolutionary strategy whereby genes replicate themselves. (Barash 1980, 3)

Although attributing agency to microentities—microorganism, genes,
sperm—is not as "Western" as some may wish to think (in fact, it is the basis
of all forms of demonology, and is apparent in countless indigenous responses
to international health programs), Keller is quite right about how a "discourse
on gene action" leads us to a devaluing, even a rejection, of embryology, a discipline which, probably more than any other, focused on the problem of dif-
ferentiation:

> If the genetic content of all cells in an organism is the same, how is it possible
> to make sense of the emergence of the manifest differences among all the cells
> that make up a complex organism? To the embryologist it seemed self-evident
> that this problem of differentiation, so deeply at the heart of their own con-
> cerns, was simply incompatible with the notion that the gene was the exclusive
> locus of action. (Keller 1995, 13)

For Keller, the shift from the language of gene action to that of gene activation was Watson and Crick's real (but unrecognized) coup, because this shift
introduced for the first time the informational metaphors that are today
supplanting the more sexually aggressive ones. Since DNA is, in fact, incapable of making copies of itself (or, for that matter, of making anything), our
attributing agency to genes is rather like Lewontin's description of the East-
man Kodak factory as the place of self-reproduction of photographs (Lewontin 1992, 33; cited in Keller 1995, 23).

Whether or not one accepts Keller's basically feminist reading—that the
shift away from genes as animating forces and toward contextualizing forces is
good—there is no doubt that the shift has been identified, and that the shift
away from gene agency leads us back to the validation of embryology. What,
then, are the problems with this view?

First is the aforementioned fact that attributing agency to personified microentities is a widespread human tendency not restricted to modern
science—i.e., it's not in the first place the obvious outcome of a penetrating

worldview designed by white, male Europeans. Indeed, to personify—to attribute volition to things—is a universal and ancient pastime that may be witnessed in any demonology. But why do scientists actually need these little personified demons at all? First, because *we all* rely upon our personificatory skill when the time comes to be creative. But there is a second important reason that has to do with the agnostic's inability to offer any explanation for why creation takes place at all. Without some personified god to whom we can attribute final causes, science finds itself actually having to invent one. This tendency is nowhere so clear as in thermodynamics, because in the relationship between hot and cold we see both the greatest expression and the greatest absence of life.

Combining intensely hot and cold molecules can produce a dramatic, if chaotic, expression of life force—so intense, in fact, that the outcome of such combining may be altogether destructive; for there is no clear reason why energy should be ordered systematically enough that it would increase or grow, let alone do so exponentially. Indeed, if anything, an expression of energy will naturally desist because of the rules of efficiency demand that energy transfer lead to energy loss; an explosion ends, a fire goes out, a kettle cools, all because of something called entropy, the thermodynamic principle by which energy gradually decreases to a level of uniform inactivity. Put simply, it isn't right that living things should continue. Because of the erosion of energy, things should, like all aging organisms, slow down and die out.

In fact, the only way in which life could be saved from entropy—that is to say, salvaged from Lord Kelvin's Second Law of Thermodynamics—was to posit that entropy did not apply to animate processes, either because heat created from the animal frame produced a mechanical effect that countered the Second Law, or because such a mechanical effect produced by the very will of the animal distinguished the animate world from the rest of nature. Darwin himself was clearly horrified by the idea that creatures gradually perfected through evolution should be doomed to entropy; and science as a whole was greatly relieved by imagining ways in which particles might combat entropy through the generation of inner stability.

However, in order not simply to proclaim that the will of God was at work, it became necessary to invent another decisive force. This force came to be known as Maxwell's demon, a purely imagined little being, whose single duty was to operate a slide that permitted only fast molecules to pass from a cooler vessel into a warmer one, thereby allowing the warmer vessel to get hotter.

This little being, as Keller points out, allowed for both free will and for environmental determinism by the novel creation of a decisive force that was not (at least obviously) "a manifest surrogate for God" (54), even though in retrospect the demon does clearly have the godlike duty of facilitating energy increase.

All the more odd, then, that the "novelty" of this idea was not immediately undermined by any anthropological critique; for such beings are the vital feature of nearly every form of polytheism. In fact, though Maxwell's demon may have allowed Euro-American science to think that it had separated itself from religion, the greatest tragedy of that poor imagined creature was the way that scientists believed it a novel resolution to the problem of energy decrease. For the necessary feature of the demon was less its will than its ability to function as a Great Reciprocator—to open and close a slide that would *enliven an exchange through the maintenance of difference*, establishing a deep difference to advance creative life. All the demon need do was recognize heat difference and allocate faster and slower molecules. Indeed, recognizing the degree to which the problem of entropy had been personified is not at all new; for, as Keller (1995, 60) notes, the whole history of "information theory" can be, and often is, read as an elaboration of Szilard's 1929 paper "On the Decrease of Entropy in a Thermodynamic System by the Intervention of Intelligent Beings," in which he tries to refute Maxwell by arguing that the demon's thinking itself results in entropy.

Is it any accident that our obsessions with computer intelligence should be mirrored in our language of computer viruses? For, try as we might to depersonify "information," we nevertheless intuitively recognize that decision-making requires energy, and energy leads either to stasis or to chaos when intentionality is eliminated. The system, then, means nothing without our assuming its ability to recognize and respond to difference. Perhaps it was just such an intuition that led Einstein to the parallel beliefs that cosmic theories should be aesthetically balanced, and that the laws of thermodynamics would outlast all other forms of scientific knowledge.

What can it mean to know that balancing difference is the foundation of creativity and, at the same time, to acknowledge that we live in a social world devoid of real encounters with otherness? Here, again, the historical record is telling; for the acute ignorance of difference is nowhere so clear as in the way in which the debate over Maxwell's demon developed between "vitalists" and "mechanists": on the one hand the mechanists argued (as did Szilard) that, since the demon had to work his partition in the face of the resistance created by faster molecules, entropy had to exist within an organism's ambient environment; on the other, the vitalists claimed that living processes differed from inorganic ones. However, little in the vitalist-mechanist debate was based on direct observation,[7] and what is so frequently overlooked is the simple fact, as vitalist James Johnstone put it, that "the movement which we call inorganic is toward the abolition of diversities, while that which we call life is toward the maintenance of diversities" (quoted in Keller 1995, 63). Fast forward to the so-called "postmodern condition" and one now has a convincing, if frightening, argument for why we so often feel immobilized, petrified, and hysterical.

So, where might we turn? Certainly not to a politically correct (i.e., reciprocally "neutral") language of equality, or to a networker's hysteria: for these only obscure the real merits of enjoying any dangerous engagement with the unknown. In fact, the only way to address this problem of biological and social entropy is to extend the boundaries of exchange actually to include the *ambient domain of reciprocal difference*—i.e., what we would in the broadest terms call the other's "social" environment. In Keller's words, "if one redraws the boundary of the living system, not at the outer skin of the organism but at the outer perimeter of a closed thermodynamic system large enough to encompass the energetic substrates required for respiration and metabolism, the problem might be said (and indeed was said) to vanish" (1995, 65).

Unfortunately, science's choice has not been to examine reciprocal exchanges of difference, but to focus on the structure of the system—to project the boundaries of life onto larger groups of relations that would have some semblance of what might loosely be defined as "organic." This is clear in Schrödinger's proposed resolution to the problem of entropy, which posits an organism drawing "negative entropy" from the world it inhabits—that an organism maintains itself by "continually sucking orderliness from its environment" (68). But this solution is problematic. All it really offers is a polite way of describing an egocentric entity that now recognizes its limitations—an organism's "concentrating a 'stream of order' on itself"—namely, the "'drinking orderliness' from a suitable environment" (69) that Keller does not hesitate to isolate as nothing more than a mammarian fantasy! Yet, setting aside Schrödinger's Freudian obsession, nothing in what he says allows us to acknowledge that studying an "ambient domain of reciprocal difference" invites us, if anything, to resurrect the dormant field of embryology. Why embryology? Because in embryology there is a logical space for elevating reciprocity over selfishness.

Are there, then, better metaphors for visualizing the selfish outcomes of embryonic imbalance? Absolutely. There are many; but a good biological one that resonates socially comes in the form of what oncologists call a teratoma, a kind of tumor made up of totipotential cells—that is, cells that are capable of differentiating into all possible specialized types. When such cells become tumorous, a teratoma overgrowth is created. Like a mad civilization made up of egocentric, self-centered, and highly specialized individuals, "teratomas are chaotic assemblies of tissues and organs, some of which appear quite normal" (LaFond 1978, 50). A chaotic tumor made up of otherwise well-formed body parts is probably, then, a much better image of the outcome of true genetic selfishness.

But, for Schrödinger, the way in which an organism frees itself from the entropy it cannot help from otherwise producing is through metabolic processes that are genetically planned. And it was this "ghost of Maxwell's demon," this only slightly veiled organizing super-being, that would soon be projected onto organizations via the intelligence systems of Norbert Wiener—where many very small agents (e.g., molecules) would function to effect decisions but do so in ways that were highly ambiguous, nonspecific, even undirected or covert.

And nowhere, it seems, is there in any of these considerations an awareness of the fact that what has been created is, put simply, a system of black magic, a game of covert and assumed intentions, a demonology, and, by any anthropological standard at least, a poor and relatively undeveloped demonology at that. Life—the *change* that occurs in *exchanges of difference*—has now gone underground; for what we see in the rise of "information" and "network" theory is a sustained belief in intentionality, coupled with a suppression of the identifiable agent of action. What unfolds is something we know well—a modern world in which things happen but for which no one is responsible, a world plagued by paranoia, a world of self-ignorance and self-hate, one that becomes, in a word, autoimmunological.

Thus, the extent to which information theory results in a deemphasis of agency and in a fueling of a network's covertness may remain as unmeasurable as it is critical. However, we have clearly seen in our discussion of illness metaphors how the power of a given metaphor to persist covertly, or indeed to survive at all, is directly proportional to its social resilience in other settings. A student who sees AIDS metaphors as an exact replication of political corruption or of the Gulf War is, in fact, illustrating for us how much *more* powerful agency becomes once its exact locus is suppressed.[8] In fact, though I accept the political motivations of Keller's argument, I diverge from her optimistic view of the benefits of employing systems and networks to describe bodily functions and cell activities. As Midgley has also surmised,

> The metaphors [of sociobiology] seem meant in some way to be taken literally; as Dawkins insists, they are "truths." And these metaphors are not just violent; they are also so familiar that they unavoidably bring their context with them when we ask how to interpret them. *This is everyday language whose proper and normal use is to describe manipulative fraud.* (1994, 8)

In fact, this is the language not only of manipulative fraud but of human oppression. Mocking the sociobiological model, she offers a telling metaphorical projection of Dawkins's "truths": "The typical middle-class intellectual is a survival machine, a robot vehicle blindly programmed to preserve the selfish individuals known as millionaires and directors of multi-national companies" (ibid., 9). True though this frightening comparison may appear to us in a dark moment, it is far from providing an adequate explanation of what motivates us to do what we do—unless, that is, we either see the world in a simplistic, and equally determined, way, or we subscribe to what one anonymous reviewer called the "pop psychology" of Dawkins's writings, which serve readers primarily as an introduction to the author's own form of fundamentalism.

So, to focus on organic relations that are context-dependent, or on genetic transcription complexes, draws our attention away from the activities of intentional agents (or, rather, from our ability to influence their activities) and toward the network—toward a "highly coordinated system of regulatory dynamics that operates simultaneously at all levels: at the level of transcription activation, of translation, of protein activation, and of intercellular communication" (ibid., 30).

While the tacit acceptance of a network's power, combined with a sense of its being beyond our influence, generates a true hysteria (even a kind of experiential schizophrenia), there is absolutely no evidence to support the idea that suppressing or limiting language actually results in the dissolution of a distasteful or dangerous way of thinking. Simply because the Balinese do not like talking about black magic does not mean that it has no currency; in fact, quite the opposite is the case. More importantly, so long as the social paradigm in which that suppression takes place is dominated by heroic values, such suppression, as we will now see, *can't* work. Simply because intentional actors have, as it were, gone underground does not mean that a belief in the system of values they stand for is any less strong.

Thus, science's so-called rediscovery of the "organism" through cybernetic theory (that is, its focus on the systemic network), or, more recently, through the embryonic nature of stem cell research, seems more like a pendulum shift than a real change of paradigm, especially given the persistent belief in the authority of a multitude of amoral agents at work within networks of power. Clearly, no amount of politically correct language, no amount of focusing on weaker and stronger relations, and no amount of "cellular equality," will transform the basic belief that someone is controlling these networks and that we, as the excluded, have been denied access to them.

It is not solely the assumption of agency without morality that renders systems theory—including immune systems theory—so troublingly hysterical. Without the moral connections that allow for intentionally risky experimentation beyond the network—for, say, creating love rather than oppression—networkers themselves have little awareness of the consequences of what they do. And though they may think that they do quite a bit, the good news is that their fear of what exists outside of their networks—their disinterest in looking at anything, or attending to anyone, not obviously powerful—renders them incapable of understanding the mechanisms of true change. Indeed, they may even develop complex theories about our rapidly changing world, theories that display no understanding whatsoever of the extent to which their ostensibly changing world is actually static and complacent. In short, networkers suck energy from existing relations because they do not know how to create energy, and they replace the reality of their own stasis with a language of supposed change.

The primary reason for this mistake has to do with the ignorance created by focusing on the center of the cell colony rather than on the periphery. It is an ignorance, for sure, that has its origin in the early Enlightenment, but it reaches its full form in the neo-Darwinian use of natural selection and in the erroneous belief that life at the center of the colony will produce a strain of blue-blood survivors far superior in adaptability to their liminal cousins who attempt to live at the colony's edge. This is fascism, for sure; but it is also a clear attempt to use the language of transformation and change as a device for maintaining stasis.

LET THEM EAT CAKE

Short and grisly had been the work of the mutineers . . . and through it all [Lord Greystoke] had stood leaning carelessly beside the companionway puffing meditatively upon his pipe as though he had been watching an indifferent cricket match. —Edgar Rice Burroughs, *Tarzan of the Apes*

In 1859 Charles Darwin published his monumental work, *On the Origin of Species by Means of Natural Selection.* Though today we less remember his competitors, no one disputes the fact that inheritance and gradualism were major obsessions of a Victorian England in the throes of an industrial revolution. At that time, the combined forces of capitalism and the Age of Discovery would come to challenge the very soul of the upper-middle classes, classes that, for the first time since Cromwell, saw their "gradualist" ways seriously threatened by "overachievers." Indeed, the very idea that the fittest survive was well-enough implanted in the general culture of Victorian England to appear self-evident to anyone of proper breeding. Saltation ("dancing," "leaping," "suddenly changing") was not only an intellectual concern then; today, still, those who feign social status are called "bounders" by the British. Dickens's Josiah Bounderby of Coketown was the precise symbol of the gradualist's nightmare. "Many deeply religious Victorians, such as Charles Kingsley, accepted Charles Darwin's suggestions at once, whereas the scientific establishment treated it with great suspicion" (Midgley 1994, 6).

It was, at least in part, a fear of bounders—of social "saltators"—that allowed the endowing of the gradualist agenda with scientific authority to meet with so much success among good Christians, despite the way in which evolution came to blows (as it still does) with Christian dogma. This particular marriage of religion and science was also the cause for Darwin's becoming the focus of heated public debate, particularly twelve years later when he applied his theory of evolution to humans in *The Descent of Man.* For Darwin survival depended upon the gradual evolution and adaptation of an organism over periods of time that could only be measured geologically, a view that would allow evolution to become the rationale for social Darwinism and, later, eugenics. The kind of sudden transformation—i.e., the "saltations"—popularized by religions and among novelists would destroy the very basis of his theory: natura no facit saltum. Nature does not saltate, it cannot suddenly transform, it does not change through "dance."

Yet, despite, or perhaps because of, Darwin's fundamental intellectual conservatism, his two most important novelties were the result of self-acknowledged intellectual saltation. Not only did natural selection "at once" strike him, but he remembers "the very spot in the road" where the link between diversity and niche capacity dawned on him. As Alan Gross puts it, insight for Darwin (as for the rest of us),

> is not a logical step that is larger than usual. It is not a logical step at all; it is a psychological state, an experience of sudden conceptual reconfiguration in the face of a pressing intellectual problem. . . . The suddenness with which we experience insight says nothing about the psychological and rational processes that underlie its possibility, processes that need not be sudden; *a fortiori*, the fact of insight cannot be evidence against the essential conservatism of personal systems of belief. (1990, 158)

"Lab work" and intellectual rigor, in other words, may lead us to the threshold of transformation, but they do not constitute it. They may sensitize us (as do our anxieties and discomforts); they may help us to recognize and reconstruct change; they may even be catalysts for change; but they are not of the same order as, or even remotely related to, the changes they presage. In Darwin's case, this preparatory conservatism took many forms: fifty-five months of observation during the circumnavigation that preceded his return to England in October 1836; the more than twenty-two years that stood between his return and his publication of the *Origin*; his indebtedness to Lyell's discoveries about so many things, including geological change.

Surely, then, the greatest Darwinian paradox of all must be the one that stands between Darwin's "private persuasion" about the continuity and gradualism of evolution and his earlier belief that evolution did, indeed, depend upon saltation—a belief that itself was also personally affirmed by the saltatory experience of eating a rare Patagonian ostrich that would later be named for him, and by the way that this very event sensitized him to the problem of speciation. This intellectual "saltating" is, in fact, not at all unlike the moment when Niels Jerne, the "father" of immune-systems theory, realized that immunity was controlled by *networks*—an idea which reportedly struck him while strolling across a bridge. Indeed, such intellectual saltating is central to making any discovery or being psychologically transformed; for, as Hampshire acknowledges, "the most profound and fruitful discoveries of truth may present themselves to a man in an apparently unconnected manner, and without any apparent source in his own directed thinking" (1965, 107).

For Darwin, the man, conservatism was not only a scientific problem but a sentimental one: so long as Darwin permitted himself "to a long exploration that prohibits early closure" (Gross 1990, 154), so too did he allow himself to see speciation—species inosculation or separation—as not degenerative, for something has to be different in order to change. How can something be simultaneously the same and different? It's the basic paradox of real transformation.

But it is when Darwin set aside the uncertainty of change in favor of his grander plan that he presented evolution as an act of faith in which universal likeness offers the teleological comfort that would allow the most conservative of upper-middle-class British gentlemen to abandon the Church of England for a belief system whose social implication was lingering just below the surface. Referring to these continuities, Darwin lays his claim: "We see in these facts some deep organic bond, prevailing throughout space and time, over the same area of land and water, and independent of their physical conditions. . . . This bond, on my theory, is simply inheritance. . . ." ([1859] 1964, 349–50 [Gross 1990, 156]). Even to the present day, advocates of evolution find solace in the apparent continuities of complex biological systems that gain meaning over many millions of years of gradual change, while hierarchical societies find similar solace in the inalienable status of their upper and upper-middle classes. What Darwin actually achieved, then, was *the reinforcement of a deep cultural prejudice at the same time as he convinced the world that he was changing it*; for the backlash of Social Darwinism—the belief that some social groups are more evolved and, therefore, "better" than others—was certainly more damaging to the human condition than the quaint notion that the world was created during seven rotations of the earth.

How incredibly ironic (that is, *unnatural*) that Darwin's theory about transformation could not be corroborated (indeed, was contradicted) by his own mental processes—as if time, and time alone, would allow him to come to terms *anesthetically*[9] with his fearful and nearly erotic relationship with transformation.[10] Darwin's own intellectual transformations, we must accept, were clearly not "natural" in any of the senses that he would employ that term for all of nature. Could he, in other words, possibly have achieved his paroxysmic, enlightening experiences without his five years of marginality amid all of the strangest and deformed things that his travels—themselves bizarre by early-nineteenth-century standards—would allow him to document? And isn't it, then, all the more important that we distinguish between what Darwin argues rhetorically to be the case for evolution, and his own attitudes about change as he understood it personally?

Although the problem of saltation would persist in the dispute between geneticists (concerned with genotypic proximate causes and evolutionary speciation) and naturalists (concerned with phenotypic ultimate causes and gradualism), Darwin knew very well that his conservatism provided the soundest basis for leading him to cathartic moments (a dinner, a walk, a spot in the road). As for the changes of view themselves, they were not, and could not be, gradual, for their paradoxical nature was embodied in transformational moments that could only be intellectualized in hindsight. This is the view of personhood that is articulated in a curriculum vitae, and, quite emphatically, not Peirce's "future self" that comes into existence within a flow of life that has yet to be formed by the "circumambient social order" (Harré 1984, 256; see discussion in Gross 1990, 144–45).

Despite evolution's major article of faith (in which complex organisms diversify), as a theory its inability to predict anything will always leave it open to being called teleological[11] (or, if one be generous, teleognomic [Mayr 1976, 2000]), and its implications for concepts of identity will forever draw our attention to an atomistic notion of persons and groups that suppresses the social settings in which identity is negotiated and ultimately achieved. These facts, we will now see, have special importance for cellular biology and for our understanding of the pathologies of infectious diseases and their vaccines.

But why turn to Darwin in a discussion of social models and microbes? Because many of the social metaphors that govern our understanding of the immune system and what vaccines actually do are based upon ongoing disagreements about what immunological diversity really means, and about the extent to which this phenomenon has a genetic basis. Darwin looms large in this discussion because to accept the notion that all immunological specificities are genetically encoded raises a fundamental conundrum: how, critics asked, "could the gene pool be maintained when any given organism was likely to employ such a small proportion of its specificity repertoire during its lifetime and when so many of the specificities that it did employ were against antigens (i.e., 'foreigners') that (who?) posed little threat to survival? In the absence of positive selective pressures, it would not take long for such unused or 'unimportant' genes to lose their identity" (Silverstein 1989, 147).

To date, immunology's answer is that each antibody is specifically structured to meet its inducing antigen, and that the number of types that a human produces, while not infinite, is unimaginably large—in fact, anywhere from 50,000 to 10^{16}, with the most frequent guess standing from 10^5 to 10^9 (ibid., 145). Alternately, families of clonotypes—that is, "specific antibodies of differing primary structure and differing affinity, but reactive nevertheless with the immunizing antigen" (146)—may reduce the number to a mere 5,000 or so. However, even where the clonotype repertoire of certain mammals seems large, a degeneracy of the immune response "appears to allow an almost embarrassingly restricted coverage of the universe of potential stimuli" (146). Put plainly, a large repertoire does not in itself ensure much, and, more embarrassing still, small vertebrate species with significantly narrower specificity repertoires than man "appear to cope very well and to survive attack by their respective pathogens with little sign of immunological impairment. . . . [even] invertebrates, apparently devoid of any semblance of the molecular immune system of vertebrates, seem to cope well in this pathogen-ridden world" (148–49). So, evolutionary issues are at the center of immunology's two major paradoxes: one involving the size and scope of the immunological repertoire, the other relating to the actual mechanism by which diversity is generated (145).

Whether, therefore, we see the thymus—the body's major generator of immunological novelty—as Jerne's mutant-breeding site ("where the immunological repertoire is somatically expanded by stepwise mutational deviations from the histocompatibility-determined starting point" [Silverstein 1989, 150]), or whether we see it as a cellular nursery school (where "students from the foetal liver have genes activated . . . that direct the production of a protein that the cells attach to their surface" [Dwyer 1995, 7]), is entirely dependent upon whether we focus on the identity of the cell as innate or as acquired within the somatic field in which its identity is realized. For the difference will indicate to us whether we come to interpret the multiple somatic field of cellular "social" relations as a negative mutant threat (i.e., a challenge to be avoided) and/or as a positive, selective environmental locus in which cellular "identity" is achieved.

One problem with the "survival-of-the-fittest" paradigm is that it is totally dependent upon agents *eliminating* that which is different (read "threatening") *and* on their realization that difference *is necessary* for adaptation and speciation. But because the difference between a threatening form of diversity and one that broadens an organism's ability to adapt cannot be established in advance—because such an evaluation is totally dependent on the precise nature of a specific "social" encounter—there is no way of avoiding evolution's teleological position.

This problem of experience—which is *psychological, attitudinal,* and *social*—is not only crucial for assessing the theoretical division between cell-mediated and humoral immunity (and even between genetics and embryology); it also unlocks for us (in its favoring the innate nature of identity over its socially negotiated manifestation) the degree to which immunology and virology are themselves bound to particular models of historical time that embody heroic cultural values in a specific narrative structure. This is why some of the most exciting work on the origins of life has focused on issues of time and memory (e.g., Morowitz 1985, 1992). It is also why vaccinology, in particular, is so significant as a field of inquiry; because it is in vaccinology that the positive outcome of an organic challenge can be observed in the lifetime of one organism—where the genetic reality of an encoded genealogical memory is no longer hypothetical. Yet, as compared to the word "immunology," how many of us have ever heard of the word, "vaccinology," let alone considered at all its deep meaning?

But the consequences may be broader still. Susumu Ohno has, for instance, suggested that the answer to the repertoire paradox "may be as applicable to the functional diversity of the nervous system and human intelligence as it is to immunity" (Silverstein 1989, 149). This is also why evolution's future adaptations have always depended, and will always depend, upon the activities *on* the "self" by an *external* agent, and why, in turn, immunological and evolutionary diversity might be better understood at the level of embryology than at the level of specificity. Though theoretical biologists have contested many aspects of Lynn Margulis's theory of cellular symbiosis, the idea that bacteria-like organisms are the ancestors of mitochondria (that is, that bacteria and our normal cells share organizational structures) is widely tolerated among scientists (Margulis 1998, 34). This, in itself, is enough to allow for some questioning of the focus on specificity over and above the more complex domain of embryology; for the latter means nothing if not the mutual, creative engendering of novel forms of life over the entire gamut of possible forms of cell-cell interaction.

The idea that immunology does not conform neatly to evolutionary selective principles—that genes may, at times, have no "self" to be "selfish" about—seems quite likely; for "selection" can have no meaning—indeed, it must, as it were, be "unnatural"—if its function is to a spit out hundreds of millions of what, for all the world, look like random mutants. In what way, under these conditions, does the world "selection" apply at all? What is being selected? What are these mutant creations "fit" for? And why, if they are fit, is "fitness" such a critical factor at all in our assessment of the value of life, unless "being" itself is a job that one is "fit" to do?

Since such large questions are rarely considered, ought we not to consider them? If, as evolutionists will still argue, cellular proliferation was meant to make an organism more adaptive, we are still faced with the fact that an infinite immunological repertoire does not actually guarantee better environmental performance than a limited one. Even though we assure ourselves that it should, and that diversity is always and everywhere "good," there is no evidence to suggest that organisms with larger repertoires fare any better when facing their pathogens. This is no small problem to be easily dismissed, and there is no avoiding the fact that repertoire size can only be made sense of "embryologically"—that is, by a full account of the *ambient domain of reciprocal difference.*

TRANSFORMATION

It is difficult to imagine that each of us began life as a single cell about the size of the period at the end of this sentence. —Neil Campbell, *Biology*

In 1955–56 C. G. Jung published his *Mysterium Coniunctionis*, a study of gender opposition in alchemy and, in particular, an examination of the *Rosarium Philosophorum*, an obscure but extraordinary alchemical text. Over the centuries, this text inspired alchemists to attempt the apparently impossible merging of opposites; more recently it has been revivified through Jung's attempt to identify "the undiscovered self." In a way, the alchemists were the first immunologists, at least in the sense that they were determined to understand the process of organic transformation, while at the same time never abandoning Aristotle's desire to understand how "what makes [the world] *one* will also be what makes a man" (Clark 1975, 47).

What is so extraordinary about the complex symbolism of the *Rosarium Philosophorum* is the degree to which it faithfully adheres to what anthropologists have learned about human change from the study of other cultures. Specifically, what we see embodied in the *Rosarium* is an understanding of human change that, despite the esoteric nature of the images themselves, embodies an awareness that transcends culture. This transcendent function can be readily demonstrated by the degree to which these images both conform to what anthropologists have observed about rites of passage worldwide and, concomitantly, by the extent to which this symbolism incorporates, and then leaves behind, the culture-specific orientation of contemporary depth psychology. For what we see is an understanding of change as a process of rebirth, a form of selective dissociation in which the framework of ritual provides a setting within which a repetition of a transformational process eventually results in a chance occurrence that allows something to become what it has never been before. Change, in other words, is a consequence of repeatedly cultivating ritual acts, accepting that a specific event may or may not carry a germ of change, recognizing the significance of a chance moment when it does occur, and allowing oneself to be dissolved by what it offers.

What anthropologists have learned about rites of passage throughout the world is astonishingly unequivocal—namely, that transformation is not a function of the fixation of identity through psychoanalysis and self-focus; rather, change takes place through mystery. True transformation, in other words, cannot be set out in advance; what appears to us to be the repetitive dysfunctionality of ritual is, in fact, a confirmation of this mystery. The ritual itself is an act of faith, a testament to the form that real change always adheres to. But the moment of actual transformation can never be known in advance; otherwise, what one becomes is only what one already is. This truth is vividly confirmed each and every time we participate in a ritual event; however, our electing to dissociate cannot guarantee that, as the Balinese say, "the god will actually descend." In scientific practice this reality is seen in bench science, where hypotheses and scientific research paradigms provide the context for "linguistic fluency." At the bench we become habituated to a certain language, a form of behavior that allows us to assimilate the "discovery" that always takes place while swimming in a lake, on a walk through the woods, or even while mundanely driving down the highway.

In the *Rosarium* version of the transformational process this dissociation is represented by the dissolution of opposites in the alchemical vessel. Here, in particular, the image identified as the "Descent into the Bath" represents how male and female, king and queen, submit themselves to a dissolution, a return to the womb—a merging of opposites in an original state in which "they are meliorated—softened—and rejoice as they dissolve" (Jung 1977, 56). Like dreams, this process of dissolution, of dissociation, of willful departure from an existing identity actually becomes the herald of transformation: "If destiny has put one in a time and place where the coniunctio is being manifested within a vessel of water, one must simply submit to it" (61). In the absence of that merging, we would only have self-sacrifice, or, worse yet, self-destruction.

But it is the merging itself that transforms human or cell death (apoptosis) into a creative and new kind of life.

Why, we may ask, is this event happening to a king and queen, and not, for instance, to Adam and Eve, or to the anonymous participants in a rite of passage whose nakedness is emblematic of the first step of transition (in which one sets aside the specific accoutrements by which one is daily defined)? The reason for the royal imagery is not that earthly privilege automatically connects one to the divine; quite the opposite in fact. The reason is that finding oneself in this transformational role is more than a function of privilege; it is a function of responsibility. As a homeless friend of mine once put it, "it's far easier for the people to go to the queen, than it is for the queen to go to the people." In gift exchange, in fact, the Queen Mother can never accept as her own those gifts presented to her when she goes to the people; for being "chosen" means that the invitation to embody the mystery of what will be created out of the transformational rite carries with it the responsibility to give back much more than has been given.

Being divinely "chosen," in other words, is at once extremely beautiful and highly demanding. Both king and queen know, as we ourselves know when we feel singled out by destiny, that if mutuality "has put one in a time and place where the coniunctio is being manifested," one cannot simply take what one wants and leave. This does not mean that king and queen are without choice; it means that they have been made aware of what they can do for the world, and that this awareness is profound.

VACCINOLOGY: A SOCIAL PARABLE

Fundamentally, we are called to choose between a memory that justifies and privileges domination, oppression, and exploitation and one that exalts and affirms reciprocity, community, and mutuality. —bell hooks, *Outlaw Culture*

In 1938 Margaret Mead and Gregory Bateson shot the footage for *Trance and Dance in Bali.* The film, completed in 1952, illustrates the epic conflict between the female witch, Rangda, and the male dragon, Barong, a battle representing the eternal struggle between good and evil. In 1952 this film stood as an important example of Mead's work on gender. Her tireless lecturing, her unusual lifestyle, and, above all, her many popular articles (especially in *Redbook*) made her into a well-known figure in American culture, despite the fact that she had been professionally ostracized by a male-dominated academic anthropology.

The exigencies of fieldwork, and the complexity and cost of producing films in tropical Southeast Asia in 1938, required that the film be choreographed to a degree that would today be unacceptable in an anthropological study. The trance dance had to be orchestrated specifically for filming, and, because Mead was interested in gender issues, it was necessary to arrange the trance dance so that women too (actually predominantly women) would go into trance. Though there is no prohibition on women attacking the witch, Rangda, going into trance, or in turning their swords on themselves, it is not a common occurrence, in part because Rangda is herself understood as an embodiment of feminine power but also because in Bali gender relations are less characterized by inequality than by what anthropologists call "dual inequality"—that is, a reciprocal inequality characterized by separate, and mutually exclusive, domains of authority. In order for the trance to succeed, it must balance the male and female, the earthly and the magical, the spoken and unspoken, the public and the private, the white and black, the so-called "right-" and "left-handed" paths. Rangda, in other words, is not a witch because she is a woman; she is a witch because the most extraordinary forms of non-earthly power have settled within her in a topsy-turvy way.

Mead's depiction of women doing, in other words, what men *usually* (though not always) do was meant to suggest to her Western skeptics that gender roles in other cultures were often reversed and that what women and men do in a society is a matter of culture rather than biology. Her tireless efforts in this regard led many to think that she did more for the popularization of women's issues that any other American of her generation. Some even regard her as *the* major postwar catalyst of the women's movement.

However, the supreme irony of *Trance and Dance in Bali* is less to be found in its effect on the way we think than in the degree to which it defined women's issues in terms of men's roles and, more significantly, in the degree to which this reworking of a non-Western ritual was at odds with its indigenous meaning. For what actually takes place in the ritual is that the human ego gives up its own heroic preoccupations and becomes a vehicle of a superhuman force; for in Bali, those who go into trance are not particularly respected for their valor. This fact is nowhere so clear as in the Balinese belief that to be hurt by one's sword is not the sign of one's actual involvement with the trance but an indication of one's disingenuous participation. To place women in the role of men, in other words, is to have missed entirely the most important bit of information—namely, the fact that the one in trance is the vehicle for an unearthly power, a power that is situationally negotiated.[1]

The trance performance is thus "embryological" in that individual identity must give way enough to allow for social negotiations with forces residing at the peripheries of the world of humans. It is therefore less important who goes into trance than how that trance is manipulated and understood socially. In Bali, *the opposite of an ego-oriented, male agent is not a female hero but no hero at all.* One need only watch the many hands of bystanders who assist the one in trance (directing, offering weapons, encouraging, fearing) to see that the true embryological view is predicated upon not gender but reciprocity—a reciprocity that takes place at the periphery of a group. Here, it is the embryo of *culture* that is replicated, not the egos of the "fittest," for those most active in the battle survive not by their personal powers alone but by the activation of those powers in a social setting in which shared values give those actions meaning. Here, equality is not a concept defined solely through "sameness." Egos exist, but they are ultimately humbled. Reciprocity is central, but it has little to do with what we would call equality; for entropy prevails when replication takes place without a genuine engagement of difference. Without radical difference no energy, no heat, is conveyed.

Biology provides a number of interesting examples of how real difference—especially real temperature difference—is enlightening. In fact, the famous Harvard medical theorist Walter Cannon described way back in the 1930s what he identified as a kind of "cerebral thermodynamics." His words, from *The Wisdom of the Body*, are still compelling:

> As we survey the arrangements which check a shift of body temperature in one direction or the other it is interesting to observe that there are successive defenses which are set up against the shift. If dilation of the skin vessels does not stop the rise of body temperature, sweating and even panting supervene. If conservation of heat by constriction of the skin vessels does not prevent a fall of temperature, there is a chemical stimulation of more rapid burning in the body by means of secreted adrenin, and if that in turn is not adequate to protect the internal environment from cooling, greater heat production by shivering is resorted to. [Studies have shown that] shivering itself has its most complete expression when that part of the brain, the diencephalon, which is the coordinating center for the sympathetic system, is intact. . . . We must recognize that

among civilized people the physiological devices for the maintenance of constant temperature may have little opportunity to function. (1932, 198)

For Cannon, the presence of central heating, warm clothing, and the absence of a stress that "inoculates" and conditions may be responsible for the biological inability to respond effectively to changes in the environment—why, that is, people are always troubled by the dysfunctioning of the "immune system" every time it rains or the weather changes. Biological stress, like social stress, is as much instructive as it may be debilitating.

Extending this perspective to the domain of cell-cell relations, one easily sees that the modern notion of equality, as a form of politically correct mock-diversity, actually enhances entropy rather than growth. To say, for instance, that fertilization is "the process by which egg and sperm find each other and fuse," or to describe fertilization in the language of equal opportunity (Keller 1995, xii) is merely to ignore the fact that millions of sperm die in their attempt to fertilize one egg. Traditionally, of course, these sperm would be defined in aggressive, heroic, "fittest" terms. Yet the most accurate model for representing this union symbolically is something much more like a Balinese trance performance: many egos attempt to fuse with divine power; the success of society depends upon pushing those egos to the limits of what can be known *and*, at the same time, limiting their heroic canonization. The Balinese model is, in other words, explicitly *antiheroic*, and its antiheroism makes it much truer to what we know scientifically than any of the models we have devised; for in it there is no conflict between entropy and replication, or speciation and survival, or individual and society.

But why should this view be called "antiheroic"? Because it allows us to recognize the millions of sperm that could have, but did not, fertilize the single female egg. For Cartesians, the cell colony is, and can always only be, its center—a place where "winners" undynamically congratulate themselves, where, to use the political metaphor, the complacent, the unimaginative (the entropic) devolve into smaller and smaller, and dumber and dumber, collectives. This is why even our most reactionary politicians now speak out in favor of biodiversity, for they have sensed that the slowdown has left them sterile. It is not that they are concerned with how relatively dynamic some cells have become at the peripheries of the colony (where, though the fatality rates approach terrifying proportions, the only possibility for real change resides). It is, rather, that they cannot tolerate the notion that those who try sometimes do not win.

The thesis now is quite clear: *the dullest survive and replicate into entropy; the most active often do not survive, but they are the transformers.* An identity that is embryologic, therefore—one where the socially negotiated sum is greater than its parts—is the only creative response to the slowing down and dying that is the sign of entropy. Otherwise, life produces only a cloned form of replication, an entropic kind of diversity in which each individual is a less diverse code of its predecessor—like a video tape which is copied over and over, the cloned gene loses its clarity, its vitality, and its "meaning." So, what happens when we apply this Balinese model to a scientific problem?

First, for the Balinese there can be no shift from an agent-oriented view of genes to a network model in which egos become meaningless. In fact, society *is only* meaningful if we understand it to be occupied by lots of microentities—male or female—with very large egos that must be, as it were, "vaccinated." Thus, a system that recognizes the relationship between creativity and a balancing of a kind of power that creates through imbalance requires by definition a focus on the environment in which relations are negotiated. "Sameness," left to itself, can only result in entropy. And egoism—traditional "male" power—is not limited simply by not invoking it; in fact the opposite may apply, since, as we have witnessed with Balinese magic, active suppression can often *increase* the power of the thing suppressed.[2] In this view, shifting our focus from the ego to the network does not in and of itself mean that we are actually embracing a new vision of anything; for one might merely be turning over the coin without assessing its denomination, its value, or the rate of exchange by which it is conveyed.

Second, for the Balinese, seeing cell activity as part of a nebulous network does not in itself enable us to transcend the ideas of fame and progress that come from traditional, historical concepts of heroism—i.e., we aren't actually abandoning our traditional male heroes by promoting hysterical networks of power; we're only saying that we don't know what the egos of fraudulent networkers are up to. We've only abandoned the idea that there can be a continuity between individual action and social good.

Third, and perhaps most damaging, is the extent to which, for the Balinese, the model of the "selfish gene" only promotes the *illusion of change* without effecting any real transformation. In Bali, an individual who is harmed in trance is said to be *too* egocentric because in being hurt he calls attention to himself—his wound being punishment for engaging in a dangerous encounter without the protection of a god. As we argue for the selfish and fraudulent nature of networks of power, so too do we deemphasize our ability both to understand the consequences of human action and to construct rituals that realign the powers of particular agents. We both undervalue and undermine, that is, our understanding of change as a compounding of the creative forces of collective marginality. Merely to recognize and actively suppress a selfish ego will only leave that ego either more or less powerful. It cannot, in itself, actually generate or create a completely different locus of agency. Realizing the utility of what Jung would have called the collective unconscious allows us, then, to acknowledge how selective dissociation is creatively managed in public ritual, and how such ego-transcending practices can be employed to evade entropy.

Fourth, and finally, is what for the Balinese would be the helplessness, the unacceptable nihilism, of the networker's view of embodiment. For while networkers accept that there are relations that should be mapped, they also accept that there are *too many relations to map*, that *no map is reliable*, and that *the experience of them cannot be embodied microcosmically in any of us*. For "network" read "immune system." For the sake of creative life, the end of both must be near.

CREATIVITY

La réunion des deux poisons est plus efficace. —Claude Bernard

A few years ago, while attending a conference on the future of immunology at the former home of the great pathologist Claude Bernard, I had the privilege of seeing on display the very curare arrows that Bernard obtained in 1844, the arrows from which he would extract the poison that one day would form the basis of surgical anesthesiology (Napier 2002). Wanting more information, I inquired about what else was known of these arrows.

On the following day, I was presented with Bernard's own copy of his *La Science expérimental*, published in 1878, the year of his death. In addition to an engraving of the arrows and a discussion of curare, I discovered, hidden in the pages of this book and written in Bernard's own hand, the epigraph offered above. In combining his curare samples (he had, by then, acquired others which are also in the museum), Bernard knew that the potency of the poison/remedy could actually be increased. What he meant, of course, was not only

that the poisons are deadly, but that joining of the two powers was more efficacious. We know this, first, because the true conjunction of two things creates a third thing that is greater than the sum of the two—that is, that life
continues, despite the forces of entropy, when the power of opposites is orchestrated productively (the greater the opposition, the more significant that
which is created).

Asclepius, the first Greek healer (*pharmakon*), learned his art from the centaur Chiron—half horse, half man, both wild and wise. And his most powerful of medicines was that made from the blood of the monstrous and terrifying
Gorgon: "What flowed from her left side he [Asclepius] used for the perdition
of mankind; while what flowed from her right he used for their salvation, and
by that means he raised the dead" (Apollodorus *Library* 3.10.3). In fact, there
is here enough of an intrinsic ambivalence to allow for this relationship to be
both dual and reciprocal, even to the degree that "the poison, the forbidden
thing, is at the same time the remedy" (Meier 1989, 100). Such was the oracle
of Apollo: "whatever wounds heals" (*ho trosas iasetai*). This does not mean that
wounding is a form of healing; it means that there is a sympathy (*sympatheia*)
of which the symptom is an expression of some homeopathic imbalance. This
kind of creation—through the distinguishing and then the merging of opposites—was always well known.

For the Greeks, then, sympathy and symptom were alike, since the *symp-
toma* involved a coincidence, a mutuality of two persons thinking or dreaming
in a like mind. "Synchronicity and identity between the dreams of two persons
. . . were always felt as having a healing effect" (ibid., 93). Sympathy allows the
symptom to be shared. It is what alchemically transforms sublimation into
something sublime. This is how for the alchemist a psychic substance gets
created "that has a nontemporal or eternal dimension to it, a kind of incor-
ruptibility" (Edinger 1994, 97): "Sublimation is an upward movement from
below. It refers to a chemical event in which, if certain substances are heated
. . . they vaporize and then condense or crystallize on the cooler portions of
the vessel; that is called sublimation or sublimatio." And this is also, of course,
how an illness is "cured"—that is, creatively reconfigured so that the subliminal, the "flaw," is transformed, as the great Baroque artist Bernini once put it,
into the sublime—"to make use of a defect in such a way that if it had not existed one would have [had] to invent it" (Baldinucci [1682] 1966 [see Napier
1992, 125]).

This is also precisely the role of novel cells: they are only generators of flaws if they fail to transform an "odd" mutation into the essential focus of something new. The question of whether any of the multiple B- or T-cells the body produces are superfluous aberrations or essential adaptations cannot be known in advance. This is critical not only in coming to terms with so-called natural selection—with the degree to which we falsely rely on teleological explanations in immunological evolution, but more directly here in realizing the undeniable and necessary uncertainty of creativity.

Why, we may ask, are such realizations important? As one immunologist put it to me: "Let's say I accept what you're saying; what am I to do, give up bench science?" Where, in other words, is the middle ground, the way forward? Well, to answer this we must confront how the very essence of what destabilizes can itself become a creative catalyst—how what appears to be a critical flaw (the generator of illness and organic or psychological destruction) gets transformed into a creative power. But how—especially in today's increasingly polarized intellectual climate of self and other—can we transcend the relentless pressures of existing networks of power at least enough to allow the moment to be generated in which the fertilization of self and other can have its day to produce the new third thing that is so essential for the continuation of social, of biological, and of emotional life?

The metaphors of alchemy provide one answer, if only because they will not allow us to see power in but one way; they will not allow us to forget its essential ambivalence. They give no space for the dangerous separation and polarization of opposite worlds, where that disjunction of self and other produces, by alienating us from knowledge of the pathogen, a yet more destructive form of autoimmunity. So, one central problem for bench science is that the very specificity of what makes for good research practice may actually reinforce the self/nonself paradigm of immunology in ways that are not productive. Conversely, research practice may make the very idea of transcending the simple model of self and nonself, of host and alien, difficult. Actually, it makes this impossible.

Networks are not only a problem for understanding the creative ambivalence of power; they also pose real problems for cognition. Inquiring as to why "the classical neural network model [of the human brain] does not provide a resolution to the question of binding of patterns," Kak, for instance, calls attention to the problem of interpreting the world as objective knowledge "a convergence of the worlds of the physical, the mental, and the mathematical" (1996, 186). Kak points out the limitations that are placed upon what we can know by a view of knowledge that so much depends on a "physical world which generates the mental picture which, in turn, creates the scientific theory" (190).

Yet we know that such distinctions between the physical, mental, and mathematical are largely artificial: when my late grandfather first introduced me to Napier's Bones, I was unaware (until I later used them) that Napier's mathematical calculating object was itself now a part of the physical world—what made his discovery revolutionary for navigation (and, hence, the building of a maritime empire) was the fact that the mathematical model became physical. His mechanical discovery, in other words, significantly modified the physical activity of calculating at sea; the discovery became an essential part of the experience it shaped. Only when one *employs* his series of Bones does one realize that a physical pattern obtains among diagonal relations *across* fields of related forms (see chapter 4).

The chances of real discovery, therefore, are limited not so much by any absence of intuitive understanding about invention as they are by what we value at the bench. Experimental science is extremely unwilling to introduce outside perspectives that might actually provide the kind of unlikely superimpositions that we know are crucial to real discovery (Rothenberg 1988, 176; Napier 1992, 190–99). And there are examples much closer to bench immunology—curiously also from the field of mathematics. In 1967, J. S. Griffin, a London mathematician, was the first to show—and through math and logic rather than bench science—that proteins could in all likelihood self-replicate (Rhodes 1997, 125). Griffin's landmark suggestion not only "provided a mechanism that might account for scrapie strains as mutations in the gene that coded for the host protein," but it transformed how proteins would come to be conceptualized in a number of slow viruses. Indeed, the very path of research on scrapie and BSE (mad cow disease) would have been unlikely without the initial perception on the part of an anthropologist, Shirley Lindenbaum, that there was a connection in New Guinea between the brain disease (*kuru*), and the practice of endocannibalism (ibid., 75–77).

However, most of modern science is built upon the artifice of *experiment*, rather than *experience*, even though what Schrödinger and Heisenberg intuitively understood in the discovery of wave mechanics was that the universe was made up of superimposed and inseparable levels of activity, that creativity is the outcome of superimposition, and that the particular is always contained in (and cannot be identified outside of) the universal (Kak 1996; Schrödinger

[1925] 1961). To give measure to the particular, in other words, we must have some sense of what it is a part of. And how one does this is by examining the ways that diverse, superimposed elements might be related. The research on creativity is quite unequivocal on this matter (Rothenberg 1988). Studies repeatedly demonstrate not only the importance of dissociation in creative discovery (the way that inventions occur spontaneously while dreaming, or walking, or driving a car), but they also emphasize the need to superimpose apparently unlikely elements—to see patterns or analogies in places where others find disjunction.

This awareness—that change is made possible by recognizing patterns through psychological dissociation—is today much more important than ever before because the rules of modern life actively discourage, and at times even prohibit, what we call "daydreaming." Perhaps nowhere is this so clear as in the scientific tendency to label arbitrarily everything, to inscribe, as Latour says, anything and everything on the window of an instrument. Harmless though this behavior may seem, it is precisely the cause of the absence of creative thinkers. While Americans can tell you at least one thing invented by Edison, and even that Einstein was at least some kind of genius, most would be hard pressed to name a single recipient of a Nobel prize in science in the last decade. Is this only because what has been discovered is too complex to know? I doubt it; for the mystification of laboratory life has not only encouraged scientists to be unaccountable to the uninitiated, but has deified the scientific fact, making a fetish out of almost any scientific inscription. The generation of a scientific fact-as-fetish—what Latour calls a "factish"[3]—becomes, then, an end in itself. With the scientist locked up in his laboratory like some medieval monk, it becomes easy for the bench researcher and his admirers to forget how essential social life actually is to creative growth. Denied a meaning that is born out of the kinds of daily dissociations that characterize everyday encounters, the scientific artifact can survive under any arbitrary aegis or label.

But this modern form of social consensus—where naming the unknown replaces the quest for knowing something deeply—is not, one must emphasize, universally valued. Indeed, resisting labels can in some social settings be understood creatively, as when a Balinese individual hesitates to label another's illness prematurely because the right "demon" has yet to show its face. Here, rather than place an arbitrary label on the unknown, one suspends early closure by withholding a name—that is, one awaits the social placement of the sufferer's "problem," at which time the illness will be acknowledged. Then, and only then, will we have the privilege of putting a *proper* name to that sufferer's experience. *The social event that defines the transformation becomes the scene for naming the pathology*, not the other way around. If someone speaks in voices, in other words, don't jump to the conclusion that you are witnessing some multiple personality disorder—especially if what you hope eventually to understand is the way in which the overt evidence of that individual's behavior relates to the collective setting in which a good and proper name can one day be attached to the transformation he so desperately seeks. Don't name this thing prematurely—though having a name to give something that is convincing and novel may get you a major prize, in the long run it will not survive (nor will you) unless that label resonates deeply at other cultural levels.

In science, this premature naming is everyday habit, and is most obvious in the unsubtle ignoring of anything the function of which is not obvious. A good genetic example, here, are *retrotransposons*, nuceotide sequences having no known function that transpose themselves via reverse transcription throughout the genomic DNA and constitute more than 10 percent of the human genome. Although they appear to insert themselves arbitrarily, their "randomness" might also function anti-entropically—that is to say, they may prove algorithmically to be the basis of a *creative* activity—because they continually resequence genetic information. Like Napier's Bones, then, the problem with sequencing or mapping the genome is that sequencing on its own will not cause one to look at a research domain differently; but seeing a mutuality emerge across different sequential domains—say, across Balinese spirits and T-cells, or across alchemy and immunology—may provide a catalyst for some genuinely creative idea.

So, to get to the particular, one needs to transcend columns to find some universal; then one needs to *begin* with some universal in order that the particular become identified by means of a binding cognitive shape—a category—that will eventually reunite that particular thing with something more systemic, even more mystical. Here is the problem of immunology's specificity in, as it were, a nutshell; immunology begins with the specific cellular interaction while ignoring the interrelations because we assume that complex relations cannot themselves be experimentally replicated.

Who, after all, takes as experimentally feasible the examination of what pathologies an illness may immunize one against? What illnesses does a cohort of similarly unwell individuals *not* suffer from?

These are not abstract questions, because we already know that clinical therapies are not always and everywhere specific. "In developing chemical agents for the treatment of malaria," for instance, "little thought is really given to the advantages and disadvantages of concentrating exclusively upon agents which are selectively toxic to the parasite in contrast to agents which are able to reverse the pathological effects of the disease, without necessarily eliminating the causative organism" (Kirby 1997, 9). The best experimental proof of the systematization of a pathology, in other words, is not to be found in the futile attempt to reconstruct complex and subtle relations at the bench; rather, the best proof may be provided through observing the way in which one complex set of relations creates a state in which another complex set of relations ceases to function, either due to the toxicity of one with respect to the other, or due to the ability of one to reverse the pathological effects of the other without necessarily eliminating it—like the plasmodistatic (as opposed to plasmodicidal) compounds that may relieve symptoms or reverse the effects of malaria among indigenous peoples without necessarily killing the parasite; or, in immunology, rather (to extend this metaphorically) like a retrovirus on a grand scale: creating enormous diversity by incorporating that which is foreign into cells by substituting foreign genes for essential virus genes.

And what do we mean by "foreign" anyway if, as is entirely likely, the nucleic acids of viruses evolve from normal cell genes (for, otherwise, binding would be a very untidy thing)? That rheumatoid arthritis could be treated with a protein derived from bubonic plague provides one wonderful example of such mutuality (Coghlan 1998). But to make matters more complex, it is also possible that some such former "selves" and former "other-selves" may not be subject to evolution at all, no matter how stable or unstable those viruses may be in a laboratory environment. The discovery of a common plant pathogen called tomato mosaic virus (ToMV) in the Greenland icepack not only aroused fears that ancient strains of other pathogens might be released by global warming, but it also challenged the view that life is a continuous struggle in which novel "nonselves" are met by new hybrids of "self": for the viruses

> put a spanner in the works of viral evolution studies, [because] instead of representing the endpoint of steady evolution, modern populations of viruses might

be a complex mishmash of highly evolved ones and others that have taken a holiday from evolution in cold storage. Perhaps there are actually ancient populations that have been recycled over and over again. . . . How can you do evolutionary studies if that's true? (Walker 1999, 4)

In this view, ancient populations are being recycled side-by-side with ever-changing new ones in such a way that development is far from unilinear—much the way RNA comes back to redefine the germline in the form of retro-transcriptase, the enzyme that reconfigures DNA in retroviruses such as HIV.

The self/nonself model is thus further challenged, since at least in one important sense the elimination of nonself may also be described as a denial of self. To begin with the environmental—indeed, the universal—is not only to acknowledge what Hindus mean by their great phrase *tat tvam asi* ("That art Thou"), but also to understand how they are capable of seeing the "self" both as another and as an overarching idea—not a mere separable person, but a microcosm of the "systemic." This is also why a projection of the universal force, or *brahma*, constitutes for Hindus the most complete form of happiness, why "artful" deeds become central ways of achieving the divine, why giving up, giving away, something (finding a way to distinguish the universal in what is given) allows one to enjoy a world that is connected to experience through the senses—to see, via connectedness (via *rasa* or feeling), the presence of the divine in one's opposite wave. Such a recursion can be evidenced in a broad range of coherent metaphors about attraction, as we can see, for instance, in the analogy of love and antibody that was utilized long ago by Freud's disciple, Groddek. Here, love "is no more than the need to enter into and remain in a relationship with the one who holds the key to our thoughts. . . . Love comes into being like an antibody, in order to neutralize the virus of terror" (Roustang 1982, 124). No doubt the rise of the age of immunology is a true sign that the virus of terror is, indeed, ascending.

SOLUTIO

Our dissolving water which is familiar and friendly . . . —alchemical invocation

In the previous discussion we observed how the absence of sympathic concerns in scientific practice can give way to research strategies that are wanting if not inappropriate, and how the absence of superimposition results in forms of science that are themselves disconnected from the very world they would otherwise hope to explain. Taking the next step, one might now ask how much scientific autonomy and the scientist's sense of self-importance influence the nature of scientific theory. Was Niels Jerne's notion of an autonomous and hierarchical immune system influenced by his private belief that he was destined to be above the common man? Were Sir Peter Medawar's views on immunological intolerance influenced by his own intolerance for the uneducated and his known disdain for anything that did not live up to his standards of scientific verifiability?[4] Can one's sense of superiority itself lead to theoretical constructs that are not only socially disconnected but unnecessarily hierarchical?

Conversely, does attending to the social setting of one's scientific research program give way to socially integrated forms of discovery? The correlation is tempting to consider. Jenner, for instance, is widely acknowledged as the father of vaccinology, yet he "discovered" something already commonly recognized by milkmaids. In this sense, he was more the father of British medical anthropology than of a particular experimental science. Indeed, that Jenner carried with him throughout his life a private respect for social forms of knowledge is clear: he never, for instance, gave up the wampum—and, at times, proudly wore the belt—sent to him by the Chiefs of the Five Nations of the North American Indians in appreciation of his vaccine for smallpox. "Brother," their letter of appreciation began,

> Our Father has delivered to us the book you sent to instruct us how to use the discovery which the Great Spirit made to you whereby the smallpox, that fatal enemy of our tribe, may be driven from the earth. . . . We sent with this a belt and a string of wampum in token of our appreciation of your precious gift. (quoted in Oldstone 1998, 41)

Were only we so humble as to honor the anonymous Amazonian who gave us curare. But to do that would have involved *wanting* to engage that person.

No doubt one of the least attractive aspects of the Age of Immunology is the way in which we are denied, and in turn deny ourselves, the experience of being entirely open about our emotional lives and needs. Unhindered by that sort of oppressively artificial world in which networkers cautiously expose any empathic expression that may be known as theirs alone, the sentiment of the chiefs of the Five Nations made possible a powerful superimposition that Jenner valued deeply. Does, then, the absence of reciprocity that is so deeply a part of immunology's elimination of nonself actually eliminate by definition a creative response of "self" to "other"? If so, can the heady arrogance of modern science be itself ameliorated by a creative solution ("solutio") in which the alchemical merging of self and other within the bath of holy water replaces something alienated with something newly created—where the combination of self and nonself leads to the creation of something new that is greater than its parts? Is not, then, the resolution of entropy implicit from ancient times in the dissolving risk required for generating a new, living thing?

How far have we removed ourselves from this quest for the Holy Grail of creative awareness? If anything, it seems today that the attempt to eliminate "nonself" has denied us the knowledge that risk is not only dangerous but the essential precondition for creativity itself. Yet there is also a moral in that same legend that should not be forgotten; for despite his ignorance of the ways of the world, Parzival eventually did find his way to the creative act through which he and Conduiramurs were physically and spiritually united, a "solution" in which two opposites became one.

Just as the basic paradigm of immunology is intrinsically destructive, so too is its antidote creative, and even procreative. "Nonself" (or "other's self," or "nonesuch self") is, indeed, the antibody of love that comes into being through mutuality—not only in order to neutralize the virus of terror, but also to recognize and reunite with an antigenic "self" with which it might create something completely new: "La réunion des deux . . . est plus efficace"; this is why "nonself" ought more rightly to be called "other's self"—that is, an expression of another's identity that becomes a reflection of something shared, a mutuality. To call another's self a "nonself" is inaccurate. "Other" is not a "nonself"; it is quite clearly a different "self"—one in whose image we see ourselves.

To describe otherness in such terms is not so metaphysically wanting, then, as it may first appear; for nowhere is the dissolution of self and other more clearly rendered than in the very structure of the antibody. In order for binding to take place, an "other" must be recognized as an extension or reflection of an existing identity, which itself is defined by the dissolution of a binary opposition.

A simple examination of the structure of an antibody will illustrate just how wanting the Cartesian self/nonself model is (figure 19). Here we see it as a Y-shaped molecule having a body or "leg" and two antigen-binding sites, or

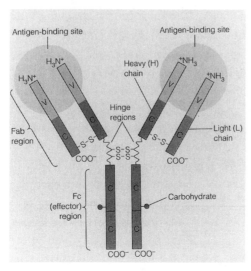

FIGURE 19. **The Antibody Molecule**
The antibody is a Y-shaped molecule having a body or "leg" and two antigen-binding sites, or "arms." In this model it is clear that the binding site is less "self" than it is a *self's creation of otherness*, its construction of difference; for each arm is a site of change, a locus of transformation, a vehicle for transforming variability into a thing which is constant. (From Becker, Reece, and Poenie 1996, fig. 24.9, p. 796. Copyright © 1986, 1991, 1996 by The Benjamin/Cummings Publishing Company, Inc. Reprinted by permission of Pearson Education, Inc.)

"arms." These antigen-binding sites constitute the *variable* domain of the immunological repertoire—the highly diversified field presented to antigens. To this variable domain is attached the single constant domain, the molecule's effector site, where the antigen, once attached, is interacted with. In this model it is clear that the binding site is less "self" than it is a *self's creation of otherness*, its construction of difference; for each arm is a site of change, a locus of transformation, a vehicle for commitment—for transforming variability into a thing which is constant. To accomplish the dual goals of binding and assimilating, each arm is variable at its binding end and constant at effector-site end: each arm, in other words, has an identical heavy chain and an identical light chain that are variable where they bind and constant where they connect to their effector. Each binding site of the molecule is, additionally, dual rather than singular, for it embodies the interactive potential of what the molecule might become—less "self" than "self-image," less person than persona, less "nonself" than, as it were, "nonesuch self."

Each antibody is, therefore, structured to perform two functions. The first function is to recognize the antigen and to bind to it. Second, the antibody reacts. Though this second function is traditionally thought of as an act of *disposal*, it may equally be described as an act of *assimilation*, or of *embodiment*, or of any of the other less common metaphors that might otherwise be applied to engulfment. Indeed, assimilation is not only a more constructive metaphor for defining this process but a more accurate one, since the interaction of antibody and antigen results in a genuine transformation.

Thus, structurally at least, an antibody molecule may be visualized as two pairs of polypeptide chains, each having two arms that consist of an identical light and heavy chain.[5] In fact, this same ability to structure a binary opposition is reflected most dramatically in research on the extraordinary diversity of the antibody repertoire, which may produce as many as 10^8 to 10^9 different molecules that can respond to almost any antigen an organism will ever encounter; for the DNA sequences that encode these molecules exist broadly across the genome and are brought together quite remarkably across what might only be described as vast oceans of DNA. Viewed this way, it is not so much that the body can create an antibody that can respond to any antigen the body encounters, but that the encounter takes place because the antibody brings life to the otherwise inert virus; for the virus will never become an antigen, in other words, if the antibody does not bring life to it.

While the model provided in figure 19 conforms to what is structurally understood about the antibody, it only begins to suggest the beauty and symmetry of the molecule (figure 20). For the molecule itself displays none of the compartmentalization of the structural model. Indeed, what we see is an interlocking of two symmetrical patterns that divide the molecule not by its two functions but by its right and left side. Like two number 9s facing back to back with their tails intertwined, the antibody's constant section is actually comprised of the merging of its binary opposition. Its constant "self," that is, is composed of the merging through a central carbohydrate, of its opposite halves, while its "other," as it were, is expressed in the individuality, the separateness, of its opposite binding sites. What this tells us is quite important:

First, it indicates that its constancy is a function of the merging of opposites, their bonding and individual dissolution, as it were. The constancy is a function of merging. Opposites attract and like dissolves like.

Second, it indicates that the specificity—the uniqueness, the individuality—of the molecule derives from its own representation of what is beyond itself.

Third, it indicates that the antibody is less a representation of a Cartesian "self" than it is the body's best attempt to construct a creative mechanism for revitalizing the nucleic acids of the normal cell from which both it and its inducing antigen once derived.

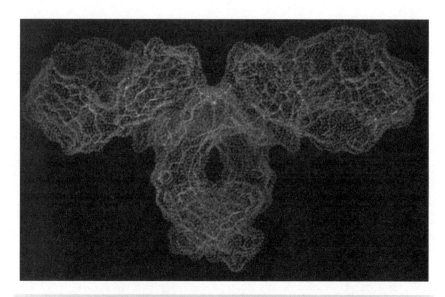

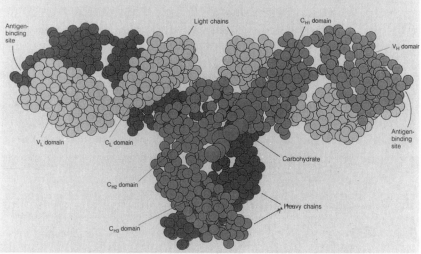

FIGURE 20. **The Symmetry of the Immunoglobulin Molecule**
The structural beauty and symmetry of the antibody molecule are here seen in the immunoglobulin (IgG) as an interlocking of two symmetrical patterns that divide the molecule, not by its two functions, but by its right and left sides. Here, the "self" is reflected in the merging of opposite halves, while the "other," so to speak, is manifested in the molecule's separate and opposite binding sites. (*Top:* Computer graphic image courtesy of Arthur J. Olson, The Scripps Research Institute, © 1986. *Bottom:* Reproduced courtesy of David R. Davies.)

If these conclusions are accurate, they should be reflected in what is now known of antigen/antibody relations, and they should also allow us to employ them in addressing the major conundra of contemporary immunology. It is to the scientific nature of the immunological "self," therefore, that our final analytical discussion should now turn.

undiscovered selves

Tat tvam asi ("That art Thou")

ILLOGICAL SELF

In 1960 the Nobel Committee awarded its prize in medicine to F. Macfarlane Burnet and Peter B. Medawar for their groundbreaking work on immunity and the role of "self" and "nonself" in both maintaining and destroying organic integrity. Medawar's ideas about acquired immunologic tolerance developed out of his demonstration that mice could "learn" to accept foreign tissue if injected with allogenic bone marrow at or before birth; Burnet's contribution was predicated on the body's production of antibodies that recognized foreignness (i.e., "not-self") but, in so doing, did not recognize "self." Their work not only defined for several decades the field of immunology but also became the basis for much of what we understand today about transplantation biology.

In the decades that followed, several complex theoretical models were developed in this rapidly growing field. Most important of these were the systemic network theory of Niels Jerne (there was, one must recall, no network of the "immune system" in the literature before the late 1960s), and the associative recognition theory of Melvin Cohn, which contested Jerne's network on the basis of both its lack of antigen-specific responsiveness and its broad experimental unverifiability (Napier 1996). This need for a systemic explanation was historically decisive: it helped account for the ideas of immunologic "memory" and the logarithmic rate of antibody formation. This it did by arguing that a random diversification of gamma globulin molecules could quickly replicate once they had bound to an injected antigen. Though Jerne's gamma globulins were soon replaced by the diversified cell theories of Talmage and Burnet (in which antibody production was stimulated by the interactions between antigens and cell-surface receptors), the idea of an immune "system" had now passed unchallenged into scientific discourse, making it virtually impossible to construct a viable theory that did not see survival in terms of the intolerance of "self" for "nonself." Indeed, Medawar and Burnet (and many of their colleagues who did not win Nobel Prizes [e.g., Fenner, Billingham, Brent]) had already implicitly codified the presence of this "system" by arguing the view that "the developing animal would be tricked into recognizing the substance as 'self'" (Nossal 1969, 99), if this event occurred before lymphoid maturation.

But despite early optimism about the role of self and nonself in understanding the nature of organic tolerance, the fundamental paradigm on which classical immunology stands or falls (the recognition and elimination of "nonself") has yet to facilitate any resolution of the field's major concerns—with autoimmunity, with transplantation, and with tumor immunology. Indeed, throughout the history of modern immunology the self/nonself model seems to have created so many intractable issues that many researchers think it ought simply to be put to rest (Tauber 1994). Most recently, Polly Matzinger has not only joined those immunologists who have made the case for revising the self/nonself nomenclature but has urged that it be replaced by a model of the immune system in which "danger" (that which damages cells and causes lytic death) induces dendritic cells to present antigens from damaged tissues to lymph nodes. In this view, the work of antigen-presenting cells (macrophages and dendritic cells) allows the immune system to become "aware," as it were, of impending damage. Indeed, Matzinger has recently taken the encouraging leap of suggesting that her model of danger may actually advance a less static notion of selfhood that does not by definition demand the elimination of the self/nonself dichotomy.[1]

While immunologists are not metaphysicians, one can readily see that this debate hinges on an idea about selfhood that is almost wholly unexamined, or if examined, blissfully uninformed by the diverse ways that philosophers—not to mention other cultural traditions—have constructed what we call "identity."[2] This lacuna is made glaringly obvious by the degree to which immunology has traditionally hinged on a recognition and elimination of biological difference, by the unsolved problems that self/nonself models have created, by the discipline's current attempts to jettison the self/nonself nomenclature, by the inability of immunologists to define "selfhood" in any novel way—in other words, by a wide array of problems all of which bear the scent of culturally tendentious parochial thinking.

At the same time, most arguments against the self are based upon the wonderful, and largely unrecognized, insight that *change* (i.e., transformation) is *the* core issue of contemporary immunology. The problem comes when immunologists place this observation against the background of a "self" that is only salient, persistent, and, in a word, "static." In such a view, because "we are constantly acquiring tolerance to our own proteins," we are changing in ways that are incommensurate with an inalienable kind of "self." Or, to put it more simply, "the self is constantly being defined anew—which is another way of saying that it doesn't really exist at all" (Richardson 1996, 86).

So, despite their apparent disinterest in metaphysics and other notions of identity, contemporary immunologists have (no doubt, rightly) identified "change" (i.e., transformation) as the core issue of immunology. The problem is, as we will see, that they have eliminated "self" because they are incapable of defining it or, at best, can only identify it tautologically as "not other."

RETHINKING THE UNTHINKABLE

Though most bench scientists would protest that such armchair speculating is a luxury they cannot afford, it is surely worth considering what might happen were immunologists to pause and consider the degree to which they are themselves (ideologically, theoretically, and practically) trapped by their allegiance to a particular cultural construction of "self." Could they benefit in any significant way from rethinking their assumptions about identity? Could a look across cultural and philosophical domains actually allow them to address more productively current issues in their field? Could, in fact, individuals raised with other cultural paradigms of the self actually be better positioned to take immunology out of its metaphysical doldrums and place it on a new ideological plateau? In what follows, I will argue not only that such an activity is productive but that it may even allow us to solve immunology's most vexing paradoxes.

What I have in mind here is the adoption of a more assimilative model of the self—one widely known in various forms in other times and across cultural boundaries. Indeed, though Maxwell's demon and the dendritic cell have allowed science to separate itself from God, they both actually adopt a way of thinking that has all of the trappings of another religious form—that one well known to anthropologists under the name of animism. This form of thinking—surprisingly like that of popular immunology—posits that the world is motivated by many forces that sometimes function independently, and that matter of any sort can be the conveyor of spiritual power. Look at any popular description of immunological invasion—indeed, read any medical school text on the subject—and you will get the picture precisely. In fact, as we have seen throughout this study, there is absolutely no difference whatsoever in the language of contemporary immunology and that of certain of the more animistic forms of Hinduism, or, say, the demonological constructs of the Middle Ages. The difficulty today is that most scientists would avoid the comparison, claiming instead that the descriptive language they use is a mere convenience, and a confusing one that is probably best avoided.

Thus, while immunologists use animistic language and modes of thinking on a daily basis, they deny the importance of this "primitive" religious form, saying that the language is only a device that makes possible the imperfect conceptualization of ideas that are in themselves very abstract; like anthropologists of the last century, and like modern Freudians, they even believe that the describing of cells as volitional agents is regressive—an indicator, that is, of not understanding what's really going on. So, rather than accepting what they say as in itself important, they in the end run from the self/nonself language that initially attracted them to the field. Instead, they deny the significance of their florid metaphorical vocabulary—in which cells recruit, mask, deceive, appropriate, and kill. The problem here is that in so doing they also fail, importantly, to understand how such metaphorical personifications (the kind that proliferate in animism) are the basis of their—in fact, of most—inventive thinking.

There is a broad literature (especially in psychology and in anthropology) that shows how much of what we call scientific discovery takes place in an imaginative domain in which projecting one's intentional self into an otherwise nonvolitional domain makes possible the discovery of some new relation or idea. We've already considered in this study some examples of how scientists make their most important discoveries by imagining themselves as a blood cell, a bit of tissue, or an organ. Isn't it time then to set aside the fear of being labeled unscientific, childlike, or regressive—time to acknowledge how genius always displays itself through the imaginative projection of intentions onto things that normally don't have them?

Why not encourage immunologists to follow the lead of other cultures and of contemporary information theorists who have little difficulty in conceptualizing experimental models of the self that rely on personification, and especially on the imaginative (i.e., "animistic") projection of intent (e.g., Kak 2002)?[3] How unfortunate, then, that immunologists do not recognize the animistic forms of thinking that are so essential to what they do, let alone express an interest in the history of those ideas that constitute the very essence of what they take as their knowledge. For something is being sensed, and whether that sensor is a "self" or a cell in some network matters less than the anthropomorphic projections that facilitated its discovery in the first place.

Denial, as the Alcoholics Anonymous slogan reminds us, is not a river in Egypt. Why not simply accept the fact that the best creative thoughts happen through animistic projection? Well, part of the answer is that swallowing the fact makes science much messier than our governments, our granting agencies, and our universities would like us to think. But the other, more serious problem is that such thinking also plays a major role in madness. What psychologists who study creative people realize is that creating is a psychologically risky business. Here, I am less referring to the large numbers of Nobel laureates who are clinically depressed than I am to the awareness that once you embark on the road of fantasy, you either discover the theory of relativity, or you end up as an outcast fixing shoes or stamping license plates. In short, not many people who value their status as members of the scientific establishment really want to discover badly enough that they are willing to take such risks.

And that's not the end of it; for the problem, alas, is further complicated by another part of the creative puzzle. This being that, in order to make any "regressive" idea work in a novel way, one needs to be successful at placing it in some new relationship between two things that had previously seemed unalike. The recipe, in other words, is as simple as it is, if not dangerous, at least potentially futile; for the majority of idle thinking is just that. Here, again, psychological research repeatedly demonstrates that the fantastic superimpositions of discovering minds either create things new and wonderful or things that are at best useless and at worst weird and maybe unhealthy.

If prospects didn't already seem hopeless enough, there's even a third problem: this being that the *dynamics of the creative act itself are entirely dependent on the successful superimposition of two unlike things that merge to create some novel outcome.* Just as stasis induces a fear of difference, so, too, does transformation depend upon risk and uncertainty. Successful engagement of difference induces amelioration—i.e., vaccinology, not immunology. That which is truly creative, in other words, *transforms* the organism. Though immunology is, for certain, an expression of life, it is life as combat rather than life as creation.

Why make so much of this? Part of the answer is that it's hard to appreciate things truly different when your immediate life is in chaos. The other answer is that anthropologists are often the worst enemies of anthropology; for traditional peoples themselves frequently talk of marrying their enemies or, for instance, about the powers of men and women as autonomous—that is, not unequal, but interdependent. It's not an idea that goes down well in a modern democracy, but it does illustrate a deep desire to take the ambivalent power that exists when hot meets cold (right meets left, black meets white, insider meets outsider) and turn it into a creative rather than a destructive experience.

Cold and hot induce the molecular activity of life. The problem is that when they are randomly brought together they also induce chaos and disorder—i.e., an expression of vitality whose lack of order eventually leads to its opposite: inactivity, decrease of motion, and the end of life as we know it. This is why the second law of thermodynamics is more important to immunology than is natural selection; for natural selection only has meaning in retrospect (where a confrontation with difference can be said with certainty to have been either destructive or positively conditioning), whereas thermodynamics asks *how* vitality (the expression of difference) is realized as a constructive or a destructive endeavor. An imbalance of difference is explosive; just enough of it moves the engines of creation quite beautifully.

Once we accept the degree to which creativity has been ignored—even suppressed—by modern immunology, we begin to see the logical problem with thinking that change indicates some threat to a self as something both prior and persistent; for the field is not at all designed to deal with creativity. And it is this covert suppression of creativity that makes it possible to build a hypothesis that is both illogical and philosophically unsound—this being the notion that the acquisition of tolerance to our own proteins (the constant redefining of the self) implies that the self either does not exist or that it is irrelevant to immunology. *However, no polytheist could ever accept this popular immunological notion, because defining the self anew is what its social role is.* A self is realized (i.e., recognized as living and therefore known) through its many *trans-*

formations. Indeed, to any philosopher or social anthropologist examining the issue, immunologists seem always to be announcing the importance of, or the end of, "self" without ever defining what in fact they might mean by it.

This oversight, alas, has profound consequences for immunology, because once examined it can be shown to be patently flawed and even logically unacceptable. For even a very superficial examination of the anthropological literature will illustrate the degree to which "selfhood" is culturally constructed. In fact, there are numerous healthy models of selfhood from other cultures that not only assimilate change but that are predicated upon it. From Native Americans, West Africans, Melanesians—i.e., throughout the world—we learn of models of selfhood that include in an indigenous category of the person the idea that a "self" is constantly being transformed by its social role (Napier 1986, 1992).

The idea of an innate, inalienable identity may be universal, but it can also be quite variably valued as compared to its social expression, its *persona*, through which an individual's identity becomes manifest. And one need not do fieldwork in a remote location to sense the importance of this shift in emphasis. Although a Japanese businessman might be as self-centered and as egocentric as his American counterpart, there is no question that his corporate identity is significantly different than what any American might understand by the word "employee." Set aside your fears of making "otherness" too exotic, and you will quickly see that there is much that can be learned by cultivating an interest in another lifeway even more removed from one's own than the world occupied by a Japanese friend.

So, change by itself cannot be the ground upon which self and nonself become inappropriate categories; this is nowhere so obvious in immunology as in the intuition that the "danger" model ought not necessarily be inconsistent with a model based on self and nonself. Where danger is inconsistent is at the levels of change and of transformation, which is why the self's prior and persistent character is such a focus of critical debate among theoreticians.

Thus, that a "self" could be identified by its social role is quite hard for immunologists to accept, even though the idea is not unfamiliar to Western thought. Any Roman historian could, for instance, verify the ancient notion of social responsibility by which a good community could, by virtue of its demonstrated orderliness, be identified as a *civitas libera atque immunis*—that is, as free from draconian overlords. That an immunological "persona" (i.e., person plus social role) is fundamental to what might be meant by immunity is deeply embedded in Western thought despite our modern obsession with stasis. Not only, then, are bench scientists failing to ask basic questions about what they mean by "self,"[4] but they are (in my view quite mistakenly) assuming that both the existence of a "system" and the role of natural selection in its creation are incontrovertible. Yet both involve, as can be plainly demonstrated, assumptions that are sometimes unrigorous.

Before making assumptions about what a "self" might or might not be, I would like to examine more directly the conundra of immunology with respect to their logical consistency—to ask, that is, if putting natural selection itself in jeopardy actually allows us to dissolve immunology's central paradoxes. To pose the question of why the immune system was created by evolution, I presently argue, is to take something that is theoretically nonpredictive (evolution) and ask why it created a set of complex relations (the immune system) that, as Cohn rightly states, is based "on experimental systems of such great complexity that many interpretations are possible and reproducibility becomes a luxury" (Cohn, Langman, and Geckeler 1980, 198). Add to these muddied waters the assumption of scientists that what we mean by "tolerance" is obvious, and one can only throw up one's hands and ask some basic questions about where this confusion all began. To do this, of course, is to recognized just how shaky are the grounds of the field itself.

CONUNDRA; OR, WHO IS NATURAL SELECTION?

Let us begin with an examination of immunology's central paradoxes. Although various arguments have been put forward to explain them away, their repeated appearance in the literature should alert us to the fact that they are far from fully resolved. In addressing them we will ask if there is any logical way by which their inconsistencies might be made coherent. And we will see that there is only one solution that satisfies all conditions for logical consistency. Startling and unexpected though it may seem, there is a view—indeed, but one view—that allows us to render logically consistent what has been observed experimentally.

Multiplicity/Specificity   For all of the difficult theoretical issues posed by modern immunology, we must be grateful that it has given rise to so many paradoxes and apparent contradictions. These have finally illustrated the truth of what would otherwise have been considered a scientific heresy—namely, that Darwin's natural selection is not a theory at all in the sense of being a view that, once accepted, can have predictive value (Napier 1996). In immunology, the continuing and near-religious acceptance of natural selection should itself make us suspicious that it is involved in much more than logical thought; and the fact that it possesses only historical or teleological value ought to set off all sorts of alarms: for we only know in hindsight, that is, if mutated variation (what in immunology is called a specificity repertoire) is superfluous or adaptive.[5] So, the argument which follows accepts as necessary science's own rigorous criterion that a theory needs to comply with empirical evidence, and have predictive value, if it is to be called a theory. Surprisingly, the argument here is in fact more novel than it ought to be, because, clearly, no one can foresee the consequences of diversity.

Scientists begin, then, wrongly—i.e., with a historical explanation (natural selection) that has no predictive value—and this they call a theory. Next they add a set of assumed relations (i.e., an immune system) which also cannot be experimentally verified,[6] and a concept of selfhood that is almost totally unexamined. Finally, they ask what such an evolved system of related "selves" can and cannot tolerate (i.e., what is self and what is foreign), and they do so without any awareness that tolerance itself can include among other things the following: a tolerance that results from indifference; a tolerance that stems from the recognition of autonomy; a tolerance that owes its existence to a love of variety; alas, even a tolerance that is the outcome of utter exhaustion. Is it any wonder that immunology is in such a muddle?

And things get worse; the story does not end with recognizing how such an unacceptably atheoretical and unempirical idea has so deeply influenced a domain of science. What we have come to know as good bench science has itself also *reinforced* (and not necessarily in a productive manner) the self/nonself paradigm of immunology. It takes little reflection to recognize that the very limited scope of controlled experimentation precludes from the outset an appreciation of how a "self" infects and is infected by that ambient life of which it is inextricably a part.[7] Indeed, what I will herein argue is that it is immunology's unexamined view of what a self might be that is almost wholly responsible for its nagging paradoxes, and that this limited view is, as well, the precise thing that stands in the way of a better understanding of what has already been observed at the bench. So, let us, then, step back momentarily.

Despite current attempts to redefine the field, immunology has always depended on the organic elimination of pathogens—if not from some self that is prior and persistent, at least from an organism that senses and responds to a foreign threat. At the cellular level, the process of rejection allows us to infer that the task of recognizing and eliminating (i.e., of protecting against) the outside world is the sine qua non of immunology—an organic event in which "nonself" (i.e., "difference") is systematically purged. Suppression of immune function allows an organism to "accept" difference, while the human body is otherwise quick to discharge difference or become itself the object of appropriation or destruction. This is, among other things, why fertilization—the maternal acceptance of the foreign—has never enough pleased immunologists as a subject of inquiry to make fetal acceptance a core subject in the discipline. In immunology, as elsewhere, we so often focus on the finality of organic death that we fail to see death's paradox—namely, in the long haul, that the recognizable end of one organism is marked by its assimilation into something else, and, in the short haul, that we autonomous beings live by harboring difference (in the maternal-fetal, in the gut, and above all, I would maintain, in the creation of antibodies). The presence or absence of an obvious vitality is, in other words, the primary way we distinguish between that which is *selfish* and that which is *selfless.* This is, as it were, natural selection's raison d'être.

But to think about death in a "vaccinological" way—that organisms *assimilate* one another to become sensitized to difference—is not merely to mystify its apparent final reality. It is also to draw our attention to the paradox of assimilation by which the "self" impresses its identity upon its environment by expressing—literally giving—something of itself. This is, for instance, why "dying" has always been used as a metaphor of both physical and spiritual love.

A construction of selfhood that focuses solely on the recognition and elimination of difference cannot cure illness, or allow us to create a mutual self that might so cure. Furthermore, it is simply not good enough to give up the self/nonself model without first attempting to redefine what a "self" might be. We will surely fail if we, as some suggest, merely "abandon the self-nonself question and focus on the rapid advances that are revolutionizing cell biology" (Schwartz 1995, 1177), to put the paradigm aside simply because it appears no longer to work. Rather, the way to address immunology's paradigmatic problems is to examine logically how the discipline defines its domain of inquiry in the first place, and in so doing to recognize that *natural selection is necessarily the unavoidable mainstay of immunology even though it cannot predict the meaning of what is observed* when an immunologist observes a cellular interaction or scrutinizes a gel—even though it is believed to have allowed our bone marrow, thymus, and lymph to create a vast and largely superfluous array of mutant cells. For without positive selective pressures, that god named Natural Selection would presumably have eliminated our dysfunctional—even useless—genetic material. This is why the immunological repertoire is deemed problematic, for the proliferation of "meaningless" antibodies defies one of the Selection God's basic commandments.

As Langman and Cohn in particular have argued (e.g., 1997a, 1997b), the only reason for antibody specificity is to make a self/nonself distinction. Therefore, specificity can only be defined in these terms. It makes no sense at all to have a self/nonself discrimination unless it is antigen-specific, and unless there is a self that is both prior and persistent. On such an identity is predicated the very concept of specificity; for without specificity it is difficult to determine what control exists to keep autoimmunity relatively low; without an immune system, there is nothing to prevent one from becoming, as Cohn says, a toxic dump site. While most immunologists accept this premise of identity, in the context of natural selection we now see that it is very flawed; for the numerical size of a specificity repertoire becomes irrelevant except in hindsight, where it makes sense in terms of our scientific god, Natural Selection.

However, as any student of immunology knows, what is more important than numbers is whether a reciprocity exists between an antibody or T-cell and an inducing antigen. This is a crucial fact that is often forgotten while being dazzled by the body's ability to produce its unimaginable array of antibodies; and it needs to be reiterated repeatedly. For, once given its due, we begin to see just how problematic are those definitions of the "self" that are predicated solely on organic "compatibility." Here, Metchnikoff's early embryologic notion that an organism's biological integrity is dependent "on the endeavor of integrating [its intrinsically] disharmonious elements by active processes" (Tauber and Chernyak 1991, 7) may be worth reviving. Though one might not easily accept his parallel contention that the human organism is fundamentally disharmonious, there is no doubt that he viewed immunity as an active search for compatibility. In fact, his belief that immunity was predicated on an organism's need to produce harmony out of imbalance also speaks cogently to the relatively recent understanding that autoimmunity is not only a debilitating but a natural process that is prevalent among the healthy (see, e.g., Cohen and Young 1991).

Compatibility ("La réunion des deux")   A tumor, an open lesion, a viral infection are each understood as incompatible with "self."[8] In examining such
relationships, such pathologies, it becomes abundantly clear why it is so difficult and unsatisfying for immunologists to transform, transcend, or abandon
this idiom of identity as a function of recognizing and eliminating difference.
However, herein is also contained the very evidence for reevaluating immunology's fundamental premise: namely, the idea that antigen/antibody
interactions are dependent on antibody specificity—Macfarlane Burnet's
recognition of "nonself," and not of "self." To cite Langman and Cohn, "the
immune definition of self can only be based on evolutionary selectable criteria" in which "components that are not exposed to immune recognition are
self" (1997b, 217).

But the major conundra of immunology invite another view that Burnet
could not have envisioned on the basis of what was then known—this being
that the immune response, rather than functioning as a self-identifying system, is, in fact, *the body's manufacture of "other" selves*, a reinvention, a reciprocal imaging, as it were, of "lost," or otherwise "alienated," former selves, a
transformation of the "self's" own nucleic history. Stated simply, the only way
that the self/nonself paradigm can work at all is to revise the construct of selfhood enough to accept what immunologists themselves have been arguing all
along—namely, that pathogens bind because they express the kin of normal
cell genes.

In fact, just as the immune system appears to have entered our consciousness by some form of unstated consensus, so too in tumor immunology has
the notion now been tacitly acknowledged that viral oncogenes come from
normal cell genes—that they are genes that have gotten loose, normal parts of
the genome that, when they escape, become pathogenic. This conclusion is
made likely by the fact that oncogenes have normal cell parts, and, reciprocally, that every oncogene has a normal cell counterpart. While it cannot be
shown (by definition) that all viruses have normal cell counterparts, such new
views do illustrate the extent to which at least certain viruses might be better
understood as "other self," rather than as "nonself." In terms of having a concrete outcome for scientific research programs, the fact that oncogenes have
normal cell counterparts allows us to understand why oncological research
is now interested not only in developing compounds that bind with and destroy cancer cells, but in modifying the proteins that influence cellular "self-
sacrifice" (apoptosis) when a normal cell is influenced by a proto-oncogene.

A pathogen may, in other words, be "other," but an "other" that is pathological because it is akin to (or the child of) a "former self." Thus envisioned, the nucleic acids of cell genes (in bone marrow, lymph, and the thymus) are the body's repertoire of potential "nonself"—that is, the body's attempt to recreate novel, different cells that might assimilate some forgotten, now "alienated," former self. In this view, *the body creates novel "nonselves" in an effort to locate and identify distant and disconnected "former selves."* Though its identity may be prior and persistent, it is only realized in its environmental encounters—especially in moments of transformation where its persistent qualities are at risk.

The argument here is not complex, and it may already be intimated in the T-cell's inability to recognize an antigen unless the latter is associated with a genetically encoded (*altered self*) molecule. It may also be intimated in *molecular mimicry*, where "a number of viruses and bacteria have been shown to possess antigenic determinants that are identical to or similar to normal host-cell components" (Kuby 1992, 394).[9] But this argument *does* require a complete revision of Burnet's view. To wit: Immunity does not produce, represent, or protect "self." In fact, the only view that actually does not create contradictions with what is known is this: that the immune response is both an identifier of a traditional Cartesian self, and also the body's generator of nonself— that is, a protein repository out of which one's ancient past and one's present meet to create or to destroy a future. Like the ancient Greek concept of time, any future immune system response is thus perceived less as a remote state than as a thing brought forward and projected in front of us.

Thus defined, the self/otherself discrimination is no different from the self/nonself one except for the crucial conceptual opening it offers to a question that is never considered. And the question is this: Why does a retrovirus return to infect a cell anyway? What motivates its return? Here, only the self/otherself (i.e., "prior," "disconnected" self) model makes possible an understanding of why this is happening at all, since it allows for both the creative embodiment of otherness (e.g., as in mitochondria) and the combative encounters with an alien world (e.g., as in immune responses), whereas the older self/nonself model allows only for the latter.

Indeed, once one accepts this redefinition one also can answer other vexing questions concerning the relationship between genetics (the germline) and experience (the soma). The great debate between Darwinians (the "Goliaths" who claim that acquired characters cannot be inherited over Weismann's "soma-germ plasma" tissue barrier) and Lamarkians (the "Davids" who cite the importance of experientially transformed [i.e., somatically mutated] genes that are reverse-transcribed and, thus, recombined with germline sequences) need not exist at all if one understands that what reverse transcriptase (the life-giving enzyme that copies an RNA base sequence into a DNA base sequence) is transmitting is not "nonself" (the outside world) but unrecognized former self (the self as it otherwise might have been). Reverse transcriptase allows for a conversation to take place between the germline and its lived expression in the physical, material world, a conversation that is Darwinian and Lamarkian alike, a conversation that is both linear and circular— i.e., one that is truly recursive; for reverse transcription is both the mechanism by which the outside world influences the germline and the vehicle by which self-tolerance is learned during development.

Viewed recursively, then, there is no need for any molecular "big bang" in which related but different genes arose "by duplication of a single primordial gene followed by mutational change in the DNA sequences of the duplicates" (Steele, Lindley, and Blanden 1998, 184). Now we can, indeed, see that environmental pressures are not selective at all; they are assimilative—reconfigured, and utilized to redefine what a potential self might be. In short, the feedback loop works much better if what is being fed back by RNA in the soma-to-germline gene feedback process is "otherself," for only in this way can the primordial "nice little story" of evolution be removed from the unilinear dogma to which Darwinism is chained.[10]

And no theory of catastrophe, nor even Eldredge and Gould's punctuated equilibrium (1972; Gould and Eldredge 1977), can change the face of the lifeless stasis for which neo-Darwinism has always stood. Indeed, one argument for the rapid growth of immunology over the past three decades may be that those involved in its theory intuit its possibilities for advancing some of the greatest issues in the history of Western thought.

Reciprocity The notion of reciprocity makes possible the very relationships that our current concepts of self lack. This is yet another level at which Matzinger's argument is totally correct (Matzinger and Fuchs 1996); where that argument may be constructively debated, however, is over its abandonment of the self as the locus of creative generation. Bearing in mind that many of our viruses in all likelihood developed out of the nucleic acids of normal cell genes (for how else could they bind?),[11] it is only logical that the immune response is less combative than it is reciprocal—the reaction of a cell to its developmental (as it were, "historical") antecedent—a conversation, to use Matzinger's turn of phrase, with the very genes that may be killing you. The function of the immune response, in other words, is not to create versions of a "self's" protection, but to generate the body's latest version of a "nonself," a reciprocal variation that attempts to balance an earlier (and, if disconnected, potentially harmful) "self." Antibodies, in this view, are not "self," but the body's creative "nonselves." Antigens, on the other hand, are new variations of earlier selves that test the body's ability to achieve developmental integration, both out of the past and into the future. Here, successfully created nonselves (i.e., antibodies that are shown to have recursive significance) become, that is, our *otherselves*. Otherselves, once recognized, stimulate the growth of the new self.

The utility of this hypothesis is, as we will now see, evidenced in its ability to resolve immunology's major paradoxes. The only way, that is, of bringing together what is observed in immunology and a functional view of a persistent "self" is to redefine that self with respect to its object, and to do so by a logical inversion of received belief. For by redefining the relationship between self and world (between antibody and antigen, between self and otherself) it becomes possible to envision a creative identity—a thermodynamics of life—which advances through the maintenance of difference.

Why thermodynamics? Because in thermodynamics vitality is expressed in *difference*.[12] The greater the difference, the more life that is expressed. In natural selection the opposite holds: one cannot say if a selective pressure is desirable or damaging (i.e., whether it advances life) until the outcome of that pressure can be viewed in hindsight. Natural selection is, in other words, only natural if one believes, as Darwin did, that God moves nature, and that nature is godly; for only if nature is itself godly, can one appeal to it as the final arbiter. This is why natural selection—despite its somewhat pedestrian name—always appears in the final moments of scientific argument; for natural selection has clearly been deified by modern science.[13]

So, is immunology completely bound up with the construction of unilinear arguments, with evolutionary notions of progress, and with our misunderstanding of energy? This, it seems to me, is incontrovertible.

PARADOX

If the human body is actually creating versions of "nonself" ("otherself"), how do we translate this realization into a language that works? How do we dissolve the old metaphors and reconstruct them in a way that conforms to what we now know? In addressing this problem, we must first note (incredibly!) that such reconstruction is precisely the role played by RNA in transforming DNA—which, by extension, also suggests that the aberrant conclusions to which the contrived path of bench science has led contemporary immunology may be as much attributed to our mistaken attribution of life to DNA rather than to the RNA that surely should own this epithet. So, now let us see how these contrivances have led to paradoxes that cannot be ignored.

Paradox 1: Identity. How can evolution function to preserve self by creating a preservation mechanism that succeeds by not recognizing self? The answer here is that "identity" is preserved in that a "self" (a continuously evolving living thing) is recognized not in specific antibodies, but is *unrecognized* (and therefore attacked) *in all of its former nucleic selves*—i.e., in antigens. An "unrecognized" self in the environment becomes the adversary in combat, a recognized self becomes for better or worse directly assimilated.

Paradox 2: Multiplicity. How is it possible that the human body continues to create a broad specificity repertoire when so-called "natural" selection demands that apparently superfluous "deformations" be eliminated? The answer to this second paradox is that natural selection is no longer a problem because the body isn't creating "self." How, as Silverstein summarizes it, "could the gene pool be maintained when any given organism was likely to employ such a small proportion of its specificity repertoire during its lifetime and when so many of the specificities that it did employ were against antigens that posed little threat to survival? In the absence of positive selective pressures, it would not take long for such unused or 'unimportant' genes to lose their identity" (1989, 147).

This is the conundrum: The human body appears to produce such an extraordinary number (usually thought to be from 10^8 to 10^9) of antibodies for inducing antigens (some threatening, some harmless) that its activities appear almost random.[14] According to natural selection, these numbers should "naturally" be limited. Superfluous—what elsewhere would be called "maverick" or "mutant"—creations are, if they have no obvious application, eliminated. But the body doesn't work this way. No argument about it; diversity proliferates. This is why the repertoire is for immunologists "paradoxical." Furthermore, in order for binding to take place an antibody must be created with a locking mechanism that works for an unknown antigen. This also makes no sense because variation, by definition, is infinite—unless one assumes that antigens developed out of the nucleic acids of normal cell genes (i.e., out of the nucleic acids of former selves), while antibodies, on the other hand, are understood as creative attempts at imagining difference—as it were, internalized "nonselves."

Paradox 3: Scope of the immunological repertoire. How can we argue that the proliferation of B-cells and T-cells is adaptive, when neither the size of that repertoire, nor even the presence or absence of the thymus itself, can be construed as an indicator of resistance? The answer to this third paradox is that repertoire scope is only relevant to the number of pathogens that can influence an organism; indeed, one may not need a thymus at all if there is no pathogen—no alienated variation of "former self"—being expressed.

Stasis is and always will be favored by a germline which, left to its own entropic devices, would evolve into a proliferation of weaker and weaker individuals—like clones whose genetic strength becomes increasingly limited with each replication. Specificity, therefore, has nothing to do with creation.

Finally, one needs to bear in mind the simple observation (almost always lost during "warfare" at the bench) that the "foreign" viruses and prokaryotes that the body deals with *are not always harmful.* Some are totally harmless; others are real mutation-transformation factories that have no clearly defined "target"; and still others seem to undermine the very notion that the body always seeks to rid itself of the foreign. So, identifying nonself is not necessarily defensive in the accepted model, unless by defense we simply mean that antibodies go after *everything* that they recognize. Let us, therefore, conclude with a brief look at how acceptance of the foreign, and compatibility with the foreign, fare in a new theory that defines antibodies as recursive nonselves and antigens as attenuated selves.

NONSELF OR OTHERSELF?

Like the motions of the serpent, which the Egyptians made the emblem of intellectual power; or like the path of sound through the air; at every step he pauses and half recedes, and from the retrogressive movement collects the force which again carries him onwards. —Coleridge

Acceptance or Rejection (Reciprocity Reconsidered)   Recognition and rejection of "nonself" is just one half of immunology's domain of inquiry; for the specificity repertoire is not the only problem for immunology (attempting, that is, to account for its near random activities). Acceptance is as much a problem, and especially the question of how a fetus that is, as it were, antigenically "foreign" to the mother can develop without inducing the same sort of rejection that attends organ transplants. Specificity (recognition and rejection) and fetal acceptance are instructive examples as much because of how we puzzle over them (how they just don't fit any accepted paradigm): in the case of the specificity repertoire, because it violates, as we have seen, the Darwinian rule that things dysfunctional or nonfunctional get eliminated; in the case of the fetus because considering it so confounds us, as stem-cell research now makes clear, that we don't even know how to look at it immunologically in any way that is satisfying, except to argue a view that is as formally unsatisfying as it is aesthetically ugly: that birth itself is a form of immunological rejection.

And because pathology and creativity are two sides of the same coin, anaphylaxis provides a more honest model for immunology than do theories created in controlled environments where results are built only upon an undiversified field. These processes were known for a long time before immunology became the examination of a presumed "system": back in the nineteenth century attention had already been drawn to the peculiarities of anaphylaxis. Indeed, if a fertilized egg is "other," then pregnancy is something of a positive anaphylactic process, since in anaphylaxis things can cause either themselves or their opposite: like the escapement in a pre-electronic watch, a cycle repeats over and over and then suddenly clicks. An awareness of this fact marks the difference between a good path and a bad one. Good things can soon become evil if one does not work very hard to sustain them. The way one does this is by utilizing positively the few things in life that for each of us are inalienable—a principle, a cosmology, a personal relationship.

And why, we must finally ask, is there so much silence about acceptance and rejection? For embryology and pregnancy (where a mother is responding to fetal antigens) the silence becomes even more telling when we look at what scientists themselves say about studying maternity; because, no matter how central and fascinating the problem may be, what we see is a clear and simple case of the dissatisfaction of science with the kind of "study" that exploring the problem necessarily requires. As one well-known researcher put it:

The maternal/fetal was a good idea, but we just didn't have the techniques, just didn't have the way of approaching the question. It's something that a lot of people have got into for a short time and then got out of—the immunological aspects of nature's most successful foreign graft—how the fetus actually survives inside the immunologically hostile mother. (Charlesworth et al. 1989, 214)

Considering the fact that eight out of ten autoimmune disorders occur in women, and that pregnant women frequently find temporary relief from their otherwise chronic autoimmune symptoms, one might in all seriousness ask if their tribulations are less a function of implicated cells that cross the barrier between mother and child than the fact that the specificity of scientific research guarantees from the start that we will never see the forest for the trees, that we will never discover in the current research paradigm a way of respectfully examining more that one relation at a time.[15]

So, do we then set aside a most fascinating question because to study it is technically discomforting? Do we simply abandon such an inquiry because it doesn't conform to the values of a scientific culture, a social setting, that is at the mercy of those cultural prejudices about self and nonself that dominate our era? Why not begin again—if I may put the question directly—with an evaluation of the artless categories that so often govern research? Why not start over by asking from the outset about the kind of limitations placed upon how we think by the culturally derived critical categories that—except for demographic accident—would have led us to think that thalassemia and malaria are totally unrelated? Why not face the deep human need to examine a mutuality, a coexistence, a *co*-incidence? That is, why not start with a quite verifiable analysis of how populations with one disease either express, or are tolerant of, what appear to us to be completely unrelated illnesses?

There is, in fact, no reason at all why a productive research paradigm could not be developed around the examination of how one system that results in what we name as a particular illness responds to the presence of a completely different, but equally identified, illness of a different sort. Why not expose one "system" to another? Why not, as in creativity itself, see how the superimposition of unlikely elements can result in the creation of an entirely new paradigm, an entirely new form of knowledge? Why, in other words, race merrily down the road of clonal and monoclonal specificity, when what we are seeking to understand is less the relation between immunal cause and effect, than the relation between the general (the immune system) and experience? Why not replace the mechanical with the quantum mechanical? Better yet, why not replace both with the higher order of creativity itself?

One might justifiably ask why immunology got itself into such a fix of paradoxes in the first place. Here, the real demon is microbiology and its destructive marriage to the experimental method. Though most of modern science is built upon *experiment*, rather than *experience*, what Schrödinger and Heisenberg intuitively understood in the discovery of wave mechanics was that the universe was made up of superimposed and inseparable levels of activity, that creativity is the outcome of superimposition, and that the particular is always contained by (and cannot be identified outside of) its context. To give measure to the particular, in other words, we must have some sense of what it is a part of. And because the experimental method by definition must control and limit the ambient environment, it actually works directly against anything that might otherwise sensitize us enough to value complex relations. For the difference between experiment and experience is that the former is completely bounded by certain self-consciously contrived contexts of observation (cf. Margolis 1993, 183).

Self and Nonself (Compatibility Reconsidered)   Every human gut is a processing *reservoir of nonself*. There is, we can now see, no inherent reason for believing that *body boundary maintenance* is the only measure of preservation. Similarly, at the cellular level, the simple equation of "self" with "compatibility" breaks down when we look at the lives of cells that display clonal continuity; one look at the lives of cells on a petri dish—where cells at the center of the colony darken and die (as evidenced by the spores they have created to protect themselves)—shows clearly that the equation of "compatibility" with "similarity," and "similarity" in turn with "identity" results only in entropy and eventual death. In fact, identity survives, if it survives at all, at a more dangerous periphery where it is contested, challenged, earned, and negotiated. This equation of "self" and "compatibility" also breaks down when we look at the vaccinological assimilation of otherness, or at symbiosis (and particularly at the relationship between animal and plant DNA): something as simple as the human gut clearly offers a wide range of synergistic activity between self and nonself *within* the body. Now, there are many other factors here, but these are, plainly and simply (anyone can see them), the central issues.

These facts lead only to one conclusion: immune responses are not what the body creates as specific markers of "selfhood." The B- and T-cells that are generated by the human organism are not the response of a "self" to its hostile environment. Instead, they are this: the repository of a reinventable nucleic history that each of us has housed within our body. What the body presents, therefore, to an antigen is not combat. It is reciprocity—and, furthermore, a reciprocity whose purest form is represented in the retrovirus, where reverse transcriptase allows the recuperation of a former self. For this if for no other reason, the retrovirus should now more properly be called *recursive*, since it illustrates most beautifully the reciprocity that obtains between an organism and the nucleic acids of ("normal") cell genes from which that organism has been distanced.

What bone marrow and the thymus create, in other words, is not a "self" that steps forward to meet an antigen, but *the body's best version of a nonself*, a reciprocal variation that—if "self" can, as it were, be recaptured—will balance a potentially harmful antigen, a former (if now disconnected) version of "self." Like the recursive retrovirus (which now becomes less a damaging aberration than the *self's expression of itself as another*), an immune response can also be defined as the *self's (body's) expression of itself (antibody) as another (antigen)*—or, better yet, redefined as *one's image (antibody) of its former self (antigen) as new self (body)*.

Put temporally, the body reciprocates with the past in an attempt to create a new future. Macfarlane Burnet said "it could be no other way" than to be a determinant of self. He didn't realize that there was, metaphysical though it may be, yet another way that would allow us to address what we now know to be immunology's paradoxes—another way that might actually also change our conceptualization of the self and its environment. This is surely not a last word on the immunological self, but the only logical way by which what is perceived can be reconciled with what is known.

When I say that my hypothesis is the inversion of Burnet's, what I propose is that we accept the obvious—that an antigen is a form of self (i.e., a unique development of former self), and that an antibody is the body's best go at nonself (i.e., a former-self inducer). Put simply, I am not trying to argue that the self/environment relationship has been changed by advances in cell biology to the degree that the self/nonself issue is now moot; but I do think that one can re-jig the terms so that they conform better to problems of the field that have been inadequately addressed. The need to make them conform is central; for the self/nonself issue may be not only the central problem of molecular biology but also of modernity, no matter how many exotic terms and new words we invoke in order to deflect or revise the basic assumptions of the field.

Thus far, I should think, there is no problem with thinking of antigens as former selves (imitators or descendants) and antibodies as the body's attempt to create novel nonselves that might re-engage former selves. But what makes the former-self (antigen)/former-self-inducer (antibody) model new and useful (i.e., not merely semantic)? The answers are simple, and may be summarized by reviewing what this new model makes possible:

First, accepting a widely recognized link with the past obviates the need to create lots of imaginary stories about the evolution of germline mutations and natural selection in primordial creatures—i.e., accepting the former-self/former-self-inducer model makes less central the highly speculative domain of evolutionary biology, a field of inquiry which (because it invents speculative stories) focuses more on novel change than on acceptance of the degree to which induction is based on complementarity. If self gets constructed out of a sorting process in which T- and B-cells proliferate in an attempt to identify now-avulsed former-selves or things very much like them—i.e., if pathogens are, at *any* level, transformations of normal cell genes (and therefore, as former-selves, genetically related)—the size of the repertoire (soma or germline) and its phenomenal mutating both make much better sense; moreover, if T- and B-cells function to induce what has become unknown, these novel cells no longer need be subjected to the unprovable hypotheses about germline mutation that evolution necessitates. In short, thinking of antigens as transformed former-selves and antibodies as former-self-inducers creates a view that is free of the fantastic hypothesizing that germline evolutionists indulge in, and that is, put simply, more economical than the Cartesian speculations of contemporary biology.

Second, if B- and T-cells are the essential mechanism for identifying former or other selves (i.e., antigens) which are now, as it were, "free," immunity becomes ideologically less dependent on not recognizing self than it does upon trying to locate former-self. This clears up the very muddy outcome of Burnet's basic idea that the evolution of the immune system thrives on self-ignorance—i.e., that evolution has worked to create a preservation system that works by not recognizing what it is ostensibly preserving. Like the first point above, this new construction is a simpler and more economical view. It makes common sense that immunity be recognized as a dynamic, and fundamentally recursive, search engine.

Third, thinking of antibodies as "former-self search engines" conforms much better to what we now know about retrotranscription than does Burnet's "self-ignorance" model. For what is the function of a retrovirus if not to restore "lost" DNA, to rewrite its past, and, as it were, to reconstruct the self's history by making possible a new identity?

Fourth, at the level of human understanding, this new construction not only helps show us the degree to which contemporary neo-Darwinism is built on unverifiable prejudice, but it highlights the role that this framework has played in the theoretical and ideological malformations of modern immunology. If natural selection is the parent of immunological identity, what cell biology shows us is that there is, plainly, *nothing natural* at all about selection, especially as it relates to a prior and persistent identity; *for that identity can never ascertain at the moment of induction if a selective pressure is ultimately destructive or constructive. All this kind of self can, therefore, do is constantly attempt to eliminate difference.* The result of this elimination may give us the notion of immunology; but, as any petri dish will show, it also gives us entropy, natural selection's and Darwin's greatest enemy.

What I maintain is that the thesis herein outlined is free of the flaws of the argument for natural selection, because identity cannot exist or grow in my model without potentially hazardous encounters. Selfish cells will always prefer cloning, and the genes of clones, as we know, get increasingly weak (that is, genetically simpler) as they replicate. The neo-Darwinians, in other words, can't be right.

Fifth, by my construction, both immunity and autoimmunity become much more simplified because they no longer have to be defined by reference to those aforementioned selective pressures that are, by definition, teleological. In my view "identity" becomes defined not merely as a prior and persistent thing, but as the outcome of reciprocal (i.e., induced) relations. Cells (and organisms), as it were, earn their identities, much as we ourselves do! As we say, no man is an island. Yes, identity is in part specific (innate, inherited), but it is not only that. As we have already said, the change in perspective is not merely semantic; it is not mere philosophical luxury because it conforms with what can be observed in real life as opposed to in genetically modified mice. If a philosophical notion bears more resemblance to what can be observed in the transformations of life than a scientific one that is artificial and largely static, the latter should be dropped in favor of the former.

Sixth, and perhaps most important, thinking of antigens as parts or developments of former self, and antibodies as the body's creative construction of what it has forgotten (i.e., as "former-self search engines") helps us to address an age-old enigma about the status of viruses as living things. Permit me, by way of a brief disgression, a "recursive" afterthought.

LIVE AND LET LIVE

One of the unexpected blessings of having an interest in science as a philosophical and a cultural endeavor is that one need not always be preoccupied in discarding everything old for anything new. Lying about my bookshelves are some dated literary artifacts that I still find interesting—old textbooks, popular magazine articles about scientific advances, and brochures that were often handed to me by well-wishing clinicians who found my inquiries about cellular identity exasperating.

Though it may be a bit of a luxury to lose oneself in a text that science no longer finds valid, I am grateful for having been subjected to these clinical ambiguities, first, because they confirmed for me not only how absent was immune-system talk a mere three decades ago, but, second, because they made real for me just how many unrigorous assumptions one had to swallow if one intended to make one's way as a scientific professional. These are two good reasons for pausing by those shelves of outdated books, but there are others.

As Latour has shown, the number of times one actually unwinds a scientific argument by tracing its lineage backwards is about as often as one hears the argument that science is impeding the progress of society and the growth of collective knowledge. Yet the archaeology of science is probably far more relevant to its future than the covering up that results when bench scientists claim to be far too busy for this luxury of idle contemplation. I say this because reviewing what people were willing to believe in, say, 1964 may be far less an indicator of how far science has come than perhaps a glaring statement of how much we are willing to ignore in order to avoid having to examine the basic precepts of who we are and what we do; for almost as soon as viral antigens were discovered, the question of their status as living things became problematic enough to be put aside as unanswerable.

Decades later, rather than confronting the same simple question (as, say, one might in an undergraduate course in microbiology), we are still asked to suspend our curiosity, if not our would-be intellectual rigor, and to accept that the very survival of the sciences of virology and immunology may even prove the issue unimportant. Here is an example from a distinguished contemporary textbook on cellular biology:

> The question is sometimes asked whether or not viruses are living. The answer depends crucially on what we mean by "living," and it is probably worth pondering only to the extent that it helps us more fully understand what viruses are—and what they are not. The most fundamental properties of living things are *mobility, irritability* (perception of, and response to, environmental stimuli), and the *ability to reproduce.* Viruses clearly do not satisfy the first two criteria. Outside their host cells, viruses are inert and inactive. They can, in fact, be isolated and crystallized almost like a chemical compound. It is only in an appropriate host cell that a virus becomes functional, undergoing a cycle of synthesis and assembly that gives rise to more viruses. (Becker, Reece, and Poenie 1996, 105)

So, how far have we really come? Here's the 1964 version of this problem from the highly popular *Life* Science Library book, *The Cell.* I choose this text because it was deliberately compiled for popular consumption by scientists and distinguished writers (including C. P. Snow). It is, in other words, an example of science's best effort to make itself clear:

> Until the discovery of the virus, scientists felt that even if life was difficult to define they could at least distinguish between animate and inanimate matter. But the virus cannot accurately be described as either. Some are shaped very much like pyrite or other mineral crystals; others resemble living organisms such as euglena. The virus has no means of locomotion, it possesses no source of power and it cannot grow. (Pfeiffer et al. 1964, 173)

So far, there is not much to be concerned about here, until, that is, we realize how today, as in 1964, putting the issue of vitality aside leads us directly back into the domain of assumed cultural dogma; for in the very next sentence we read that a virus "can *reproduce* but not until it has *commandeered* a cell. It can *reduce* a healthy, productive cell to a mere nursery that fosters a new generation of viruses" (173, my emphasis). Indeed, only on the previous page we learned:

> A virus can *invade, enslave* and *destroy* a cell with frightening efficiency. Like a tiny tadpole, its head full of DNA or RNA, the virus drifts until it hooks onto a cell. It *bores* into the cell and, like a hypodermic needle, *injects* its nucleic acid. The cell helplessly relinquishes its machinery to the *invader,* which *reproduces* at breakneck speed. In about half an hour the dead cell ruptures and releases a flood of new parasites. (172, my emphasis)

How, we might have demanded (not only then but now), could a virus *commandeer* a healthy cell, *reduce* it to a nursery, and *reproduce* itself at breakneck speed if it is inert and possesses no means of locomotion? If viruses have no power, no mobility, and no ability to reproduce, how can they continue to commandeer, reduce, invade, enslave, destroy, bore, inject, and reproduce? In short, they cannot; they never could; and they never will. So why do we continue to use this language not only in popular publications but in scientific texts, in medical lectures, and at the bench?

One answer is that what we are really doing in these instances is reifying our cultural prejudices about identity through the guise of microscopic parable. As the same popular text hopefully stated back in 1964, "there is a growing feeling among biologists that immunological studies may soon provide significant insights into the factors which make each organism a distinct individual" (175).

Yet what in fact has happened is rather different. While physicists seem less and less willing to dirty their hands with messy mechanical experiments, cell biologists, blaming the physicists for too much thinking, have seized the bench as a bastion of applied anti-intellectualism. Don't idle over unanswerable questions, we are advised. As an interviewer was told by a noted Australian bench immunologist: "There is a correlation between reading the literature and mediocrity in scientific work" (Charlesworth et al. 1989, 118). Remarkably, this is not only a belief that one has to go it alone if one wishes to discover something new; for many, the anti-intellectual nature of bench microbiology involves being openly "contemptuous of scientists who imagine you can do science by having bright ideas in an armchair with your feet up, and even of scientists who regularly read the scientific literature" (ibid., 116–

17). Where, we may ask, does the daydreaming Einstein fit into such a picture? What space exists for that Swiss patent officer who later wore bedroom slippers around Princeton and a homemade hat while sailing his little boat with my similarly eccentric grandfather?

And what happens when scientists themselves fail to take an interest in the glaring cultural assumptions that control their thinking? Not only do they more or less guarantee that nothing unexpected will be found, but they also limit their ability to recognize the unexpected when it is plainly before them; for one of the obvious outcomes of the fact that a virus cannot live without a living cell is that the virus cannot *do* anything. This fact can, to revise the focus of Burnet's own claim, "be no other way."

So, what can be said about viral "life"? What can be said is that the so-called immune self (i.e., our antibodies) must *attract* those potentially pathological viral antigens. Horrid though this idea might be to an evolutionary survivalist, it does make good sense, because that antibody—as the body's best version of "lost- or former-self"—is the mechanism by which a living thing allows itself to explore the boundaries of life, to engage that danger which is the precondition for real change.

Though the antibodies we create may still be "self" (if only because it is we who make them), what we do by creating them can no longer be understood either in terms of defense, or in terms of recognizing and eliminating danger; for there can be no active danger to be defeated if the virus is not alive and has no motivation of its own. An obstruction on the footpath of life is only hazardous to us if we decide to take a walk, and the reasons a body might take a walk are as numerous and complex as the sum of experiences that will come to bear on its recognizing who it is through each new engagement along that unknown path of events.

The organism does not, then, as Schrödinger once thought, *draw life* from the environment; *the antibody, quite clearly, brings life to the virus*; for the very thing that allows us to attribute life to viruses in the first place is the Darwinism that requires that we avoid threatening encounters, and especially those dangerous encounters we may well not survive. And the only reason we have not allowed ourselves to see viruses as wholly inert is the fact that our religion of natural selection has habituated us to ascribing intentions to anything that alters an organism that on its own should strive to remain unchanged.

In neo-Darwinism there's no "reason," in other words, that a healthy organism ought to seek out something that might harm it; and because organisms just don't spontaneously endanger themselves in a "naturally selective" world, all we are left with is the idea that viruses are aggressive killers, when, in fact, they are inert until a cell brings life to them. So counterintuitive is the concept of "inviting danger," that when cells systematically engage in encounters that kill them we refer to their activities as suicidal.[16]

This idea—that viruses may be expressed only when a cell "wears" them—no doubt appears quite odd to those of us stuck in a Cartesian world. And it's too bad, really. Were we at all curious about other models of personhood, we might well have recognized earlier on how knowing those models could enhance our ability to revise contemporary immunology. Indeed, even though much of the world's diversity has been eliminated by modernity,[17] anthropology still offers numerous examples that normalize what to us seems like an odd microbial model.

In West Africa, for instance, orators ("griots") do not possess the words that they commit to memory, for

> the words that constitute history are much too powerful to be "owned" by any one person or group of people; rather these words "own" those who speak them. Accomplished griots do not "own" history; rather they are possessed by the forces of the past. . . . Only these griots are capable of meeting the greatest challenge: imparting social knowledge to the next generation. (Stoller 1997, 25)[18]

Similarly, we saw earlier in this study how masked rituals depend upon the idea that identity gets realized (i.e., known) when a mask-wearer brings his or her life force to the inert mask object that now becomes the catalyst for transformation. In such ritual performances, the character (like the cell once it meets its virus) "takes over and gives life to the song and movement" (Herbst 1997, 69). The performer plus social role—i.e., the character, the persona—brings life to the mask (or even to several masks in succession), each of which possess a unique quality (a "protein") that must be assessed and (hopefully) balanced by the person (the "cell") who/that wears it. As the Balinese say, some masks can, indeed, kill one, especially if one happens to have misjudged the preparatory requirements for its use. This ritualized mask is the opposite of Descartes's mischievous mask, really; and this reversal in thinking allows us to see that the volitional language we employ to ascribe intentions to viruses is only a conceptual response made necessary by our Cartesian notion of the self.

Viruses, then, look and are shaped as if they were inanimate because *they are the keys to exploring those borderlands at which one's identity as a living thing becomes contested and eventually defined.* Identity, in this sense, is as much what we will come to make of it in a performative setting as it is a prior and persistent quality. It is more active than latent.

Descartes's "I think therefore I am" must, then, carry with it its corollary: "If I am not active, I cannot exist; if I do not explore personae that are risky, I will not grow and be transformed. I will know nothing of life." What the strange arrival of contemporary immunology suggests is that it is perhaps time to examine how, in moments of transition, our identities are shaped and "known" to us through risk, and, in particular, through challenging encounters with difference. Life, liberty, and the pursuit of happiness are as much a privilege as they are a right, but if we ignore our charge as humans to create, it is we who die out.

How, today, we might reasonably ask, could an Einstein publish a major piece in a scientific journal with no citations or references to previously published materials? In the era of institutionalized co-authorship such an event seems virtually impossible, even though everyone knows that scientific discovery is largely the outcome of dissociative thought—i.e., of daydreaming. Yet, if the cell colony can subdivide, creating other universes (heaven? hell?), its form will continue to grow. It is only on the petri dish of the known world where those spores that are the preamble to cell division and replication become protective devices that kill off the colony at its center. And it is only by willfully engaging the dangerous periphery that knowing the self becomes possible.

I feel very strongly that I am under the influence of things or questions which were left incomplete and unanswered by my parents and grandparents and more distant ancestors . . . as if I had to complete or perhaps continue things which previous ages had left unfinished. —Jung, *Memories, Dreams, Reflections*

further in grandmother
grandfather hold my hand
as I go on through this life
try to understand
the beauty of your faces
I will never see again
but I know you are with me now
leading me further in
—Greg Brown, "further in"

Caveat Lector *Although the strictly "immunological" book I have written is now finished, the argument it creates—that social entropy can only be revitalized through personal growth—lacks any direct demonstration. It would, therefore, be remiss of me not at least, if even inadequately, to provide some intimation of how the general theoretical argument might be translated into a system of personal belief.*

While I certainly offer without apology what follows, I will say that not everyone who has patiently considered my line of thought to this juncture should continue. This final section has little or nothing to do with positivistic arguing; critically speaking, it offers nothing—i.e., no thing—*that would delight the specifist or, indeed, the postmodernist. Those who think of themselves first as scientists, or as philosophers, or as anthropologists, would do well to put the book down at this juncture. What follows is, as it were, "amodern"; for the opposite of a theory of immunology is not just another theory about cell-cell relations, but an exploration of a cognitive alternative through which liminality, difference, and binary opposition are engaged in ways that are basically different than immunology's model of recognition and elimination.*

The alternative to egocentric elimination by warring "males" is not a world of warring egocentric "females," but a world in which warfare, specificity, and egocentrism give way to a distinctly different notion of power. The Balinese examples previously offered are instructive because the "immunological" eat-or-be-eaten egocentrism of kings and warriors (i.e., the kshatriya *caste of earthly rulers) is balanced by, and in fact is subordinate to, the domain of magic in which the caste of* brahmana *priests transcends such pedestrian concerns in favor of an embryological balancing of the cosmos. Here, specificity is secondary: ego gives way to anonymity, identity is replaced by mysticism, and naming has less power than does metaphor. In the* brahmana *domain personal experience must be the only true guide to cosmic awareness because life means little if the self fails at actively engaging the eternal—if life, that is, is not a mythic integration of one's own history with the ancient, the primordial, and the archetypal. Here, beauty resides in assuring some absolute connection between microcosmic and macrocosmic, not in the simple glorification of the individual. In the* brahmana *view, history means nothing if it cannot be echoed in what one believes oneself to be engaged in now.*

For the brahmana, *then, a book on immunology would mean little without some exploration of the mythologizer's own domain of symbolic meaning. So when, in chapter 4, I introduced the mathematical inventions of John Napier, it made no difference at that point in the book's argument that he was an ancient member of my ancestral clan; nor did it matter that his role as one of history's greatest advocates of mathematical specificity advanced significantly the kind of Eurocentric patriarchy—of progress and expansionism—that much of the past century has worked to redress. Nor would it have been apparent in (or relevant to) the earlier parts of this study that the scientific agenda he so enthusiastically embraced was also, in his own mind, connected to his anti-Catholic sentiments. In fact, in his own day, Napier was much better known for his writings against the papacy and its matriarchal love of the Blessed Virgin than for his having invented logarithms.*

At the risk of appearing self-indulgent, what follows is a demonstration of how that which is self-generated (i.e., autogenous) can work toward transcending entropy. What I offer is merely a catalyst—a willing demonstration of how the study of "nonself" has generated in my own life responses to entropy that are sometimes general, sometimes individual, but always marginal; for it is in the creative encounter with liminality that the assimilation of other allows in each of us a constructive embodiment of difference.

The opposite of a study based on the intellectual values brought to focus by the Enlightenment is not another sort of analytical specificity—another complaint about what is wrong with modern life—but something stated in subjective generalities: not the words of an ego-oriented "male" world, nor an ego-oriented "female" world, but a world in which the ego is dissolved by its own recursive mythologizing.

This final section, then, attempts to illustrate subjectively how both entropy and the deadly specificity of "immunological" thinking get transcended through creative self-fashioning.

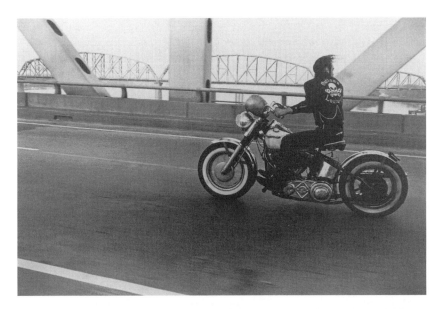

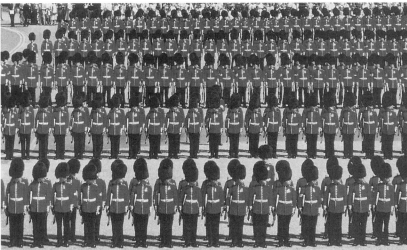

FIGURE 21. **Margin and Center**
Danny Lyon's photograph *Crossing the Ohio River, Louisville* (*top*) provides a suggestive intimation of the social, psychological, and physical risks associated with "crossing over," while the depersonalized "cloning" exhibited in the postcard of the Household Brigade (*bottom*) represents the safety and the entropy of the fearful hiding within society's self-replicating center. (*Top:* Photo reproduced courtesy of Danny Lyon.)

From the beginning I fully know of it.
Long ago one was thinking of it.
Long ago one spoke of it.
I am indeed its child.
Absolutely I am Earth's child.
I am indeed its grandchild.
—Navajo Blessingway

FROM LIMINAL TO MARGINAL

> *Any Templar appointed by God's hand to be master over a foreign folk must forbid the asking of his name or race and help them to their rights.* —inscription on the Holy Grail, Wolfram von Eschenbach, *Parzival*

Palm Sunday marks the day of Christ's triumphant entry into Jerusalem. A week before his resurrection on Easter, and a mere five days before his crucifixion, we celebrate the entry of the great "outsider" into society's center. It is the very day which symbolizes the moment when one at the margin makes his bold move to transform the still and dying center, even if the outcome of this event is as of yet unknown to those who witness it. Christ's crucifixion, which symbolically honors—even makes noble—the many would-be liminal transformers who fail to survive the changes they hope to stimulate, seems on this feast remote and unlikely. Lent's forty days of fasting are nearly over, and everywhere we see and hear reminders of rebirth and renewal. The spring branches (palms, olives, pussywillows) are themselves pure emblems of creation, birth, resurrection. The festive procession itself marks the chosen moment for change. It is the time throughout the world when, at the full moon, the rites of spring signal the rebirth of all that is natural. Persephone returns from Hades, fertility rites are everywhere present, and the Earth itself is reincarnated. In the words of the Song of Songs,

> Arise, my beloved, my beautiful one, and come!
> For see, the winter is past, the rains are over and gone.

The flowers appear on the earth,

... and the song of the dove is again heard in our land.

It's almost as if Christ walked from the periphery of our petri dish to the core of the colony. Think of walking from the margin of the circle of society to its center—from the unpopulated countryside into the bustling din of a crowded assembly of people. Think of moving from the periphery down a pie-shaped road that is broad at the margins of the circle and that narrows to an eventual vanishing point at the center of the colony (figure 22). Here we see the time-honored relationship between nature and culture: the outside and the inside, the bush and the village, the wild and the settled; here also we see the fragile mechanism by which the two are connected: by which the center is transformed by the outside; or the center transforms the outside; or the outside is captured and, as it were, "crucified."

At the margin the scope of what might be considered one's range of motion—that is, the variation in experiences that might be considered a part of one's chosen "path"—is considerable. As one travels toward the center (figure 22, *bottom*, area 1)—into the middle of the complacent culture—a number of things take place, but three tendencies are especially insidious for would-be cultural transformers. First, since the road itself gets narrower, the range of what can be understood as "different" decreases radically, because the clones inhabiting the center have dedicated what little remains of their identities to homogenization. Convincing themselves that they are breeding a "fittest" race, they single-mindedly work toward ignoring or victimizing genuine difference, while simultaneously exoticizing the familiar. Here, the smallest variation gets labeled as extreme: the field of medicine becomes obsessed with shape-changing growth hormones (that homogenize the small and the large) and behavior-modifying drugs (that lull our passions into complacent conformity). Andy Warhol mischievously thrills at a future in which we all look the same, while Erving Goffman complains that this homogenizing tendency leads to the worship of a monolithic ideal against which we all secretly fall short. It is the darkest side of the familial tendency to nourish—to desire to hurt that which is different because one cannot oneself experience it.

Second, since true difference must be eliminated in favor of homogeneity, the accoutrements of marginality become appropriated and cloned by the center as a false representation of its own supposed diversity—where the liminal gets ameliorated by the center (figure 22, *bottom*, area 2). The graffiti

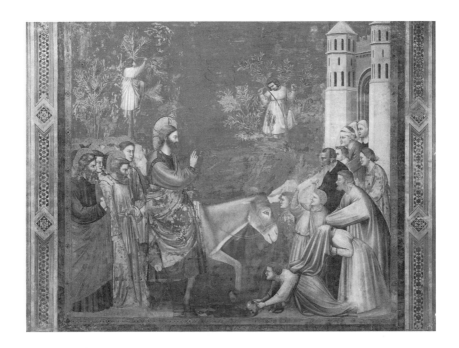

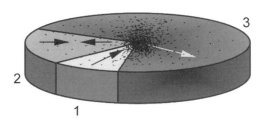

FIGURE 22. **From Periphery to Center**

The entry of Christ into Jerusalem (*top*) provides us with the best example of an entire religion being centered around the honoring of a victimized transformer. Like cell colonies, societies are also most alive at their peripheries where they are contested, challenged, and defined. In the diagrammatic representation of the relationship of the periphery to the center (*bottom*), we see the constrictive nature of movement from margin to center (as the breadth of "difference" becomes smaller). (*Top:* Giotto di Bondone [1266–1336], entrance of Christ into Jerusalem, Scrovegni Chapel, Padua, Italy. Copyright Alinari/Art Resource, N.Y. *Bottom:* Drawing by Carolann Davis and Andrew Napier.)

artist has his work appear not on a subway train but for sale in a gallery frame. The punk's pierced body becomes common boardroom chic. The regimented potluck dinner replaces real epistemological and cultural variation. For the once-liminal transformer, the normalization of what was previously danger-ous induces a sense that "magic" is no longer possible.

Third, and most common (figure 22, *bottom*, area 3), as one approaches the center, the spores made by cloned and dying cells to protect themselves not only converge upon, crowd out, limit, or openly destroy variation, but they set up a reflective wall of people that, to extend the image, cannot be seen over— a wall which functions to force the once-marginal transformer to see himself in the mirrors worn as masks by the Cartesian cells at the colony's center. As he reaches the center, the transformer's reflection gets closer and closer; his image in Veronica's veil induces the realization that the diversity of the world around him is merely a reflection of how he sees himself. Since, at the colony's very center, the domain of what might be accepted as "meaningful" has al-ready been drastically reduced, the scope of potential experiences that are considered feasible also gets smaller and smaller. In fact, only those with extraordinary transformational skills seem capable of surviving the colony's onslaught. This is why Christ's crucifixion can be viewed as a eulogy for the multitudes of would-be changers who get nailed in the process. This is why successful movers of the center are often described as threatening deceivers— for instance, as "shape-changers" among the Navajo Indians, or as "vampires" among Eastern Europeans who, let us not forget, believed that the vampire's ghoulish power was evidenced in its image not being reflected in those very mirrors held up to it by society. In this third relational form, the center often destroys the periphery.

But for those of us with less than supernatural abilities, the dilemma of de-ciding when to make the move from margin to center is quite complex, deci-sively subtle, and potentially hazardous. The homeless person who, after twenty years of shivering in doorways, comes into a clinic for help, may (if he escapes being drugged into conformity) never return again to that or any other clinic if the initial encounter fails. For there is so much invested in one moment—so much pride given up in the decision to walk the road inward— that even the social workers and therapists who are there to "help" the home-less may find the expectations of these "aliens" unfeasible if not entirely unac-ceptable. How, then, does that which is marginal influence the core of the empty vessel of culture? How can the decision to move from the outside in result in a positive rather than a negative transformation? How might the out-come of the dangerous journey from outside in be influenced by the very moment one selects for, as it were, "walking into Jerusalem"? Let us examine another time-honored example that we considered briefly in chapter 6.

In a quite extraordinary extempore lecture, the late Joseph Campbell compared Eliot's "The Waste Land" with its model, Wolfram von Eschenbach's early-thirteenth-century *Parzival*. Each concerns the challenges of the human soul trying to create meaning in a "land of people living inauthentic lives, doing what they think they have to do to live, not in the way of the spontaneity of love or of an affirmation of life, but dutifully, obediently, and even grudgingly, because that is the way people are living" (1981, 21).

Campbell's intention in comparing the two ages was to remind us of what we have herein identified as our immunological—and, when self-destructive, "autoimmunological"—historical moments: moments when, as Wilde once said, humans proceed to "kill the thing they love"; when a society, through neglect of its own mystical needs, punishes what it should have honored; when "a people's own inherent spirituality [is] cut down by an order of values radically out of accord with the order of nature itself" (ibid., 22). At such times, the spiritual courage required to risk social—even eternal—damnation in the interest of human love "typifies the heroism of anyone of that period thinking to live a life of his own. It has," Campbell continues, "something to say to us also of the power and courage of a perfect love in any age" (21).

For von Eschenbach (as for Eliot and Campbell), one who is alive can only respond to the conditions of a pathological era by an extraordinary compassion—a combination of disinterest in convention, of trust, and even of fasting. As so many shamanic initiation rites illustrate, a deep knowledge of the marginal—the borderlands—is required at such moments, and achieved through entrusting oneself to some "life-force," some eternal urge that is greater than convention, something we must allow to take and guide us. For Parzival, it was his horse that symbolized nature's vehicle of liberation; for once he gave himself over to nature, he was capable of finding his way—a relaxing of the horse's reins being the specific act of submission that allowed him to be carried to the castle of the young orphan queen, Conduiramurs (*conduire amour*). There, Parzival

> was received with interest, relieved of his armor, bathed clean of its rust, and
> that night, in his bed, awoke to find the young queen kneeling at his side.

"Lady," said he, "are you mocking me? One kneels that way only to God." She replied: "If you promise to be temperate, I shall lie then by your side." And neither he nor she, states the poet, had any notion of joining in love. Parzival lacked, in fact, all knowledge of the art, and she, desperate and ashamed, had come in misery of her life. In tears she told him of her plight. A neighboring king . . . had sent an army . . . to appropriate her land, when he would himself arrive and, in the good old way, make her his wife. (24)

At dawn on the following day, Parzival rides out to slay the king, an amazing feat for an unintended hero—in fact, an antihero (indeed, a simpleton) whose mother had earlier dressed him as a clown—a "shape-changer"—until, through combat, he was able to obtain the armor of a victim knight. When Parzival returned to Conduiramurs he found her dressed as a married woman:

She embraced him before all; her citizens paid him homage, and she declared him to be her lord and theirs. That night they were again in bed together, but, as Wolfram says, "he lay with her so decently that not many a lady nowadays would have been satisfied with such a night." Yet she thought of herself as his wife. Two days and two nights more they were together in this way, until, at last, enlacing legs and arms, they found the closeness sweet, and that old custom, ever new, had become theirs. No priest confirmed the marriage. It was confirmed in love and was itself the sacrament of love. And neither lust nor fear, but courage and compassion had been its motivations; indifference to social opinion having been prerequisite to its occurrence at all. What their world would have called good marriages had been by both rejected; and thus Parzival's first great step away from the Waste Land of the way of the world had been accomplished. (24–25)

Without attending here to the many magical elements of this legend—its initiatory rites, its numerical symbolism, its supernormal values and ways of seeing—one can still openly identify how Parzival's liminal wandering, like that of mystics modern and ancient, allowed him to transcend his fear of nature—how, that is, his self-imposed fast becomes the primary vehicle for risking his own being in order to redefine from society's periphery what a human relationship might be.

In *Sensuous Scholarship*, Paul Stoller describes the same process by means of an enigmatic encounter in a restaurant; there, a random event (the chance opening of a book) leads to a similar story of abandoned social convention. The story he recounts is one in which, during a discussion of fieldwork with a friend, a book of Sufi legends is arbitrarily opened to one about a saint named Mojud who arrives at his calling in a most unintentional and liminal fashion:

> Mojud was a moderately prosperous official in a Kingdom, who foresaw a promotion to Inspector of Weights and Measures. One day, however, Mojud saw the image of Khadir, the guide of the Sufis. Khadir told him to quit his job and present himself by the river's edge in three days' time. With much ambivalence, Mojud quit his very desirable job. His peers thought him crazy, but soon forgot about him. Three days passed and Mojud went to the river's edge where he saw Khadir, who ordered him to tear off his clothes and jump into the river. "We'll see if someone saves you."
>
> Mojud dived into the river and was swept downstream. Since he knew how to swim, he didn't drown, but the river's current carried him a long way. Eventually, a fisherman scooped him out of the water.
>
> The fisherman asked: "Why have you been in the river? You could drown."
>
> "I'm not sure," said Mojud. Having pity for the hapless survivor, the fisherman took him in. Mojud learned how to fish and taught the fisherman how to read and write. After five months Khadir appeared again and ordered him to leave. Mojud left reluctantly and walked along a road, where he encountered a passing farmer who wondered if he desired work. Mojud said yes. In this way, he spent two years with the farmer, during which he amassed savings. Khadir again appeared and told him to leave the farmer and use his savings to become a skin merchant. Although he liked his life on the farm, he journeyed to Mosul, where he became a well-known trader. After he had saved quite a bit of money, Khadir came yet again. This time he demanded that Mojud give away all his money and travel to Samarkand, where he would work for a grocer. Not knowing what to expect, Mojud obeyed. In Samarkand Mojud began to show signs of spiritual illumination. He healed the sick and advised the wise. As time passed, increasing numbers of people, old and young, rich and poor, came to him for guidance. In this way, Mojud, now a great Sufi, founded the Naqshbandi Order. (Stoller 1997, x–xi [after Shah 1970])

Mojud, in other words, achieves his calling by a trial of initiation in which the goal is not known at the outset. All he is aware of, in fact, is his phenomenal involvement. His ability to heal others is arrived at not by "education" but by addressing (quite unconventionally) his deepest need for experience, and by addressing that need through "fasting" from the conventional rewards toward which human intentions are normally directed. Mojud becomes, as it were, a *sadhu*, a renouncer, a holy pilgrim—one who lives out a life of marginality and accepts his peripheral existence because it is the only way for him to redefine the relationship between his spiritual yearning and his physical presence.[1]

As Eliot clearly envisaged in "The Waste Land," our contemporary age is also marked by the deep need to alter our destiny or face being victimized by it. But how, like Mojud, can we enough dissociate ourselves from our everyday desires—can we set aside, for instance, the consumer gluttony to which we have become so accustomed—that like him we might each facilitate our own becoming? Odd, isn't it, that an age characterized by both symbolic and real obesity should also be so characterized by anorexia? Odd, perhaps, until we acknowledge that anorexia is, in Mojud's terms, less an eating disorder than a drastic response to a society whose mouth is agape in anticipation of the silver spoon. Indeed, the very word, anorexia, supports this interpretation; for in Greek, it is opposed to *orektos*, meaning "longed for" or "desired."

In this view, anorexia is less the denial of nourishment than a sometimes fatal attempt to facilitate change, an "absence of desire" the goal of which is to take control of what seems uncontrollable, to redirect, even if harmfully, one's own destiny. Perhaps were our counselors and therapists more aware of this deep need they might themselves accept that fasting and liminality are the preconditions of transformation, preconditions that only become more exaggerated in an immunological era. The fasting of St. Francis or of any Buddhist monk shows this clearly, provided we find a way of stepping enough outside of our entropic world to see just how its laziness galvanizes responses that are increasingly exaggerated.

Perhaps, then, what distinguishes our era at the level of transformation is that we have offered no river of mutuality into which the impulse to separate is met by an impulse to merge, no mechanism of acknowledging separation as a valid way of achieving mutuality, no space where the initial risk is accompanied by a knowledge that even under conditions of extreme liminality one can have faith in another; for why else should so many of us impose upon ourselves such a dangerous abstinence except in the waning hope of yet achieving something greater—a mutual love of another, a dissolution into oneness? Referring to what he calls Schopenhauer's "beautiful essay" ("The Foundations of Morality"), Joseph Campbell asks:

> How it is that a human being can so experience the pain and peril of another, that, forgetting his own well-being, he moves spontaneously to that other's rescue? How is it that what we generally take to be the first law of nature, self-preservation, can be thus suddenly suspended, so that even at the risk of death one moves on impulse to another's rescue? And the answer that [Schopenhauer] gives is this: that such a move is inspired by a metaphysical truth and realization, namely, that we and that other *are* one, our sense and experience of separateness being of a secondary order, a mere effect of the way in which light-world consciousness experiences objects within a conditioning frame of space and time. More deeply, more truly, we are of one consciousness and one life. (1981, 29)

Is it any wonder, then, that the answer to Schopenhauer's "light-world" is a balancing of it with the darkness of the underworld—that is, Blake's "Marriage of Heaven and Hell," a cosmic regeneration where, "walking among the fires of hell, delighted with the enjoyments of Genius, which to Angels look like torment and insanity" one finds the particular giving way to the union of opposites where divisiveness is transcended in the experience of I and thou?

These experiences cannot, it is certain, be known by a self alone. Nor can their realities be understood and embodied without another. This is why love and invention are identical—why Parzival's wandering could only end as it did, in Campbell's notion of the transformation of a physical union into a metaphysical one:

> Though It is hidden in all things
> That Universal Self does not shine forth,
> Yet is seen by subtle seers
> Of subtle mind and subtle sight.
> (*Katha Upanishad*, 3:12)

Yet how does one learn to find the universal in the particular? How does one create a space where the particular can grow into a creation that is genuinely new? And how does one even begin to recognize the subtle signs of creative possibility while struggling to survive in a world that discourages transformation and the kinds of real risks that catalyze personal change? This is where the prior and persistent self becomes its own enemy, where depth psychology excuses us from confronting our own destinies, and where, as we will now see, our obsessions with self erode the possibilities for both love and creativity.

Put in Balinese terms, the problem of creativity—of why positive transformations should prevail over negative ones, of why life should ever prevail over pathology or entropy—always involves theology because religious transformation and illness are structurally identical, even if one more often has a positive and the other more often a negative outcome. Arguably, our intellectual examining of life is no less theologically based, even if science since Darwin at least has resisted acknowledging the fact. For, though we have lengthy and intellectually satisfying answers for why organisms pack up and turn to ash (indeed, all of medicine can be viewed as an explanatory mechanism for why living things fall apart), we do less well with understanding why a thing should live. While pathology dedicates itself to why living things die, science has more or less handed over to religion the spiritual question of why life prevails.

But why should the knowledge that something will remain ineffable itself settle, and at time defeat, our intellectual curiosity? Of course, it shouldn't. Nor should it bar us from acknowledging how our setting aside what is unanswerable often leads us unknowingly to offering scientific solutions that are covertly, and even naively, spiritual. Though the singular function of Maxwell's demon may have convinced scientists that they had remained agnostic, such animated specificity is, as we have seen, exactly what makes polytheisms work.

Try as we may, it thus seems as if each time we attempt a scientific explanation for why things ought to live and grow in an entropic and pathogen-ridden world, we end up in introducing some decisive entity that does nothing if not display our ignorance of forms of religious understanding that have been fully developed elsewhere. Maxwell's demon, to put things bluntly, is a poor substitute for a Balinese demon. Matzinger's danger model likewise possesses anthropomorphic qualities despite her intended goal of transforming immunology's self/nonself paradigm. More overtly still, Irun Cohen has argued that immunology needs yet a new demon—an "immunological homunculus" or "little man" to provide a cognitive paradigm for understanding how clonal selection is restricted and activated (1992a, 1992b; Cohen and

Young 1991). So how far have we come from Maxwell's basic "rediscovery" of an anthropological commonplace? If immunology is any test, not very; though now at least we can hope to acknowledge that our deepest and most creative explanations of why life persists are to be found in the domain of what some would call religion.

TIME AND TIME AGAIN

You know it's going to happen, so you remember it. —Harriet Napier's definition of déjà vu (at age 9)

In the *Fioretti*, the anonymous accounts of the life and deeds of St. Francis of Assisi, there is a chapter[2] devoted to the manner in which this saint of all that is natural passed Lent on an island in the middle of Lake Perugia, surviving his forty days on a mere half a loaf of bread. The story is one of transformation: Francis goes to visit a friend on Carnival Day (Shrove Tuesday), the traditional moment for both pagans and Christians when the inversion of all that is "normal" marks Winter's death through Spring's rebirth. Not coincidentally, as we will see, the friend of Francis lives next to Lake Perugia, in the middle of which is an uninhabited island. The following evening—that is, the night of Ash Wednesday—Francis is rowed to the island. He carries with him two loaves of bread to sustain him during his forty days. He asks his friend not to return until Holy Thursday.

> So the friend went away, and Francis remained alone. And finding no building where he could shelter, he went into a very dense thicket where thorns and other bushes formed a kind of arbour or grotto, and here he spent the time in prayer and contemplation. . . . eating . . . nothing but a half a small loaf [which he consumed] out of reverence for the fast of Christ the Blessed, who fasted forty days and forty nights without taking any bodily sustenance. So by eating half of this loaf he avoided the venom of vainglory, and at the same time followed the example of Christ in fasting forty days and forty nights. (Sherley-Price 1959, 41)

Francis, as it were, gained the indulgence of the Lord by not indulging himself. He avoids that which is potentially venomous by the near homeopathic consumption of grain at the seasonal moment when fertility goddesses around the world are emerging to celebrate the carnivalesque and carnal

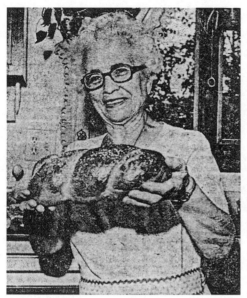

FIGURE 23. **Sowing New Life**
My late grandmother, whose family
came from near Pergusa, Sicily, inherited the ancient practice of giving bread.
Throughout peasant Sicily and aboriginal
Italy distributing loaves is understood as a
statement of one's commitment to sowing
goodness, creativity, and life. While doing
this is primarily seen as a female indulgence—one of caring and forgiveness—it
is also recognized as a quenching of male
desire. This latter idea is particularly true
at Carnival time (e.g., in contemporary
Sardinia) where men cross-dress in black
and are given loaves of bread to wear as
phalluses. As my grandmother used to say,
"You can have the best dough, but if you
don't have a hot hand your bread will
flop." (Copyright Charles Stueben/
Pittsburgh Post-Gazette, 2002. All rights
reserved. Reprinted with permission.)

transformation into new life (figure 23). Ash Wednesday, the ashen marking
of the forehead which all Hindus recognize as *naman* or the act of "naming,"
here symbolizes the birth of a new identity by the Catholic patron of all that is
wild and natural.

And how does he do this? By going out, by crossing the water, by marking
his transformation after carnival through an "inoculation" of wheat, an ingestion of minute amounts of grain product. While the crossing of water has always been a sign of significant transformation, it is the island in the middle
that marks the liminal "threshold" moment. And why, moreover, do we call a
doorway a threshold? Because this is the place where, when grain is separated,
it begins its new life as seed or as bread, where wheat is accumulated for making future bread, where the beating of the stalks produces the very seeds from
which flour is made. Life returns at this time, it is "reinvented" through marking or naming, through "vaccinating" the old self in honor of what it might
become. In keeping with the fertile occupations that are more commonly the
prerogative of spring goddesses worldwide, Francis brings bread to the transformational moment. The future is created by reinventing the past, since
one's sense of being, of "presence," is the outcome of an intimate embodiment

of both the old and the new. On this island of paradox, then, we simultaneously rediscover the key to new life and create that new life.[3]

But why make such a big thing of going back? In part because our obsessions with heroic narrative reaffirm for us a sense of time as a solely linear, historical, "specifying" process. We conceptualize change as entirely unilinear to
the degree that it takes an Einstein to bend the trajectory of time even imper-
ceptably; rarely do we allow it to dip at all, let alone circle back on itself in a
truly recursive way. Today, what few rites of passage survive tend to move us
from one stage to the next along life's path with little or no sense of time's recursive qualities. In turn, what this unilinear view of change invites us to do is
name the world around us far too quickly; to specify without context; to ap-
prehend, to fear, and ultimately to eliminate difference by rushing to categorize it. The perceived flow of life's narrative itself induces the belief that our
concepts of "progress" and "history" are universal, without recognizing the
way in which meaning is enriched by going out and coming back, or by going
back into the past and coming forward.

Today, more perhaps than before, the inclination to forget the past is seen
in the senseless process of naming things and experiences without any reference to their broader potential correlates. Man is a namer, an identifier, a la-
beler—but in our specified and masculinized world, we fail to remember the
biblical lesson that names mean nothing if they are, like the newest star or
hurricane, mere arbitrary references to a list of yet unused words, or to the
number on a particular test tube. William Powers by contrast says this of
Lakota Indian cosmology:

> Although the creation of the universe is seen by most people as a theological
> statement about first causes, one may look at the same stories profitably from
> the point of view of classification. The creation story in any culture is an at-
> tempt to put the chaotic universe that surrounds humans into some kind of or-
> der, and part of the mechanism used to accomplish this is the simple act of
> naming everything. (1986, 153)

Put, however, in Lakota terms, one cannot make sense of the past without employing it in a responsible "recursive" way that has meaning for the present.
Similarly, one cannot venture out onto an island of isolation and expect to return unharmed if one has not, first, accepted the delicate and dangerous

"naming" of one's time and place of reentry, if one has not literally "prayed" (i.e., thought recursively) about constructing one's reentry along an ellipse that is timely. Synchronicity here is the only thing that allows one to avoid a fiery descent. For the Lakota, one cannot embark on a vision quest without remembering one's obligation to reframe what is innate and primordial. The "quest" must be brought back, discussed, and reinterpreted by the priests or priestesses who devote their energies to reintegrating and recharging the still center. This is why in Hinduism priests who are close to earthly rulers (i.e., who gain power from politics) are always held with suspicion; for they are more likely to neutralize the powers of the margin in the interest of leaving the center untransformed.[4]

Although knowledge is, as it were, within each of us (i.e., not something external), it at best means nothing, and at worst it is harmful to us, unless we strive to recognize it through transcending the mundane. Likewise, among the Navajo, the act of realizing beauty becomes in itself a means of creating a link between nonhuman and human worlds. Beauty must be brought to life and lived; it is not a static, external byproduct or quality, but something that must radiate from us. Though the Navajo, like the Lakota, are keen observers and classifiers of the natural world, they do not look for beauty in observation itself; rather, each generates beauty and "projects it onto the universe" (Witherspoon 1977, 151); indeed, "the creation of beauty and the incorporation of oneself in beauty represent the highest attainment and ultimate destiny of man" (151). The work of culture, therefore, is to allow a seeker of new beauty—a "creator," a specialist in what we might call "the sacred"—"to do what society cannot do for itself" (Powers 1986, 176): to venture into the marginal where wisdom resides.

Such a goal of necessity requires separation because it is only by going out that one can come back: it is only in the domain of separation that creativity can begin, because it is here where the dichotomy between life and death can be mediated (ibid., 176). This is not only why we find rebirth and eternal return as primary themes of curing and of love, but why the deep illnesses of societies, as well as the concrete illnesses of individuals, must in the end be addressed by those who can take the journey of separation and find the path of reentry. Indeed, "if the collective group, society, could mediate its own concerns over life and death, there would be no need for ritual specialists" (176). What the specialist understands is that pathologies are transformable—that the deadly tumor is not only a pathology, but a form of uncontrolled growth.

What to everyone else looks like "an illness that can't be cured" is to the specialist "a compulsion to create that needs to be focused." What the specialist tries, therefore, to do is give shape to the compulsion to create that others can't control and that they therefore see as "incurable." The specialist understands that irregularities have potential, that antibodies need to appear random, that hysteria or "attention deficits" are actually the necessary basis of true change.

We all know in our heart of hearts that the center is a place of stillness, a place of waiting for a journey out. Groups, as Fredrik Barth (1969) has eloquently shown, define themselves by interaction with other groups at their borders, while the sacred itself is created anew by superimposing extremes; for "what happens at the extremes is essential. We must free ourselves from familiar ideas: we tend to put the essential at the center and the rest at the periphery . . . [but] that which encompasses, is more important than that which is encompassed" (Dumont 1970, 76); and when that which encompasses is the very catalyst for transforming an entropic center, we begin to see the paradox in the divine potential of every human being—we begin, in the words attributed to Empedocles, to see that God and those who can embody the divine are like a circle "whose center is everywhere and whose periphery is nowhere." Society, then, is of necessity also a circle, but one "whose central cells are, as we say, *nowhere*, and whose peripheral ones are *everywhere*."

Center and margin, village and bush, culture and nature, security and danger: these are all binary categories that are mitigated by those who attempt the creative crossing.[5] They are models of the petri dish of culture that directly challenge biology to think more "embryologically." Because our individualism is "center-focused," it not only dissuades us from living in beauty, but it also desensitizes us from recognizing the many ways that the margin and center are dynamically related: first, in the rare moment when an outsider, an "other," "possesses" the center and induces transformation; second, when the center appropriates and defuses the power of the unfamiliar by reshaping it; and, third, when the naming process simply alienates and destroys anything different. The first is love; the second, vaccinology; the third, immunology. This last is where we are now. The second we still see in the curious (the bohemian brought to the art gallery). The first is what we deeply need.

If pathology is a form of uncontrolled growth, why, we may rightfully ask, have Westerners not only so thoroughly separated illness from the domain of religion, but actually developed "immunological" relationships that first destroy difference outside and then turn us against ourselves? The answer is simple, and it is this: that we have yet to accept the deep consequences of Copernicus's great discovery—we have, namely, yet to see ourselves in any place but the center. It is a view, surprisingly, that is not universal:

> Whereas Euro-American science and theology understand humans to be the sine qua non of all living things, the Lakota see humans as the most humble. For whites, the humans were the last to inhabit the earth, and are therefore a crowning glory of all that preceded them. For the Lakota, humans were last, and that makes them newest, youngest, and most ignorant. (Powers 1986, 154)

What are the concrete effects of being last? What are the effects of knowing that in the organization of the world other systems antedate and are senior to ours? One only has to envision oneself in such a world to realize that being placed in a position of relative immaturity implies not jumping to conclusions about how the world is organized. After all, if there is a continuous relationship between the abstractions of nature and the classifications and categories that are part of human culture, Adam's job—the act of naming—cannot be properly accomplished without attending to how things might be understood by the swallow, the black-tail deer, or the meadowlark. This is not an act to be mistaken for poetry; it is a quite explicit mechanism for acknowledging one's "grandfathers" and "grandmothers," for a recursive returning to the past,[6] a bringing of the past forward, a deliberate *slowing down* when one is tempted to name the new prematurely.[7]

Identifying one's world must be accomplished carefully: don't rush to put a number on a test tube or a kind of cell, for you may misplace it easily in the broader scheme of things. Be conservative in what you call your world; bring your past forward into the present and you will also find that you have done what you can to place yourself favorably when the moment arrives to risk your next vision quest. For a future that is made up simply of goals to be reached, objectives to be met, and competitors to be overcome gives rise to a world that is just like the cloned gene that loses its chromosomes at its ends. It becomes attenuated, simpler, weaker, and eventually dead at the center—a so-called Terminator that kills others and even itself in a final attempt to cling to its unilinear mission; for at the center there is no deeply felt need to remodel the past at the margin where a new and yet-unknown future must be attempted.

This is not a hard concept to appreciate, but it does require a particular outlook on experience that is challenging and unfamiliar to modernity.

Put simply, placing humans at the center of the universe, or at the end of the Great Chain of Being, makes naming things too quickly an irresistible urge. Placing humankind at an exclusive center shifts the locus of wisdom away from the marginal places where it truly exists. This is why we all need to start replacing competition with thoughts of others, with embryology, with tolerance and generosity, even with goodness—why science, in the absence of artful living, will wallow in its own entropy. This is why we need to take ourselves away from the center, why we need to go out in order to come back, and why we must go back in order to go forward. This is why (scientists take note) real invention will not, and can no longer, take place only at the bench; why we rightfully see creation more in the worlds of the Navajo, the Lakota, or the Balinese than in our own. It is this recursive continuity to which so many traditional peoples refer when they succeed in creating "beauty"; for creating "beauty" in one's life is not merely a stimulus for birth and rebirth, but a necessity for meaningful discovery.

Conversely, to use one's intellectual skills to rush forward with one's inscribing tools in hand—to label and overspecify—may be the very ugliest aspect of our humaneness. There are many parables of the failures of such activities. Lewis Carroll's mapmakers (see chapter 5) provided one such example, but by extension any unilinear, marching forward (any "blind progress") can lead us not into a land of "exquisite specificity" but into a frightening domain of disharmony where a human being exists as what Metchnikoff, the founding father of immunology, once called "an ape's 'monster' . . . an abnormal, sick creature subjected to medicine" (quoted in Tauber and Chernyak 1991, 22).[8] It doesn't take a Luddite, an enemy of technical progress, to recognize this problem. All one need do is look closely at the outcomes of specificity.

ABOMINATIONS

As Lord Morpheus would have it the great stories always return to their original form.
—Michael Bristol, "Designing a Better Virus"

The "Black Hole" is a salvage yard in Los Alamos, New Mexico, the purpose of which is to recycle the castoffs of nuclear destruction. It is owned by a

retired defense industry employee who frequents government auctions in order to stock his vast establishment with all manner of bizarre and outdated
devices—things which we know were once meant for serious destructive purposes, but which now are the objects of applied fascination for artists, electri-
cians, and, well, anyone with an ability to accommodate the unthinkable. Two
dollars will buy you a cable used to detonate a nuclear bomb—that is, if one
can find the box that stores them beneath weird gauges, sensors, and plastic
sheets that gather what little rain falls in this part of the world (but yet leaks)
through the roof. Some people come in and out—others more or less "live"
there—but nobody leaves without being offered a five dollar can of fake plutonium[9] and a lecture about the nuclear holocaust that ends with the dramatic
appearance from beneath the counter of a soccer ball with its twenty hexago-
nal surfaces numbered to illustrate the shape of the actual detonator (figure 24).
Here it all is, the end of our enlightened existence, and the final testament to
the elimination of nonself. For the atomic bomb is an elaboration of a geometric principle built around one of nature's most powerful shapes, the icosahedron.[10]

From his impromptu counter-turned-lectern the proprietor will tell you
that you have to create a future that fully acknowledges current realities—
that "you have to begin from where you are"; that there is no sense in evoking
nostalgic sentiment about a world in which the objects that surround you in
the "Black Hole" did not exist; that these things are a part of us now, and we
have to do something about them. At this old store in a town of new-age
nightmares a mere twenty-sided object not only represents, but is, the very
shape that can name, without question, when the doors of the Enlightenment
will finally close.

Odd that the basic icosahedron has also long been known as "'nature's favorite shape' . . . because it is so common in viruses" (Stewart 1998, 70) (figure
25a). Odd, too, that the icosahedron is the precise shape that is honored by an
ancient alchemical monument put up in 1663 on the grounds of Holyrood
Palace (figure 25b), the official Scottish residence of the reigning monarch.

Do look at this emblem; for it is in effect the physical symbol, to recall
Descartes, of the "enlightened" elimination of difference—not the *formal relations* the isocahedron embodies, but the *form itself*—a devotion to a *specific
abstraction* of a sort that the Enlightenment favored, rather than to the *abstract
relations* that the shape embodies. Permit me this digression:

While it may be the very love of the *specificity of the shape* that was recog-

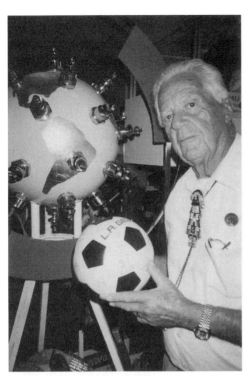

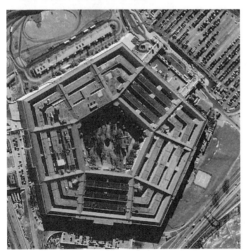
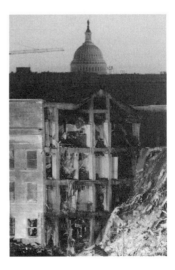

FIGURE 24A. **Ed Grothus, at "The Black Hole," Los Alamos**

A lecture on the icosahedral shape of a nuclear bomb may be taken in on most days at "The Black Hole" in Los Alamos, New Mexico. Ed Grothus runs this former supermarket, now filled with detritus salvaged from nearby nuclear labs. In addition to the business, Grothus is the founder of the First Church of High Technology, an adjacent A-frame building dedicated to "turning wine into water—heavy water, the isotope." Grothus calls his church a "church of destruction" with Los Alamos as its "holy temple." (Photo by author.)

FIGURE 24B. **The Virus of Terror**
The terrorist bombings of September 11, 2001, show horrifically how one power symbol (the Pentagon, shown before and after) becomes itself the victim of that amorphous social "virus" now known as a terrorist "cell." (Reproduced courtesy of spaceimaging.com.)

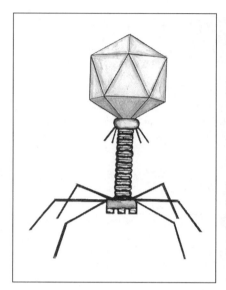 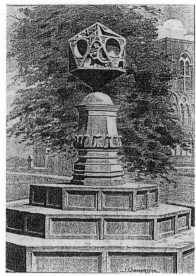

FIGURE 25A. **Mature Bacterial Virus (Bacteriophage)**
Though viruses assume many shapes, the common blueprint is an icosahedral DNA capsule mounted
to a stem through which that DNA is drawn into a host cell. (Drawing by author.)
FIGURE 25B. **Sundial, Holyrood Palace, Edinburgh, Scotland**
Put up in 1633 by order of Charles I, the Holyrood Sundial stands, according to Fulcanelli (1960), as
the emblem of royal support for a secret society of freemasons and alchemists (the Order of the Thistle)
who considered themselves the descendants of the Knights of the Round Table. Why a sundial in this
shape? Because the march of the sun stood for intellectual clarity, and the form of the regular
icosahedron was the crystal shape controlled by the subterranean spirits (*gnomes*) that guarded the
secrets of the precious metals. The form was thus understood since Gnostic times as the symbol of
gnomon, the "spirit of intelligence," a key to esoteric knowledge. (Drawing by J. Champagne.)

nized in, and honored since, the Enlightenment, the seeds for this reverence
are more mystical and much earlier. They were already well known by the
Greeks (the icosahedron is one of the five "platonic" bodies of the neo-
Pythagoreans),[11] but they were probably recognized earlier still.[12] Though
these shapes are very common (the soccer ball is an Archemedian solid), in the
Enlightenment there was a definite shift from a focus on the relations they
made possible to the idolizing of the shape itself. Up until that time, it was the
proportional relations that were the keys to unlocking those component parts
that were though of in quite spiritual terms.

   Leonardo of Pisa, the thirteenth-century mathematician who invented
what we now call the Fibonacci sequence, was literally entranced by the rela-

tions made possible as the result of the numerical inventions of the Hindus and Arabs. What he did was to recognize that there was a *formal relation* between numbers each of which (after the number 3) was the sum of the previous two (i.e., 1, 2—then—3, 5, 8, 13, 21, 34, 55, etc.). Similarly, recognizing the relations of those same numbers made it possible for John Napier to discover logarithms at the dawn of the Enlightenment; for Napier, as for Leonardo, the formal relations themselves had mystical properties: unless one sees how these numbers function relationally, they are simply meaningless. Seen, however, *together*, they offer a window onto something that verges on the divine; for they can provide a structure for some of nature's most beautiful shapes—like the numbers of spirals that are expressed on sunflowers, or the shape of the nautilus shell. Even today, though the experimental method has quelled embryology, sentiment around these relational abstractions runs very deep: "there's an even chance that the supreme creator, if such a being exists, is a mathematician" (Gunn 1997, 23). Leonardo's love of numbers was religious, and Napier, let us not forget, was an alchemist who was deeply involved in magic, as well as in, among his many other occupations, an antipapal demonstration of the mathematical perfections of the biblical book of Revelation. He really did object to the embryologic fascination of the Vatican with the Virgin Mary!

The beauty of the nautilus rests, then, not in its individual chambers but in its part-whole relationships that increase logarithmically. Like the famous Golden Section, the chambers of the nautilus are sized by dividing "any object in two so that the ratio of the smaller piece to the larger is the same as the larger piece to the whole" (ibid., 24). By using Fibonnaci numbers as a tool, one can see the Golden Section logarithmically made real in growth and form (figure 26).

What made the discoveries of Leonardo and Napier compelling, in other words, was not the specific numbers that might be inscribed by some computer operator on the window of an instrument, but *the generality*—i.e., what they allow us to conceptualize embryologically. For each, focusing too much on specificity produces something like Frankenstein's monster, an agglomeration of "stitched together" categories that bear no relation to one another.

What one gets through excessive inscription, to extend the analogy, is a nautilus made up of unrelated objects—a malformation, a teratoma,[13] a dysfunctionally growing tumorous mass of teeth, nails, and other deformed body

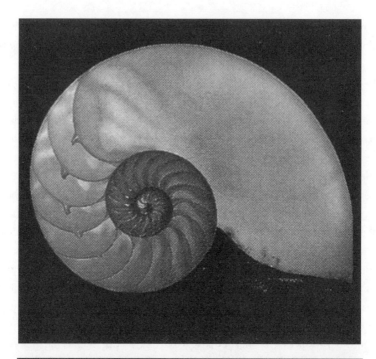

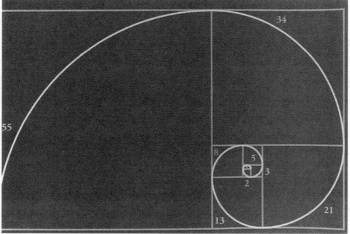

FIGURE 26. **Spiral in the Golden Section**
A Golden Section is achieved when any ratio of a smaller piece to a larger one is the
same as the larger one to the whole. Here the nautilus expresses this relationship
parabolically as what mathematicians call a *Napierian logarithm*. (*Top:* Photo by Heather
Angel, used with permission. *Bottom:* Diagram by Trevor Bounford,
www.bounford.com, used with permission.)

parts. Either that, or one gets a Scottish version of the Frankenstein monster. And one must wonder, really, if Mary Shelley's fabricated creature wasn't itself an altogether "Holyrood" invention of a most maniacally specified sort.[14]

So why the importance of this shape and other polyhedra for the Enlightened destruction of difference? Because they are there for a *reason*: each is a so-called "minimal-energy" shape—an embodiment of energy conservation, an efficient solution, a thermodynamic dream, a weapon of progress, a line of least resistance. The numbers of their faces

> play a special role in the structure of a virus—just as Fibonacci numbers play a special role in the structure of a plant. In fact, magic numbers are the numbers of identical protein units that can be fitted together in an almost regular way, to form a nearly spherical surface. . . .
>
> It would be difficult to find more compelling evidence than this patterning of DNA, RNA, and viruses to show the importance of mathematical patterns in making life possible—certainly earthly life, the only kind we know. DNA plays the role that it does because of a simple geometric pattern, the double helix. In a sense, it's more a *logical* pattern, for the key feature is not the helix, but the complementary pairing of bases. It is this pattern, which exists as much in the abstract as in any physical law, that evolution used as a basis on which to create life on Earth. On its foundations, other patterns were erected, in particular the quasi-mathematical enigma that is the genetic code. (Stewart 1998, 70–72)

Thus, the minimal-energy shape is an abstraction designed to win out—to be named and replicated, to recruit allies and eliminate alternatives: in short, the shape honors itself, as it does in Edinburgh, as a trophy of its abstract nature—a key to its power. Is it any accident, then, that the isocahedron, and the spiral or helical coil to which it is formally related, are nature's favorite "viral" shapes? Yet again we find ourselves arriving at a uniform truth that appears to have been articulated since prehistoric times (figure 27).

Is it any accident that in these shapes particular numbers, like uncommitted genes in sequence,[15] have no specific meaning? Like the genetic double helix that has been deified by modern science, or the mystery of the similarly helical number "9,"[16] we create an emblem of the Fibonnaci coil without recognizing that its power resides (as does that of DNA) more in the relations it encompasses than in the numbers or genes which make up its component parts.

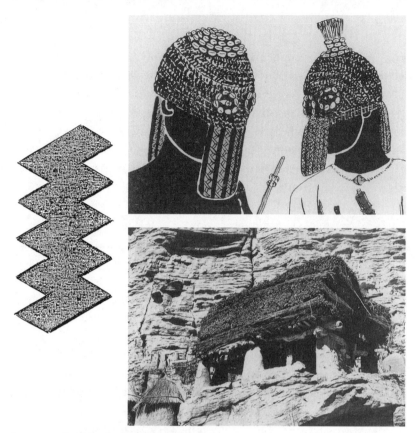

FIGURE 27. **Realizing the Symbolism of Words**

The coil reflected as an unfolded icosahedron (*left*). The icosahedron and the coil are nature's favorite viral shapes because they are essentially the same thing.

Among the Dogon of Mali, the first human garment was made of coiled fringes, its helical threads being "the chosen vehicle for the words which the Spirit desired to reveal to the earth. He [the spirit] endued his hands with magic power by raising them to his lips while he plaited the skirt, so that the moisture of his words was imparted to the damp plaits, and the spiral revelation was embodied in the technical instruction. . . . Thus clothed, the earth had a language, the first language of this world and the most primitive of all time. Its syntax was elementary, its verbs few, and its vocabulary without elegance. The words were breathed sounds scarcely differentiated from one another, but nevertheless vehicles. Such as it was, this ill-defined speech sufficed for the great works of the beginning of all things" (Griaule 1965, 20). For the Dogon, these first words are not only vaporous lines of rising desert moisture but the first covering of the womb (the "mouth") of the earth; for when Dogon ancestors speak, what comes forth "is a warm vapor which conveys, and itself constitutes, speech" (20). Like water, this vapor has a sound which follows the path of the helicoid line before dying away. Dogon skirts, masks (*top right*), and even ritual houses are thus frequently constructed of coils, for each of these reifies "the first act in the ordering of the universe and the revelation of the helical sign in the form of an undulating broken line" (20).

The ideal ritual space, as in the men's ritual hut or *toguna* (*bottom right*), is made of eight ancestral posts set out in a coiling sequence with a massive low roof of woven ("coiled") millet stalks. The roof, or "head," of the building thus becomes "a sea of words" touched by all who enter. For the Dogon, man is the original specifier or "namer." (*Left:* Drawing by author. *Top and bottom right:* Drawing and photo by M. Griaule, © Publications Scientifiques du Muséum national d'Histoire naturelle, Paris.)

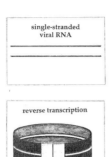

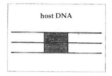

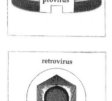

FIGURE 28. **Creations of the Golden Ratio**
Reverse transcription creates the pentagonal virus (*left*). The protein capsid of a retrovirus is typically icosahedral and contains two copies of the viral RNA genome and molecules of reverse transcriptase. The pentagon is related to the Golden Ratio as follows (*below*): "Any diagonal of a regular pentagon in ratio to its sides is golden [such that BC/AB = a Golden Ratio]; and extending any side of a pentagon gives the golden ratio [that is, AD/AB]" (Balmond 1998, 187). (*Left:* Drawing by author. *Below:* Drawing by author, after Balmond.)

Despite the sometimes selfish preoccupations of those who sequence genes or patent molecules, it is clear that the viral powers of the helix and the icosahedron both stem from the way in which these forms *dissolve* the very boundaries of the specific, of that which can be named, of identity. For the helix and the icosahedron are essentially the same thing—a proviral unwinding of genetic material—because the Golden Ratio provides the template for a kind of geometric reverse transcription (figure 28). Like the process of circumambulation, movement in one direction around a given thing (say moving clockwise) results in the thing circumambulated progressing in the opposite direction (in this case counterclockwise). Slice around the inside of a grapefruit half tomorrow morning and you will see the relation precisely.[17]

What we "see," then, is not a *thing* but a thing realized as a *relationship*, something only arrived at by the simple process of subdivision of a line so that each larger part is to each lesser part as the whole is to the larger part. At the risk of appearing metaphysical, it is a thing possessed—a thing that is nothing without its "other," bent slightly by its opposite—where identity becomes relational, and, in so doing, finally gives way to its own becoming.

So why the icosahedron as nuclear detonator? Because the Golden Ratio allows for a focus on a thing as a multiplication of powerful relationships. Indeed, this is also true at the most mundane level: what, for instance, gives even the common soccer ball its shape is not the twenty hexagons but the twelve pentagons; for any diagonal created within a regular pentagon is in ratio to its sides Golden, and extending any side of a pentagon gives, alas, a ratio that is also Golden. The pentagon, in other words, bends the otherwise flat pattern, and its "Golden" nature assures that its overall shape will focus its energy in the most efficient manner.

The pentagon and the spiral—the basis of the Golden Ratio of a line and of a soccer ball—are thus two versions of the same thing; for the helical shape is merely the outcome of a distortion that would prefer to be planar.[18] If this weren't interesting enough, it is the truncated nature of this particular icosahedral shape (of twenty hexagons and twelve pentagons) that itself causes the moving soccer ball to curve madly as it spirals through space.[19] As Balmond points out in his remarkable book on the spiraling number 9: "No wonder the pentacle is deemed to be magic" (1998, 187).

How much more "magical" can things get? In short, much more. It may well be, for starters, that it is not the outwardly facing base pairs of Watson and Crick, but the stacking of ever-growing pentagons (created by facing base pairs inward) that, in fact, gives DNA its correct dimension and true form (figure 29, *left*). Indeed, the combining of the helix and icosahedron have even been implicated in the shaping of carbon molecules, producing (of all things!) a pentagonal nautilus (figure 29, *right*). More mysterious still is the fact that— like Wittgenstein's rope, Vygotsky's chain complex, and Needham's polythetic class[20]—this shape (known as Kroto's "icospiral") becomes scientifically unloved *precisely because its loose ends defy closure* (Balmond 1998, 123)—i.e., because it is *unspecified*—that is, living and growing!

Thus, the nautilus shell unfolds and folds within itself creating an endless relation of chambers, none of which can be understood in isolation. Within the nautilus, identity cannot be named—a fact so well understood by Jules

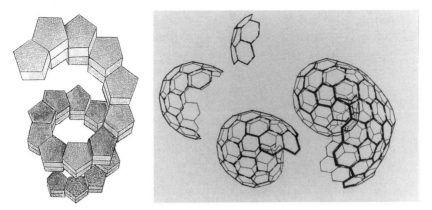

FIGURE 29. **The Pentagonal Secret of Life**
By turning the pairing of bases (of adenine with thymine, and guanine with cytosine) inward rather than outward, British artist Mark Curtis has created a model of DNA that (unlike the original 1953 model of Watson and Crick) actually conforms to sound geometric principles (*left*). In Curtis's model, the inward pairing of pentagons makes possible a spiral of the known dimensions of DNA. Though the model will not always conform to "ordinary" DNA, it provides a structure that is both functional and sequence-*specific.*

Though its significance is still highly contested, the combination of the icosahedron and the spiral has produced what is now called the "icospiral" (*right*)—a nautilus-like shell form that "combines the two most bioemotive shapes, the helix and the icosahedron" (Aldersey-Williams 1995, 122). (*Left:* Drawing by author, after Mark Curtis. *Right:* From Aldersey-Williams 1995, p. 122. Copyright © 1995 by Hugh Aldersey-Williams. Reprinted by permission of John Wiley & Sons, Inc.)

Verne when he named his submarine *Nautilus,* and captained it by a man named Nemo—a specifier, a "Captain No One," a being without relations (figure 30).

Discovering logarithms and recognizing Fibonnaci numbers—in short, seeking new kinds of relational understanding—are searches for what phenomenologists call nothingness (no-thingness), searches that require diverse kinds of obsessive compulsion that, when enacted successfully, get renamed as spiritual exercise.[21] And let us not forget the Lakota injunction that to name is an inferior, but necessary, condition of social life; it is not an end in itself but an acceptable compromise, a sometimes inadequate but socially important way of addressing the structure of the universe. In the commodified world of seventeenth-century Europe, that which would otherwise have been spiritual got reduced to something already avulsed from empathic relations. By the dawn of the Enlightenment, our theorizing had literally run away with us. The possibility of controlling the universe suddenly went to our heads, as the eighteenth-century obsession with the reshaping of nature made clear. And in

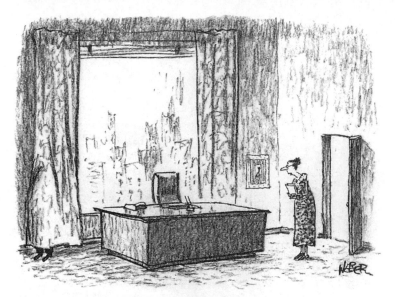

"No man is an island, Mr. Napier."

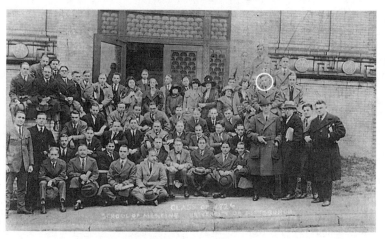

FIGURE 30. **Is There Anything in a Name?**
As Bernini said, a great work of art transforms a flaw into the central focus of a creative act. The invention of logarithms, of the decimal point, and of what is arguably the first true calculating machine allowed John Napier, the sixteenth-century Scottish mathematician, to transcend the ghost of "Mr. Nobody" (i.e., *nay per,* "no person") (*top*). Traditionally, the surname Napier meant "nay peer," "no peer" (i.e., "no equal").

My paternal grandfather, and childhood best friend, was not (as was John Napier) an alchemist, but a gifted chemist, whose response to being stigmatized (ethnically insulted) ended in his throwing a medical school professor down a staircase. Though the man was unharmed, my grandfather never graduated from medical school. Instead, he turned to his other love, applied chemistry. Here we see him in his medical school graduation photograph (*bottom*), taken just before the "incident" that made him a medical nobody (*nay per*). (*Top:* © The New Yorker Collection 1997 Robert Weber from cartoonbank.com. All rights reserved. *Bottom:* From author's collection.)

the absence of any deep contact with the phenomenal world, the idea of dealing with the past in an embodied, creative way, alas, disappeared. The only recourse left was to find the "others" (the "outsiders") and hurt them—to develop strategies that allowed for the recognition and elimination of their identities as "nonselves." Well, there was another recourse: to dissect ourselves into a horrid kind of specificity.

MARGINAL MARY

Not that faire field

Of Enna, *where* Proserpin *gathring flours*

Her self a fairer Floure by gloomy Dis

Was gatherd, which cost Ceres *all that pain*

To seek her throught the world; . . .

—Milton, *Paradise Lost*

If each human exists on earth as "an ape's monster," is it a fair assumption to conclude that paradise is, as Milton would have it, forever lost? That Milton should associate the abduction of Persephone (Proserpin) with such loss raises less the question of why her abduction by Hades (Dis) should so obviously symbolize the masculine ruination of the earth, than it does the question of why that lost paradise should lead to the tireless wandering of Demeter (Ceres). Because Demeter's love knows no end, because she never stops trying, the strength of the mother—ancient and Miltonian—is a recursive one: the search for Persephone is a search not to reconstruct lost unity, but to construct unity recursively. One has to remember before one can forget. Persephone will, forever more, be subjected to the one-dimensional linearity of Hades' emotional (phallic) needs; though she has been vaccinated by the taste of death, she will return each growing season to defy the common belief that the deadly Hades will defeat life. Persephone, in contemporary language, defeats entropy.

At the geographical center of the island of Sicily there still today can be seen the lake—traditionally believed to have no earthly inlet or outlet—through which Hades abducted Persephone into the underworld (figure 31). In the preclassical era, long before Syracuse vied with Athens as the center of Greek culture, this lake, Pergusa, had already been acknowledged as a center of ancient goddess worship. Indeed, this mysterious legend about fertility and seasonal change not only accounted for the widespread worship of a feminine

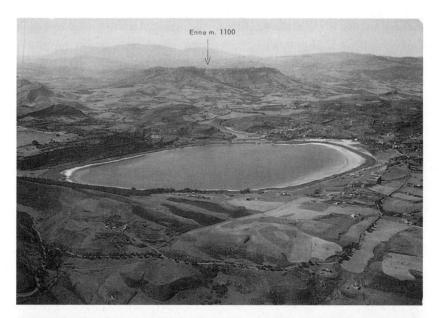

Enna m. 1100

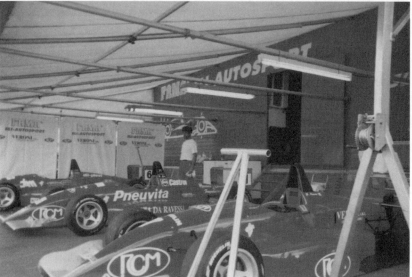

FIGURE 31. **Pergusa**

The still lake, Pergusa, the "umbilicus of Sicily," is the primordial site of Hades' abduction of Persephone (*top*; the plateau of Enna appears in the background). Today Lake Pergusa is surrounded by a high-speed automobile racetrack (*bottom*, pit area). In circumambulating this most symbolic site, do "boy-racers" honor the Goddess, Persephone, or attempt to contain her wrath? (*Bottom*: Photo by author.)

goddess in ancient Sicily but was also the source of Greece's most important feminine cult in far-off Athens. That the greatest Greek cult of the feminine—the worship of the wheat goddess, Demeter, at Eleusis—had its basis in a Sicilian rather than a Greek tradition of fertility is plain. For Lake Pergusa had been a site of earthly feminine worship since neolithic times, and the depth and pervasiveness of its cultural meaning is evidenced in its sharing the prefix of its name with a number of other words having to do with the underworld, with transformation, and with identity. Persu (phersu), for instance, was long ago recognized by Altheim (1929) as some kind of "leader" of Etruscan funerary rites. And Persephone spends half of the year with Hades, god of death.

Thus, while we tend to think of the worship of Persephone as a "Greek" invention, her origins are clearly more ancient. Indeed, mainland Italy has its own geographically centered lake, whose name, Perugia (yes, the lake of St. Francis), lends credence to the idea that the Greek legend is but an assimilative reworking of an ancient pre-"Greek" myth concerning creation and fertility. That we must not trivialize its significance is clear from the ancient use of its prefix: for per- (persona, personare, Perseus, and even Percival [Parzival]) is also the basis for our word, "person," having since prehistory been synonymous with identity and, more specifically, with a person and his or her contextualized, social, even anonymous, role.

It is thus no accident that the name of St. Francis's lake (Perugia) shares its prefix with Persephone's lake (Pergusa). For per-, our "person," was also once an identifier—but one who understood identity as a recursive act that brought the past into the present. Indeed, the later masculinizing of what "naming" might mean (in the archetypal shift from the feminine use of Per- [Persephone] to the masculine use [Perseus]) goes hand in hand with the attempt to sterilize their wildness and power—to replace, as it were, nature with culture. The Christian fathers, in other words, knew exactly what they were doing not only in construing Adam as "man the namer" but in assuring that we would remember how Francis, the masculine patron saint of the wilderness—"the man who could not get killed," as Chesterton put it—spent Lent on an island in Lake Pergusa eating a homeopathic dose of bread; for Francis, like Merlin before him,[22] was a wildman, a "seer" who endeavored to make nature masculine.

That Persephone is so clearly the embodiment of recursive femininity, of embryological awareness, is obvious in the extent to which patriarchal Greece felt compelled to overcome her. This they did by giving Perseus, their great masculine culture-hero, the prefix of her name: by the Classical period, by the era to which the West would come arrogantly to attribute the birth of civilization, Perseus was widely thought to have begun the Mycenaean patriarchy by slaying the "female leader" (Medusa). Temples depicting this act were especially found at new frontiers of Greek culture in Asia Minor, along the shores of the Black Sea, and even in Sicily itself—i.e., in the very places where this new image of authority was propagated—and coins minted especially for foreign trade were favored with images of the gorgon head. Per-, in other words, was both an indicator and an emblem of a kind of identity that today is most unfamiliar, one distinctly at odds with the patriarchal version we have inherited from the Greeks by way of the Enlightenment.[23]

How right, then, that this should also be the time when the *specific* names of great tyrants and authors should also supplant those of the gods themselves as conveyors of wisdom and truth. It can, in other words, be no accident that both civilization and identity begin, as we have come to know them, with the fathering of the line of Mycenaean kings by Perseus. Like the pagan spirits appearing as gargoyles on medieval cathedrals, the previous order gets put down by demonizing, as it were, the gods of the folks from across the river: their powerful spirits become our devils; their heroes our villains; their ancestors Ham's fallen descendants.

Though no longer applauded, this earlier, embryological form of female power is still known. It persisted, and still lives on, in the environs of Lake Pergusa; for, in nearby Enna, just a few kilometers from the lake, there stood until just after the Second World War a most extraordinary statue of the Virgin and Child in the cathedral built on the site of, and out of some stone from, the ancient temple to the Great Goddess—by Greek times now "Demeter"— and her daughter. Up until the papacy removed this scandal, the locals had been worshipping Mary and Jesus in the form of an ancient idol of the Goddess and her daughter![24] Mary is Demeter; Demeter is Persephone; and Persephone some prehistoric form of Mother Earth.[25] It's not that Jesus was a woman; rather, that procreation, re-creation, reincarnation—the retroviral—were all embodied in the feminine. Like the Lakota honoring the classificatory ambivalence of power,[26] the need to reaffirm life in an otherwise volatile Sicilian world overrode any recognition of the kind of unilineal history that male patriarchy (Perseus for the Greeks; David for Christians) represented. In such a world the new year was itself understood as a historical recapitulation of what it means, and could possibly mean, to be human—where fertility and reproduction are a part of accepting the nonspecific and universal nature of an event's "embryological" meaning.

Why should we be surprised that recursive thinking has had, as it were, such an underground existence? After all, even much later, in seventeenth-century Rome, we see the worship of Mary in a church built on the ancient shrine whose name openly acknowledges the mother goddess, Minerva (Santa Maria Sopra Minerva), and in Sicily at the same time we see at the Baroque Cathedral of St. Mary in Syracuse (Santa Maria del Piliero) the most beautiful conflation of an ancient mother goddess shrine into the actual structure of the cathedral (figure 32). Here, the local spring to the underworld is honored in a continuous architectural program: viewed from the side, one sees the ancient Doric temple to Athena (i.e., Minerva) emerging from the very walls of the cathedral: here, as in Enna, one finds remnants of the ancient shrine recon-structed for Christian purposes, but with no concessions to its feminine obli-gations. Fifth-century B.C. columns honor the prehistoric site, and immedi-ately adjacent to these columns we find seventeenth-century Baroque versions of ancient Greek architectural form. For at least 2,500 years, the "identity" of this site and its resident spirit have assimilated at its borders all like spiritual forms. The feminine goddess stands—as she briefly did in seventeenth-century Rome—as the all-inclusive "Mother."

While those who have studied Greek religion and the origins of Western civilization have often been chastised when they locate these "origins" in a transition from nature worship to patriarchy and "enlightened" specificity (i.e., to the birth of the intellect), there is surely something to be said for the idea. After all, the very concept of intellectuation is an outcome of certain culture-specific notions of individuality. There is without doubt a clear differ-ence between the most famous of Greek thinkers—say, a "Homer" who is widely recognized as an inspired genius—and a Virgin Mary whose Annunci-ation—whose circumstantial chosenness—exemplifies the way in which com-mon goodness and basic desire can transcend self-centeredness. The first, in the least, downplays its antecedents—in fact, it may argue, as would a patent attorney of some new idea, or a Classicist speaking of Western thought, that no antecedents exist. The second draws its meaning from a long line of asso-ciations regarding how the truths of the past are brought forward. In the first case, power devolves by claiming sole ownership; in the latter, power is an inchoate sensation whose morality is determined by the way in which one

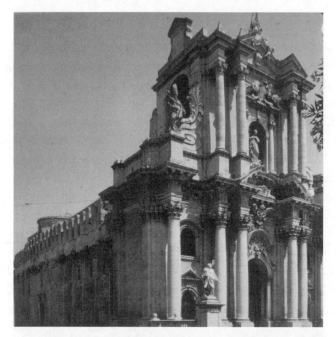

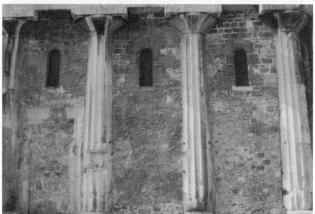

FIGURE 32. **Santa Maria del Piliero, Syracuse**

Though the facade of this cathedral is Baroque (1728–54), the structure is built around the remains of a Doric temple (to Athena) dating from the fifth century B.C. Here, in other words, we see quite remarkably how the identity of the Virgin Mary is associated with her acknowledged ancestors, her "identity" being recognized as an extension of what, to the mind of a specifist, would appear as "nonself"—i.e., as at best a loose association of a specific name to an ancient one with which she could be aligned. Instead, Mary's authority derives directly from Athena by way of her Roman equivalent, Minerva. Archaeological investigations, and a nearby sacred spring, both attest to the fact that the worship of local earth goddesses is much more ancient than what is already astonishingly visible. (*Bottom:* Photo by author.)

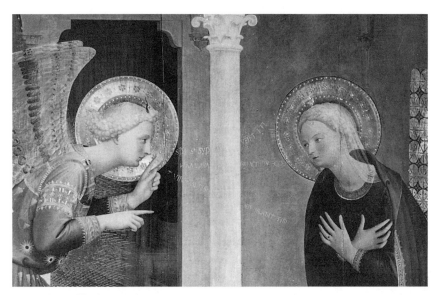

FIGURE 33. *The Annunciation*
In this beautiful fifteenth-century example of a popular theme, we see how human desire is directed in the service of goodness. At the dawn of the Renaissance it was popularly believed that certain images of the Annunciation had power in themselves, and, furthermore, that this power derived from an ancient iconographic lineage. Frequently, the encounter of Mary and the angel occurs at a basilican crossing, the Christian location of the ancient notion of the conjoined male and female powers. In this case the word is made flesh as it crosses a column that clearly divides the figures. The words of the angel are transformed into creative life as they physically transcend the symbolic threshold that the column represents—spoken first by the angel in Latin prose, but returning to him from the Virgin both inverted and backward. (Fra Angelico [1387–1455], *The Annunciation*, Museo Diocesano, Cortona, Italy. Copyright Alinari/Art Resource, N.Y.)

responds to uncertainty. The first is moved by reason, the second by desire—a sensibility quite stigmatized because it "impels us toward an object in anticipation of pleasure" (Edinger 1994, 48). This is where the maternity of the Virgin Mary, and especially her Annunciation, correlates desire to a specific action, because the naming of desire allows us to understand it as "an assignment of a difficult task" (48) (figure 33).

Although Mary's maternal desire and her Annunciation are really the same thing, how they are experienced depends on what psychologists would call "the level of psychological development" (ibid.)—or, to put it philosophically, the degree to which one can create by reaching into the past in that healthy, good way that only desire can facilitate. Again, Mary is Minerva; Minerva is Demeter; Demeter is Persephone; and Persephone is Mother Earth herself.

Or, as was briefly accepted in that brilliant moment of the Counter Reformation, Mary is Divine Wisdom who was initially "incarnated in the Egyptian Isis, then in the Greco-Roman Minerva, and ultimately, in its purest exponent, the Mother of the Lord Herself" (Heckscher 1947, 180). It is, of course, not coincidental that the Counter Reformation was also a time for extraordinary "annunciations" of desires, manifested as spiritual exercise.

As lived and believed in the traditions of the Navajo or Lakota, our "annunciation" as humans is to recreate beauty by focusing desire on goodness. The question of how we can, or whether we at all can, tap these awarenesses in a post-Enlightenment world, remains open; for merely to acknowledge and assign gendered ideologies to particular historical or cultural moments offers nothing in the way of resolving what one does now. Nostalgia about the past can provide no answer; nor can reactionary responses that are realized in anger. That these can never be healthy is, as we saw in chapter 4, made abundantly clear by the reciprocal nature of hegemony, especially as such collusive relationships are understood (by, for instance, Gramsci, Leotard, and Fanon) as enslaved reactions to existing conditions—as the dynamic "combination of force and consent variously balancing one another, . . . an active and practical involvement of the hegemonized groups, quite unlike the static, totalizing and passive subordination implied by the dominant ideology concept" (Forgacs 1988, 423–24).

How, then, is collusion with the oppressor transcended? Although the "Madonna" of Enna attests to an ancient time in the central Mediterranean when the tribute to some feminine or androgynous force was central to the conceptualization of human nature, simply romanticizing such practices (or, worse yet, mimicking them) provides no guidance in itself with respect to how one might gain similar sensibilities in an immunological age. How, to put it directly, is one moved today to leave the still center in search of new meaning? How does one engage in a personal reconstruction that does not seem self-indulgent? How does one transcend the collusive relationships that constantly encode experiences as a struggle against tyranny? The temptation, of course, is to embody the opposite of what is offered. This is anorexia—literally "the absence of desire"—a strategy that can never work because, in avoiding basic human needs, it induces a fear of one's own curiosity, an autoimmunity in which the need to be different results in being enslaved to the values one would otherwise hope to have transcended. If society is perceived to be "all wrong," and people are "right" to think it wrong, all that is meaningfully left is either an actionless sense of nostalgia and guilt—a moment of inactivity that at best merely offers the illusion of a better life—or a psychological condition that thrives on the fantasy of what might otherwise have been. Of course the two are identical. The pain of shunning desire leaves pain itself as our only source of meaning.

No wonder we force ourselves into deluded encounters with difference that aren't actually encounters. No wonder our sense of what is different gets constructed around a repeated failure to tolerate destabilization. No wonder there is no discourse in anorexia (or in feminism, for that matter) in which giving oneself over to desire becomes both the only and the best way of remolding the tyranny under which we perceive ourselves to live (figure 34).[27]

Is such new living possible? Of course it is. One only has to take the step toward bringing the marginal to the liminal—allowing the periphery to function as a catalyst for transformation (for crossing the *limen* or threshold, for the "possession" of love)—in order to sense what is possible. One only has to see—as we saw with the great Baroque artist, Bernini—the beauty in those very flaws, to make them the center of one's art, to discover through living one's desires a pleasurable way of illustrating that nothing is inevitable.

I believe that unless one can tap some powerful sense of empathy—one that is generated emotionally and physically at a very deep level—there is no way to distinguish the uncertainties that lead to indecision and self-neglect from those that are essential for transformation. Though cultivating one's personal myths is today considered self-indulgent (because one's spirituality can never be emblematic of anything greater than the private sphere), there is no other means by which the dangers of true transformation can be constructively orchestrated. In other words, positive growth depends completely upon recognizing, risking, and acting—upon binding one's past and one's actual, physical present in a way that "annunciates" a future. Otherwise, one can never know what might have been feasible.

OTHERSELF HELP

I was fully aware of the fact that despite the strong impression made upon me by the stranger and what he said, the decision rested solely with me. I agreed . . . then I heard a voice from far away saying that this was the only remedy; actually we had not realized at the beginning that we would otherwise have been incurable. —dream account, C. A. Meier, *Healing Dream and Ritual*

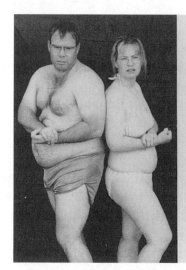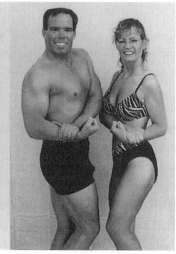

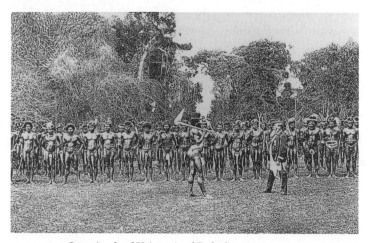

FIGURE 34. **Intentional and Unintentional Embodiment**
Anorexia literally means "the absence of desire." How do we understand the popularity
of the "self-help" genre in contemporary America, if not by reference to the wholly
self-conscious manipulation of what we might otherwise hope to become (*top*)?

Among cultures with highly supple notions of body-image boundary (e.g., among
Melanesian inhabitants of island New Caledonia, *bottom*), one could find until quite
recently the physical goals of the modern American fitness industry achieved through
the much less self-conscious act of seeing oneself in another. As ethnographers have
repeatedly shown (e.g., Weiner 1988), the animistic projection of self into a local moral
order (of merging self and other) makes possible the near glorification of human desire
in ways that are all but unknown today. What the Enlightenment worked directly to
promote was the idea that unselfconscious transformation was "undesirable" because it
was dangerous. (*Top:* From *Body for Life*, by Bill Phillips [New York: HarperCollins,
1999], 15. Reproduced with permission of High Point Media. *Bottom:* Photo by Cliché
Hughan, 1878.)

The primary theme of this book has been that creativity (the opposite of entropy) is a marginal phenomenon, and that marginality, and only marginality (despite its very high price), makes possible creative change by inducing a constructive embodiment of otherness. Though always a dangerous endeavor, assimilating otherness may, in turn, be more creatively managed when understood as former self, as a "none-such" self that appears different because its distance now makes its identity non-obvious (figure 35).

This assimilation is a social, as well as a psychological and a phenomenological, process. Because it is social, the context in which that "other" is assimilated is critical to the nature of the outcome it induces; for transformation can as readily be negative as positive. This is also why anything can be a catalyst for transformation; some Balinese can be transformed in a trance induced by a simple household object, if that object is symbolically contextualized. There is no inalienable "soul" here, only a soul whose inalienability is evidenced in its repeated demonstration. Identity is not something one owns,

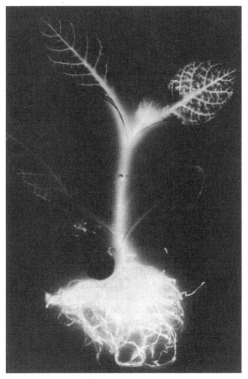

FIGURE 35. **Tobacco Plant Expressing Firefly Gene**
As an extraordinary demonstration of the assimilation of "nonself," we see here a tobacco plant whose transformed cells now literally glow in the dark. What makes this transformation possible is the presence of the same organelle in the tobacco plant and the firefly luciferase. Difference, in other words, can only be assimilated where similarity is already present. What might our world, we may ask, otherwise have been? Indeed, what might it become? (Photo by Keith Wood.)

regardless of how one behaves; indeed, there is not identity at all save for the one that gets earned, or the inherited one that gets realized through earned social action.

In fact, in some cases anthropologists have recorded very clear evidence of how identity is *only* a social construction—even to the point of arguing that there is no indigenous category of the person, except for what the Romans called the *persona*—that is, the corporeal self plus its social role. Anthropologists fear the racialisms that have arisen in the past when the social argument—that others may not subscribe to the same emotional domains as we do—is taken up by a tyrant and abused. But this is no reason to whitewash the role played, as it were, by the embryo. If we stand that afraid of essentializing culture, are we not merely giving way to the fear that we may be incapable of enjoying it?

Perhaps my favorite examples of an explicit attention to the social articulation of identity come from the accounts of the great ethnographer and missionary Maurice Leenhardt (1930, [1947] 1979) during his nearly forty years of living and working with New Caledonians. Leenhardt cites numerous instances in which what a person is can only be ascertained through how that individual embodies and lives out a particular worldview; for the physical, New Caledonian person cannot be separated from what he or she embodies. A single example makes the point: after long instruction, Leenhardt one day inquired of a close friend whether the notion of the spirit brought by missionaries was finally clear. "Not at all," came the brusque objection, "we have always known the spirit. What you have brought us is the body" (1937, 195). Elsewhere in his studies, Leenhardt shows how an attention to, and a belief in, other realities not only makes his subjects into keen observers of cultural difference, but actually provides each New Caledonian with mechanisms for bringing those other realities—those domains of "nonself"—into one's own life: stories abound where spirits themselves wear the same masks we wear to invoke them, and our dreaming, in turn, exists as a specific technique not only for entering another world but for allowing that other world to comment on our own.

Moving to a Native North American setting, we find a wonderful example of this assimilating of dreams into daily life. "As I was going about hunting," an Ojibwa man recounts,

> I came to a lake. A steep rock rose from the lake shore. I climbed up this rock to
> have a look across the lake. I thought I might sight a moose or some ducks.

When I glanced down towards the water's edge again, I saw a man standing by the rock. He was leaning on his paddle. A canoe was drawn up to the shore and in the stern sat a woman. In front of her rested a cradle board with a baby in it. Over the baby's face was a piece of green mosquito netting. The man was a stranger to me but I went up to him. I noticed that he hung his head in a strange way. He said, "You are the first man (human being) ever to see me. I want you to come and visit me." So I jumped into this canoe. When I looked down I noticed that it was all of one piece. There were no ribs or anything of the sort, and there was no bark covering. (I do not know what it was made of.)

On the northwest side of the lake there was a very high steep rock. The man headed directly for this rock. With one stroke of the paddle we were across the lake. The man threw his paddle down as we landed on a flat shelf of rock almost level with the water. Behind this the rest of the rock rose steeply before us. But when his paddle touched the rock this part opened up. He pulled the canoe in and we entered a room in the rock. It was not dark there although I could see no holes to let in any light. Before I sat down the man said, "See, there is my father and my mother." The hair of those old people was as white as a rabbit skin. I could not see a single black hair on their heads. After I had seated myself I had a chance to look around. I was amazed at all the articles I saw in the room—guns, knives, pans and other trade goods. Even the clothing these people wore must have come from a store. Yet I never remembered having seen this man at a trading post. I thought I would ask him so I said, "You told me that I was the first human being you had seen. Where, then, did you buy all of these articles I see?" To this he replied, "Have you never heard people talking about *pägítcīgan* (sacrifice)? These articles were given to us. That is how we got them." Then he took me into another room and told me to look around. I saw the meat of all kinds of animals—moose, caribou, deer, ducks. I thought to myself, this man must be a wonderful hunter, if he has been able to store up all this meat. I thought it very strange that this man had never met any other Indians in all his travels. Of course, I did not know that I was dreaming. Everything was the same as I had seen it with my eyes open. When I was ready to go I got up and shook hands with the man. He said, "Anytime that you wish to see me, this is the place where you will find me." He did not offer to open the door for me so I knew that I had to try and do this myself. I threw all the power of my mind into opening it and the rock lifted up. Then I woke up and knew that it was a dream. It was one of the first I ever had. (The narrator added that later he discovered a rocky eminence on one of the branches of the Berens

River that corresponded exactly to the place he had visited in his dream.) (Hallowell 1955, 97)

I have offered this incident in full not because it demonstrates the consequences of "animistic" thought but because it illustrates how a reciprocity between *empirical forms* (daily living, daily dreaming) helps to cultivate some deep awareness of the effects that an apparent nonself can have once we attend to its presence within us. For dreams (unlike our interpretive psychoanalytic categories), as so many cultures recognize, *are* another kind of reality, not a coded representation of something else. At times a reality of gods and ancestors, in other moments a place where those who have left the earth await their return—in the most general sense, a domain where emotions are cultivated in hypothetical realms of interaction. One recognizes immediately how attending to dreams allows us to cultivate our love of the natural world: Persephone's descent into the underworld becomes, to cite one example, significantly more meaningful if we see it as an extension of the dream passage from this world to the next. And, though the kind of embodiment made possible by synchronizing dreams with ritual practice is absent today, the *awareness* of such correspondences and their qualitative uniqueness is not restricted solely to ritualists, the mentally challenged, or to tribal peoples; for there are many legends that describe this "crossing over," and that, in turn, alert us "from the center" to the need to take risks by engaging one's perceived opposite.

At the level of human biology, I think almost immediately of the folk tale of Beauty and the Beast—not the simplified legend, but the more psychologically complex version developed by Cocteau in which the Beast is explicitly the underworld *daemon*, the spirit of darkness, Persephone's Hades, who, as it were, "sees" daylight—that is, his only salvation—in the most unconventional of all unions (figure 36). "My night is your day," he tells Beauty in darkness. "Outside it is morning." I am reminded of a dream I once had in which my deceased paternal grandfather, my childhood best friend, stands "on the other side" of a road waving me across. I fall into his waiting arms, and he chuckles lovingly and almost silently. Our job as humans in not simply to absorb and virally transform nonself, but to attend to how our very bodies might look and feel from the "other" world that "nonself" inhabits. This is the source of our creativity and future life; in cultivating an awareness of the view from the other's side, we sensitize ourselves to the need for loving difference.

For Cocteau, Beauty, like Conduiramurs, sees her destiny in the Beast;

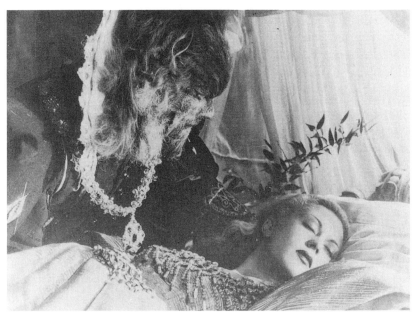

FIGURE 36. **Beauty and the Beast**
"My day is your night; outside it is morning," says the Beast to Beauty in Cocteau's extraordinary 1946 commentary on the reconciliation of "otherness." (From *Beauty and the Beast: Diary of a Film*, by Jean Cocteau, trans. Ronald Duncan [New York: Dover, 1972]. Reproduced courtesy of Dover Publications, Inc.)

when she looks in, or through, a mirror, she sees his anguish. She is clearly not the Beast herself, but both her identity and his survival depend upon their complementarity; for here the Beast (masculine form of the feminine, *la bête*) stands with his hands smoking—the ancient "smoking gun" of a recent kill, the signal that he is a visceral being—a fighter and predator who, except for meeting Beauty, would saltate uncontrollably, destroying himself and perhaps also what little innocence that might remain the world. In Cocteau's dramatic representation, the deference that the Beast shows for Beauty resembles that of Parzival (*Per*cival, our archetypal male "person") for Conduiramurs (the conduit, the vehicle, the container of pure love). In the absence of any appropriate social convention, it is ceremony, respect, and deference that replace the chaotic terms society offers to describe the love it cannot provide. No doubt at times the Beasts of the world do collapse, accepting the stigmas that society places upon them—that they are "mad," or "autistic," or "attention deficient," or "anorexic." But if they are vigilant, their search for complementarity will be rewarded; for it is only the love of beauty and beast that will change the inauthenticity of the world they have been destined to inhabit. By loving the Beast, Beauty allows him to transform himself, for she is his "other self" as much as he is hers. In love, one takes on the potentiality of the other; they love mutually, in dynamic balance. This mutuality is what the French acknowledge when they describe the body as *la terrain*, the somatic landscape in which pathogen and antigen coexist in dynamic balance. It is only through the positive creation that love makes possible, and that in turn defines what love is, that the liminal can productively transform the center before it passes back recursively into the before-and-after life.

What might be meant by the "before-and-after life" can now be understood in the context of *reciprocity*, not simply from the standpoint of activity (life) and inequality (difference): that desire itself can govern memory, present-day experience, and what is yet unknown to us is our best indicator that entropy can be undermined. In fact, what distinguishes these experiences of time is the kind and degree of one's involvement (that is, the kind and degree of one's capacity to love the risks that are unique to each domain). In other words, a deadly kind of event is only different from a lively action by degree— a complacent attitude, that is, transports a lively action into a deadly one, a negotiated identity into no identity, an interest in learning from "other" into a subliminal ruination of "other," a productive relationship into an opportunistic one (or, at least, one that damages through lack of commitment).

Everything discussed thus far has, you may have guessed, to do with *reciprocity*—the formal relationship of self and other. Reciprocity, therefore, is both a formal relation and a first condition for the constructive experience of marginality.

A second formal relation is that of *correlation*. It is the co-relativity of two things to one shared experience that allows us to develop a unity of opposites, of outer and inner, of dreams and daily life, of self and other. It is co-relativity that makes possible the sense that we unconsciously share a past and a future. This relationship has sometimes been romantically identified with a thing called collective unconscious, or archetypal awareness, or, in anthropology, with the cultural category. Correlation is essential for *mutuality*, for the awareness that change takes place when one is positively possessed by another. Ritual is the traditional medium; ritualizing is the modern alternative.

Finally, there is a third and perhaps deeper formal relationship between self and other—this relationship (because it takes place through selective dissociation) is as difficult to name as it is to describe. If "man is a namer," then this formal relationship is "everyman"—unnameable. In that it is "everyman," it comes very close to what has been called *synchronicity*. This, however, is not a satisfactory term, not only because it tries to "name" an inchoate phenomenon but because it implies that specific links exist, even if they remain unknown to us. In fact, this emphasis (seen, for instance, in the specific labeling [naming] of the occult) distracts us from the relationship's most interesting and psychically valuable feature—that is (namely!), that symbolic awareness must be actively cultivated in everyday life if we are ever to reach any awareness of the great diversity of ways in which thoughts can be embodied in meaningful, creative action. This bringing to life—or "realization"—is the only way in which our mutual intuitions become mnemonically real and creatively true. It is, therefore, not only because our symbolic perceptions cannot be named that they must be lived, but because their mutual embodiment facilitates an awareness of "a dimension of reality that can only be reached indirectly" (Progoff 1973, 13), that can only be reached by doing something symbolic in a way that includes someone else. Certainly they can be thought about, but they must be acted upon. It's not a question of feeling or not feeling a sense of urgency about one's life; it a question of choosing life over an alternative that is unacceptable. In this way, if you are living, you are doing it well.

Central to this book has been the belief that there is no knowledge of these three forms outside of marginal spaces. One cannot *presume* understanding here. Doing so evokes the passive entropy of contemporary life—the hidden secret by which the inert center of the colony erodes the true integrity of the periphery that it cannot itself realize—the writing about liminality, rather than the living of it. In European (that is Judeo-Christian, intellectual) thought, the idea that we are mostly what we do disappears during the Enlightenment, but it can be recovered in remembering the traditional consequences of a failure to reciprocate. In the pre-Enlightened Middle Ages, for instance, an "outlaw" was someone "without the law"—someone stripped of legal protection, someone who, unlike today's criminal, had no claim on civil liberties and no right to protection, regardless of how badly he or she may have been treated by others. The price one pays for not being demonstrably involved in the work of culture was, then, to become a cipher, a nonentity, worthless.

Yet, today, we somehow think that doing nothing liminal is acceptable, provided we haven't broken any of the laws that we have developed to protect us from one another. In fact, we really don't have laws of engagement—no requirement that we demonstrate our willingness to reciprocate once others have invested themselves in us; for such regulating, we believe, would encroach on our freedom. Even our so-called "good Samaritan" laws—that require citizens to assist one another at accidents, and that protect us legally from any untoward consequences of our goodwill—are largely unenforceable. It is this complete ignorance of what we crudely refer to as the moral economy—the domain of empathic reciprocity—that has left us to pay with our profound unhappiness. We even deeply believe that we are living in a world of rapid change and transformation because we sense distantly that the expression of personal change is living evidence of what is most alien to us. In fact, what may be the only identity that is distinctly ours is the very rhetoric of self-doubt that has paralyzed us. We describe our world as fast moving and hectic, yet is seems to be so incapable of creation. Our static hysteria may now permanently replace the great pleasure of living.

Having lost, or at least discounted, the knowledge of how to contextualize (and, therefore, embody) the sense of "self," we are left with only misperceptions of what constitutes change—misperceptions that are as naive as they are unflattering. What has been identified as the meritorious flexibility of those who today succeed may, in fact, only reflect the complete absence of self-knowledge that is the concomitant of the Age of Immunology—an age in which the organism attempts, as does the thymus, to survive, as our scientists would have it, through its own self-ignorance. Without some concrete nurturing of the phenomenal world, in other words, there can be only an inelegant response, a total flight, from the diverse possibilities that otherwise make life worth living.

"We have now discovered that it was an intellectually unjustified presumption on our forefathers' part to assume that man has a soul," Jung once said. Jung's startling comment, arbitrarily settled on here by the random opening of his *Modern Man in Search of a Soul* (1933, 176), still, more than half a century on, perfectly illustrates the core issue of modernity. Its content is the crux of our problem; its random appearance is precisely what Jung had in mind in writing, at certain professional risk, his introduction to the *I Ching*: namely, that an apparently nonrational—but selective and contextualized— act can help initiate indirectly a new way of approaching a deeper kind of reality than those to which we normally have access, a reality that can only be

reached by doing something symbolic in an inventive way that includes someone else. Here, every episode of personal growth is based not upon the occult
labeling of the unknown, where uncertainty itself is subjected to yet another
mystical canon, but upon something very antithetical to modern life, this being the idea that in order to change one has to cultivate a genuine curiosity,
yes an enjoyment, of difference—not the difference that is fed up to us at
some cultural potluck, but a curiosity that generates a willful approach to danger. This means also, of course, cultivating an aversion to the bright lights, the
domain of superficial accolades that we are all tempted by, and that some of us
end up living for.

Despite having retained some intuitive understanding that transformation
and growth are important, we have so lost any real curiosity for the unknown
that we actually believe that replacing one standard with another will, in fact,
free us from ourselves—free us from the rhetoric of failure that dominates a
culture at war with itself. This is why our (especially literary) theorists go on
about "revising the canon"—why, that is, academics in particular focus so
much attention on replacing one set of standards with other, no less rigid
ones—without realizing that it is the reciprocity between the canonical and
the acanonical that is really important.

This is also why we have become so embroiled in the notion of political
correctness: for here, more than anywhere, we are embarrassed by the degree
to which we have merely fought to replace one unfair system by another that
is equally draconian. Our appropriation of the concept of "fairness" as a personal right rather than a social obligation causes us to rebel at what we think is
unfair; but our belief in the idea that personal identity is inalienable keeps us
from seeing the merits of negotiating with difference. What replaces quickly
becomes as uncurious about difference as what is replaced. Our liberal academics become as reactionary as their rivals do because they never genuinely
question their own dogmas. Nor do they ever value the process by which they
negotiate those dogmas (and their own identities) in a diverse world. Instead,
they assume that their education itself excuses their lack of curiosity—as if
their laziness about demonstrating their curiosity was justified by the canonical symbols (diplomas, fellowships, and named chairs) that they can marshal
forward. They are thus never so excited than by the prospect of some badge of
merit that would pave the way for less and less emotion work—never so vexed
or fatigued than by the prospect of having to negotiate with difference.

We are, likewise, surely aware that this lack of curiosity is not something that can be placed solely on the shoulders of the uneducated. Quite the contrary; lethargy thrives precisely in the places where its existence is rigorously denied. Take psychoanalysis, for instance; here, in the very discipline that is purportedly devoted to understanding differences of thinking, we have perhaps the most deeply entrenched absence of curiosity:

> The idea that literature, or any other discipline like boxing or songwriting, could modify psychoanalytic theory—that it could be a two-way street—has always been problematic for psychoanalysts. There is, of course, no reason to think a psychoanalyst's interpretation of a boxing match would necessarily be more revealing than a boxer's account of a psychoanalytic session. But psychoanalysts have worked on the rather misleading principle that psychoanalysis is useful or interesting only if it is in some sense right, rather than believing that it is another good way of speaking about certain things like love and loss and memory. . . . Great theorists, unlike great artists, whether they intend to or not, always make us believe in progress. (Phillips 1994, 79)

The issue to which this passage alludes has, of course, nothing to do with paying attention to the heteroglot nature of experience, or to honoring diversity, or to celebrating it (whatever that could mean), or to reforming cultural canons. A boxer may or may not have anything at all to say about psychoanalysis: he or she may equally be so caught up in the embodied meaning of the pugilistic spectacle that it would be unfair to induce yet one more contest of identity. But sustaining the thought that boxers might redefine the boundaries of what is relevant to psychoanalysis requires its own kind of gymnastics—its own humor, tragedy, irony, even subtleness. All of the curious traits, in other words, that are eroded by self-righteousness.

A country doctor I know once described this self-righteous ignorance quite succinctly. Asked by a public radio interviewer how he felt about not enjoying the same professional respect as his subspecialist colleagues who held distinguished university posts—that is, about being treated as "only" a general practitioner by his professional peers who occupy "important" medical school positions—he replied without hesitation:

> You see, the problem is that . . . I am smarter than they are, but [my colleagues] they'll never know that [the idea that somebody in my line of work could be smart]. Because the thing is every time they interact with me they interact on

their terms. For example, if I talk to a cardiologist, no matter how much I know, he knows more about cardiology than I do. If I talk to a gastroenterologist, he knows more. He doesn't realize how much I know . . . because our only interaction is on his terms. And, so, from the point of view of doctoring, he doesn't see me as a smart person. And he may recognize at some point that there's a lot that I do that he can't do; but there's no way he could realize how much you have to know to do a good job at what I do.

The limited sense of curiosity the specialists displayed is much more insidious than it may at first appear; for any engagement with difference can only be transformative if the terms of transformation—the vocabularies of change— are negotiated through an interaction in which some risk or chance allows for the creation of something new. Here, as ritual indicates, it is easy to be more concrete. One need only look at the universal need for rites of passage, in which two or more individuals come together and negotiate the very terms by which they merge, to see that real change is not a thing made possible at the bench or on the analyst's couch. Initiates do not, in other words, bounce off of one another and stand alone celebrating their ignorance and isolation.

Make no mistake: there is categorically *no* evidence that personal change ever has been, or ever can be, facilitated intellectually. Assuming that the soul is always there creates, as Jung (I believe) rightly felt, an ignorance of context; as we ignore context, so too do we create a world without soul. This is why the real and imaginative creations of nonself within self (that is, the idea of pathogens as former selves, or antibodies as attempted versions of otherness) are so important for new growth. Uniqueness (identity) in this view becomes an extension of our experience with others; it is not innate, or at least not *only* innate.

It may be undeniable that the projection of identity into difference can give life or death. But it is up to us to decide for love rather than for its opposite; for it is indeed quite possible that the cultural forces that we promote to address our collective suffering may also be the precise forces that continue to cause suffering. The potential dangers are particularly acute if these prescribed techniques result in the sentimentalizing or romanticizing of something very serious. Protecting oneself from self-absorption is thus best accomplished by constantly crossing over from self to other: from center to margin, from specific and general, from certainty to ambiguity, from microbiology to embryology, from immunology to vaccinology, from the named to the unnamed, from male to female. Taking a deliberate journey into the dangerous peripheries of what may be known is essential, for a risk can only result in growth if it is carried out in the interests of basic desire and the love that is its ultimate goal.

In this examination of how self is created by, and in turn creates, nonself, we have had occasion to consider many cases in which the past has been symbolically relived by a present in anticipation of desiring a good future. While so many of these symbols have been explicitly feminine—particularly in the symbolism of maternity and in shrines to goddesses—I have not presented this study as a study of gender. Though male and female are our most basic and best understood forms of difference—because the body is the only thing of which we have both objective and subjective knowledge—it is less their physical gender than their embodiment of difference that makes them such extraordinary examples of self-in-nonself and nonself-in-self.

Let us not, therefore, forget the many examples that may seem less obvious, but that are no less ubiquitous. In human anatomy, there is the maternal-fetal, but there is also the human gut that brings nonself into symbiotic relation to self, regardless of gender. In the domain of infectious diseases we have not only the deep belief that pathogens can evolve out of normal cell genes; research suggests that even the humble parasitic worms that once populated the guts of most humans may actually help to control autoimmunity by establishing a focus for cells that, in a sterile antibiotic environment, turn on the body's own tissue (Newman 1999). At the cultural level, in settings where a form of social "embryology" prevails, we see the overt recognition of how self is largely identified by its acceptance of nonself. In these cultures we see not only other paradigms of living, but new paradigms for science. Likewise, in the literature on healing, we have countless examples of an illness being taken on by a healer in order to absorb and neutralize its pathogenicity. Faith healers worldwide become physically ill with the diseases of their patients, Hindu priests absorb and dispel pollutants, Navajo medical botanists claim that they cannot treat an illness they have not had, Balinese curers become therapists as a way of acknowledging their own instabilities, and Greek fire-walkers complain of not recognizing that a life-threatening incident was actually caused by a personal failure to attend to God's calling. The awareness of how self is defined through the assimilation of difference is so universal that an extended list of examples might be drawn from almost any part of the world.

What is called for now, however, is merely to recognize the extraordinary power of this tendency—to acknowledge how the act of creating, where unlikely elements are superimposed as a means of bringing life to new forms, more or less defines what an antibody is. Let us then never fail to remember that the antibody, like the great discovery, is created through a superimposition of unlikely elements, a superimposition that results in a creative response to a situation that might otherwise seem impossibly destabilizing. One must always leave in order to come back. Though this awareness may lead us to imagine a future that is predestined, we each decide to accept or to reject what is possible and feasible. Pathogens certainly do cause illnesses; but our illnesses are also caused by our reacting to what we think of as pathogenic. Desiring life over entropy makes a good beginning. In the experience of such true desire life triumphs in the eternal need for the marginal.

Notes

PREFACE

1. "Le Moi se confirme, mais sous les espèces de l'Autre: l'image spéculaire est un parfait symbole de l'alienation" (Genette 1966, 22).

CHAPTER ONE

1. One of the finest ethnographic accounts I know is Loring Danforth's book on Greek firewalking and religious healing (1989), in which he offers diverse and moving examples of how the sickening powers of life's most trying events are positively rearranged through transformational experiences.

2. This procedure is widely evidenced in the "shaman's apprentice" genre of anthropological writing; however, it is perhaps most clearly and eloquently expounded in the descriptive writings of Paul Stoller (e.g., 1989).

3. It is worth noting that our word "normal" has its origin in the Latin word for measure or rule (*norma*).

4. As Chase reminds us, "The knowledge that certain contagious diseases, such as variola (from the Latin for spotted) or smallpox, confer on their survivors long-lasting or permanent immunity to reinfection with these select diseases—and that, at least in the instance of smallpox, such immunity could be transferred to healthy people by inoculations of biological matter from people suffering from smallpox—was well established in many parts of this planet for more than two millennia before Jenner was born" (1982, 42). Chinese doctors blew dried smallpox scabs into their patients' noses via bone tubes. In the Middle East, Asia, and Africa people "swallowed smallpox scabs and/or had the crusts or lymphs implanted in their veins by skilled inoculators or variolators, who opened veins with sharp needles" (42). Russians were rendered immune in their saunas by the pounding of smallpox pus or lymph into the skin with massaging brooms, while other techniques are known to have been employed in Africa, Greece, Turkey, and in the American colonies, where the famous Boston witch-hunter, Cotton Mather, learned a successful technique from his African slave (42).

5. See, for instance, the discussion of *paling* (the "nausea" of disorientation in Bali) described by Herbst (1997). A taxi driver once told me, in the middle of the jungle and late at night, to move *kadja* ("toward the mountain") to make room for a new passenger. The "mountain" was nowhere to be seen, but all knew its location.

6. The literature on African divination is enormous. Beginning with the work of Sir E. E. Evans-Pritchard in the 1930s, anthropologists have taken a detailed look at how divination functions to balance benevolent and malevolent forces.

CHAPTER TWO

1. This is not to say that anthropologists have at all neglected immunology. But, aside from the cultural critiques of a few researchers (e.g., Haraway and Martin), the discipline has yet to apply its cross-cultural knowledge base to specific problems of the field.

2. It is important here not to confuse the "nonpropositional" with what Berlin has called "bad metaphysics" (1968, 34)—that is, the use of accepted convention to lay claim to things that allegedly transcend normal experience. See my discussion of Berlin (Napier 1992, 3).

3. This is rather like pointing out to a friend who has suddenly started wearing cowboy boots the fact that he had recently been watching lots of Clint Eastwood movies.

4. Note the subtle manipulation of language here to conform to the stereotype—e.g., "to report" not "to have"—even though elsewhere the same authors admit that there is a "high incidence of cervical cancer among Latin American women, most of whom report monogamous behavior."

5. Much of the critical literature on immunology and virology has focused on the ubiquitous and oppressive character of how immunological illness experiences are culturally defined, and on ways in which "the body at war with itself" functions to reinforce oppressive political views (e.g., Martin 1990, 1994; Scheper-Hughes 1990; Haraway 1989).

6. For discussion, see Charlesworth et al. 1989, 119.

7. See, e.g., Rothenberg 1988.

CHAPTER THREE

1. See, for example, Ortner's criticisms of anthropological practice (1984), or Stoller's challenge to anthropologists regarding the sensuousness both of what they purport to study (1986) and of how they go about representing their own experiences (1997).

2. The distinctions among autoimmune diseases are becoming less, rather than more, clear. Increasingly these disorders are recognized as "a spectrum of diseases ranging from ones like Hashimoto's thyroiditis, which affects only tissue of the thyroid, to generalized ones like systemic lupus erythematosus, in which antibodies react with antigens widespread throughout the body. All the autoimmune conditions can be placed somewhere along this scale" (Joneja and Bielory 1990, 108).

3. See, e.g., Scott 1985; Magagna 1991.

4. Patients frequently describe the unwillingness of doctors to accept either a disgnosis that the patient him- or herself proposes, or to acknowledge a diagnosis arrived at in a previous clinical encounter. The patient says to the doctor, "When I first came down with lupus . . . ," and the doctor snaps back: "Did I say you had lupus?"

5. It is really quite surprising when one considers how infrequently we question our admiration of those who "get on with life" without thinking too much about it. See my discussion in 1992, 48.

6. As Goffman says, "Even where widely attained norms are involved, their multiplicity has the effect of disqualifying many persons. . . . In an important sense there is only one complete unblushing male in America: a young, married, white, urban northern, heterosexual Protestant father of college education, fully employed, of good complexion, weight, and height, and a recent record in sports. Every American male tends to look out upon the world from this perspective. . . . Any male who fails to qualify in any of these ways is likely to view himself—during moments at least—as unworthy, incomplete, and inferior. . . . The general identity-values of a society may be fully entrenched nowhere, and yet they can cast some kind of shadow on the encounters encountered everywhere in daily life" (1963, 128–29). See Napier 1992, 140.

CHAPTER FOUR

1. D'Arcy Thompson 1961, 22–26, citing Sir James R. Napier, "On the Most Profitable Speed for a Fully Laden Cargo Steamer for a Given Voyage," *Proceedings of the Royal Philosophical Society, Glasgow* 6 (1865): 33–38.

2. Although Samuel Cunard was a Canadian, his reputation was largely built upon the reliability of ships and engines manufactured in Glasgow by Robert Napier, the so-called father of Clyde shipbuilding.

3. Eisenhower's 1954 state of the nation address, in *Public Papers of the Presidents of the United States: Dwight D. Eisenhower* (Washington, D.C.: GPO, 1954), 374.

4. Of the total gross tonnage (some 444 million) registered under so-called "flags of convenience," more than 55 million is registered in Liberia alone (Pleydell-Bouverie 1993). Setting aside the loss of human life and of natural habitats caused directly by the avoidance of safety regulations, and the fact that business elites who engage in convenience shipping are the only beneficiaries of the practice, one might legitimately ask if American taxpayers ought to be responsible for protecting multinationals when the multinationals themselves have chosen other national allegiances.

5. Kula, as a Melanesian system of symbolic prestation, is not unlike any other system of negotiated value (bartering, bribery, etc.) in which the nature of the interchange between exchange partners is itself the setting in which value is established. Value is, therefore, completely relative and flexible. Kula is simply the most complex and highly developed example we know of such a system of exchange.

6. An argument most elegantly and repeatedly made by James Lovelock (e.g., 1988).

CHAPTER FIVE

1. "One cannot say what a man is trying to do unless one knows what he expects to happen" (Hampshire 1970, 111).

2. A similarly direct attack on the self-imposed institutional and disciplinary constraints of social research may be seen, for instance, in the work of Paul Stoller. See, especially, his *Bad Sauce, Good Ethnography* (1986) and *Sensuous Scholarship* (1997). This argument was, of course,

made long ago in philosophy and is now, more or less, a central concern of the discipline—as in the work of Paul Feyerabend (1975), or in Thomas Kuhn's famous debate with Karl Popper over the nature of scientific change. Though most philosophers are unwilling to accept Feyerabend's argument that discovery is wholly a matter of chance, Kuhn's views have been more widely received because of his contention that paradigmatic change is the result of the cumulative impact of anomalies on relatively resistant theoretical models (see chapter 4).

3. Arguably these concerns were already apparent in early cybernetic theory (e.g., in Hughes's *Networks of Power* [1983]).

4. In a forthcoming piece ("The Writing of Passage") I argue that the canonical notions of fame to which we subscribe are less the product of experiential embodiment than they are the result of the valuation of history and what Latour refers to as our obsession with "inscription." In more "magically" motivated worlds, fame may be both avoided and feared. Commoners in Bali, for instance, often express a complete disinterest in being famous.

5. See, e.g., Lloyd (1966) on polarity and analogy, and Needham (1979) on the use of binary opposites in symbolic classification. On the role of structural polarity in affecting transformation, see, e.g., Leach 1961, 1964.

6. For discussion, see Napier 1992, 45–49.

7. See Smith and Wise's *Energy and Empire* (1989). To say that the debate was not strictly scientific is not to say that the study of entropy was not experimental. In fact, much of the work on entropy (particularly in Scotland) was focused on developing the most efficient forms of locomotion.

8. In reading Midgley's work, I was interested to see that she had also experimented with replacing the military metaphors of molecular biology.

9. See Susan Buck-Morss, "Aesthetics and Anaesthetics: Walter Benjamin's Artwork Essay Reconsidered" (1992).

10. On Victorian anxieties concerning gradualism and evolution, see Beer 1983 and Keller 1995, 51–54.

11. Although most evolutionists claim that natural selection is not a kind of teleology (that is, that it does not employ any final causes to argue for a particular, predetermined, end), in fact, it is highly teleological. Any teleological argument requires that ends are immanent in nature, that nature's actions are directed toward an end, and that its shape is, therefore, purposeful. According to natural selection, it is clearly the case that the survival of the fittest is immanent, that survivors are purposely shaped for survival, and that the end of fitness is to survive. For the counterargument, see, e.g., Mayr 2000.

CHAPTER SIX

1. This is a common theme in the literature on trance. For a compelling Christian example, see Danforth 1989. Here the extraordinary feat of firewalking is repeatedly attributed in rural Greece to the demands of St. Constantine, rather than to individual motives. Though contemporary firewalking comes (in the form of New Age healing) to be a vehicle for self-empowerment, the traditional activity was always accomplished by allowing oneself to listen to the saint's calling.

2. A contemporary example of the same kind of reaction can be seen in the introduction of helmet laws for motorcyclists. In places where the laws were repealed (on the grounds that they

violated civil liberties) riders began to wear them less than they had before the mandatory laws were first implemented (because not wearing a helmet now becomes a symbol of one's freedom).

3. I thank Bruno Latour for his timely introduction of what he calls in English the "factish": "Le mot 'fétiche' et le mot 'fait' ont la même étymologie ambiguë. . . . Le mot 'fétiche' semble renvoyer à la réalité extérieure, le mot 'fétiche' aux folles croyances du sujet. Tout les deux dissimulent, dans la profondeur de leur racine latine, la travail intense de construction qui permet la vérité des faits comme celle des esprits. C'est cette vérité qu'il nous faut dégager, sans croire ni aux élucubrations d'un sujet psychologique saturé de rêveries, ni à l'existence extérieure d'objets froids et anhistoriques qui tomberaient dans les laboratoire come du Ciel. Sans croire non plus à la croyance naïve. En joignant les deux sources étymologiques, nous appellerons *faitiche* la robuste certitude qui permet à la pratique de passer à l'action sans jamais croire à la différence entre construction et recueilllement, immanence et transcendance" (1996, 44).

4. I am referring here not only to Medawar's open cynicism for psychoanalysis, for example, but to his lack of interest in evidence—even evidence brought forth by his own students—that did not support his scientific views. In fact, Medawar's best-known book, *Pluto's Republic* (1982), got its title from an encounter Medawar had with an uneducated neighbor, who, upon learning of his interest in philosophy exclaimed: "Don't you just adore Pluto's *Republic?*" As an aside one might note how criticizing common ignorance—what the the British call "clever clever"—can come back to haunt one. Not to be forgotten is the Oxford paperback edition of Medawar's *The Limits of Science* (1984), which Lewis Thomas labeled "his latest and . . . most wonderful book": on its back one reads from his distinguished Oxford editors that "Sir Peter Medawar, who won the Nobel Prize (with Sir MacFarlane Burnet) in 1960 for his work on tissue transplantation, is the author of *Plato's Republic.*"

5. This pair is centrally connected by a single disulfide bridge and noncovalent associations, while the two heavy chains of the leg or body are glycosylated and joined by one or more disulfide bond. In this model, an antibody may be thought of as a molecule consisting of a constant domain (if you will, an assimilating "self"), and two variable domains of recognition—two binary, dual, and identical sites of interactivity at which creative difference is attempted and expressed.

CHAPTER SEVEN

1. While this book was in press, Matzinger published an article in *Science* that actually described the reciprocity of her danger model in terms of self-renewal (2002). Though immunologists have yet to familiarize themselves with notions of selfhood derived from non-Cartesian traditions, their willingness to consider that the self may be otherwise defined is heartening.

2. Tauber, for instance, notes that "in his first clonal selection theory (CST) paper (1957) Burnet did not expand upon what the self *is*. Even in his later theoretical work, Burnet almost scrupulously avoided the term" (1994, 157).

3. Although the integration of virology into computer language would constitute a separate study, it is worth noting here this profound use of personification within information technology. Note, for example, how readily the notion of a computer "virus" has been assimilated into everyday discourse.

4. Although the question has been broadly considered theoretically and historically (e.g., Tauber 1994), what has yet to take place is any real examination of the many ways in which "self" has been conceptualized across cultures.

5. Charles Fort once summed up the atheoretical dimensions of natural selection quite nicely. "Darwinism: the fittest survive. What is meant by the fittest? Not the strongest; not the cleverest—weakness and stupidity everywhere survive. There is no way of determining fitness except in that a thing does survive. 'Fitness,' then, is only another name for 'survival.' Darwinism: that survivors survive" (1941, 23).

6. "Cohn's reservations about Jerne's network are, one could argue, as much comments on the limits of scientific verifiability as criticisms of Jerne's theories. 'The absence of a network theory of antigen-specific responsiveness which has both molecular level plausibility and the potential to be mapped onto known cell-cell interactions' is, as Cohn et al. (1980) point out, inevitable given the fact that most of the relevant arguments are based on the massive accumulation of highly variable observations, 'on experimental systems of such great complexity that many interpretations are possible and reproducibility becomes a luxury.' 'God,' [they] conclude, 'has become a problem of cellular immunology, alas!'" (Napier 1996, 337). Or, as a recent *Science* article put it: "As one dissects the immune system at finer and finer levels of resolution, there is actually a decreasing predictability in the behavior of any particular unit of function (a gene, a cell)" (Germain 2001, 240).

7. Though the most outspoken advocate for this position is probably Lynn Margulis (e.g., 1998), it is not only embryology and symbiosis that do not see the germline in anything like the tidy way that bench scientists often do. Setting aside the environmental factors variably influencing retrotranscription, and the fact that most parasites are backmutants of their hosts, we now have to accept that, as we have noted in chapter 6, even climatic factors may prove crucial. As noted in chapter 6, for example, viruses found in polar ice packs "put a spanner in the works of viral evolution studies," because "instead of representing the endpoint of steady evolution, modern populations of viruses might be a complex mishmash of highly evolved ones and others that have taken a holiday from evolution in cold storage" (Walker 1999, 4). How can one do evolutionary studies, then, when such new findings in virology amply demonstrate widely variable moments of evolutionary stasis and change? Well, one can't—at least not without rethinking many developmental assumptions; for these new studies undoubtedly do "put a spanner in the works."

8. See, e.g., Leslie Brent's *History of Transplantation Immunology* (1997).

9. "In one study 600 different monoclonal antibodies . . . were tested to evaluate their reactivity with normal tissue antigens. More than 3% of the virus-specific antibodies tested also bound to normal tissue, suggesting that molecular mimicry is a fairly common phenomenon" (Kuby 1992, 394).

10. The fact that many invertebrate organisms possess totipotent stem cell lines via which somatic mutations might gain access to the germ line ought at least to alert us, though, to the need to question just what cellular commitment actually means to a vertebrate immunoglobulin system.

11. Although this idea has only recently become commonplace, its origins in theoretical biology go back at least to the 1920s (Margulis 1998, 51). As a model of the symbiotic relationship between a host and a potentially dangerous guest, however, the idea can be found in our very earliest civilizations, and certainly within many of our first written documents.

12. Let us not forget that the success of Maxwell's demon was, like the dendritic cell, the consequence of its life-giving ability to balance otherwise oppositional molecules.

13. One finds examples of this deification everywhere. Here is one from the well-respected science journal, *New Scientist*. In an otherwise level-headed discussion of the consequences of information technology on modern life, one learns that even the chaos of modern information systems is subject to the Natural Selection deity. "The Internet makes it very difficult to police rogue traders because buyer and seller often do not live within the same jurisdiction. . . . It's clear what all this means: the underlying order of life is breaking up. Most of us are blind to the change. Drugs, crime and terrorism, once localised problems, are now organised globally. Unemployment among the semi-skilled workforce will increase as more production jobs are automated. These and other precursors of social fragmentation are the consequences of our traditional power structures becoming impotent. *Natural selection will decide which parts of societies will degenerate and which mutate into stable survivors in the new environment of the Information Age*" (Angell 2000, 45 [my emphasis]). Indeed, one wonders what this omniscient Natural Selection being is not involved in. Simply substitute an all-seeing God for each time the words appear and any such statement can be read as good old-fashioned Judeo-Christian dogma.

14. Estimates run from 10^5 to 10^{16}. Furthermore, "because most antigens have many epitopes [i.e., amino acids or sugar residues that are antigenic determinants] and a given epitope can be recognized by more than one lymphocyte, the number of lymphocytes that can respond to a given antigen is much larger than the number of cells possessing a certain antigen receptor" (Becker, Reece, and Poenie 1996, 788).

15. An even broader challenge to the specificity of laboratory research is offered, for example, by Cone and Martin (1998), who argue that changes in diet caused by global systems of food marketing may block immune mechanisms by which one becomes accustomed to local allergens. See, also Lappé (1994) on the relation between the spread of disease and the disruption of local environments.

16. This process, called apoptosis, is defined by those who study it in precisely those terms—that is as "cellular suicide."

17. Estimates are that within the next century that at least one half of the world's languages (currently about 6,500 in number) will disappear (Lewis 1998).

18. See also Connerton 1989.

EPILOGUE

1. A wonderful explication of the experiential dimensions of such marginality may be seen in Hesse's novel, *Siddhartha*, which, though often mistaken for an explication of Buddhist ideology, actually provides an excellent exegesis on Tantric asceticism.

2. Which, like the tale of Mojud, I encountered by a chance opening of the text.

3. The ancient alchemists knew this process well, not only in their many references to merging, dissolution, and invention, but in the very nature of how these things work, if you will, "recursively"—crossing to an island after which a future is only possible by "going back." And they even understood this combining of the linear and the cyclical geometrically and mathematically.

4. The *purohita*, or king's main priest, may be envied for the earthly power to which he has

access, but for Hindus he also represents the lowest form of spiritual power (of *brahma*) because he has polluted himself with earthly rewards.

5. Because we all at times feel that the center is a still place, we also have within us an intuitive sense of why being "on the fence" may be productive. This is why in the Middle Ages the witch was visualized as sitting on the fence (the *hag*), the boundary that separated the culture of the village from the wildness of nature (see, e.g., Duerr 1985, 45).

6. Stoller (personal communication) notes how among the Songhay of Niger, "every magical incantation begins with a genealogy of text. N'debbi gave it to Baru, Baru gave it to Sido, Sido gave it to Jenitongo, Jenitongo gave it to Adamou, and Adamou gave it to me. What was in their minds is in my mind, what is in their hearts is in my heart."

7. "Among the Lakota, foods newly introduced by whites at the end of the nineteenth century were avoided, and were even considered inedible because of the way they looked or smelled. They were eaten only after they could be transformed into acceptable, edible foods through the ritual process of naming. One case in point is cattle, which the Lakota initially avoided because of their stench. They could not understand how the white man could eat such a filthy and odiferous animal. Over time, however, cattle were hunted as if they were buffalo, and they became partly acceptable because they had become transformed into an ersatz buffalo—a *ptegleska* 'spotted buffalo cow'" (Powers 1986, 145).

8. For a discussion of Metchnikoff's views of human disharmony, see Tauber and Chernyak 1991, 21.

9. Which apparently got the owner in hot water when he sent one to the President of the United States!

10. The soccer ball is a truncated icosahedron, very much like the so-called "buckyball" (named after geodesic dome advocate, R. Buckminster Fuller), the carbon molecule which won its discoverers the Nobel Prize in Chemistry in 1996. This is a 32-faced polygon, consisting of 12 pentagons and 20 hexagons. In the plutonium detonator all 32 sections merge at a central collision point. The beauty of the "buckyball" resides in its structural capacity to function as a vehicle for carrying a wide variety of proteins. The implications for the pharmaceutical industry are obvious. Now, it seems, science arrives late with its own proof of the ancient homeopathic idea that the very thing that kills also cures.

11. "The number of regular polyhedra (solids with equal sides, equal regular faces, equal solid angles, inscribable in a shpere) far from being infinite, is limited to five" (Ghyka [1946] 1977, 40). These five are the tetrahedron, the octahedron, the cube, the icosahedron, and the dodecahedron.

12. This is particularly likely given that the pre-Pythagorean focus of Indian geometry was on converting the circle into a square of identical area. See Rao and Kak 1998; Seidenberg 1962, 1978.

13. Other types of tumors show similar characteristics. A dermoid, for instance, is a fluid-filled, congenital cyst or tumor whose walls sometimes contain hair, teeth, or other dermal appendages.

14. For, by 1832 Jeremy Bentham, the famed utilitarian philosopher, had achieved his own autogenous demystification by being the first man who was not a convicted criminal to donate voluntarily his own body for medical dissection; and the entire country was thoroughly scandalized in 1828 when two Scotsmen by the names of Burke and Hare were apprehended for murders carried out in order to provide the Edinburgh anatomist, Dr. Robert Knox, with ma-

terials for the dissecting table. It seems, by this time, as if Scottish specificity had gone too far (Marshall 1995)!

15. In our enthusiasm for mapping genes we so often forget how uncommitted they may be in advance of environmental stimuli.

16. Cecil Balmond (1998) has written an entire book that celebrates the number 9 as the most beautiful and enigmatic of all numbers, in part at least because of its spiral shape and the geometric concepts it, therefore, embodies.

17. If you are right-handed, for instance, the clockwise slicing with the right hand induces a counterclockwise rotation of the grapefruit with the left.

18. For readers interested in the complex geometry of icosahedral molecular structures, see Aldersey-Williams 1995.

19. When a soccer ball is initially kicked the airflow passing around it is characterized by low drag and massive turbulence. But when the ball begins to slow down—entering a laminar phase (of smooth air flow)—a side force (aviatory lift, the Bernouilli principle) cause the ball to curve (i.e., spiral) radically.

20. While many authors have described the unsettling symbolic nature of categorical boundaries (e.g., Douglas 1966), these authors, diverse though their interests have been, are especially notable for their analyses of the transitional structures of linguistic, developmental, and cultural categories. On the categorical representation of growing classes of things, see Napier 1992, 54.

21. Or as a kind of mental condition that gets destroyed when the possibility for reciprocity is eliminated. See, for instance, the sad story of the moronic twins, David and Michael, who spoke to one another in a complex language of increasingly large prime numbers until they were "cured" of this by being physically separated (O. Sacks 1985).

22. On wildmen as bringers of special knowledge, see Napier 1986, chapter 2. On the relationship between Francis and Merlin, see Markale 1995, 165.

23. It is also the ancient South Indian (Tamil) for "name" (Napier 2001).

24. Though the Madonna of Enna is virtually unstudied, the mixing of gender in Christian iconography has been well documented by Bynum (1982).

25. This is why Enna has been from ancient times recognized as what Cicero called the "Umbilicus Siciliae," there being evidence not only of neolithic shrines but of necropoleis that imitate rock-cut grottos already in the 9th—8th centuries B.C.

26. "There is a strong relationship [in Lakota] between thunder, lightning, spider[s], dragonflies, turtles, lizards, and other unlikely classificatory bedfellows because they all have the power to protect as well as to harm human beings" (Powers 1986, 159).

27. I would say, here, with the exclusion of hooks (1994).

References

Aladjem, Henrietta. 1999. The Challenges of Lupus: Insights and Hope. Garden City Park, N.Y.: Avery Penguin Putnam.

Aladjem, Henrietta, and Peter H. Schur. 1988. *In Search of the Sun: A Woman's Courageous Victory over Lupus.* New York: Scribner.

Alberts, Bruce, et al. 1989. *Molecular Biology of the Cell.* 2d ed. New York: Garland.

Aldersey-Williams, Hugh. 1995. *The Most Beautiful Molecule: The Discovery of the Buckyball.* New York: Wiley.

Altheim, Franz. 1929. "Persona." *Archiv für Religionswissenschaft* 27:35–52.

Angell, Ian. 2000. "Battle Stations." *New Scientist,* 4 March, 44–45.

Ashton, John, ed. 1994. *The Epidemiological Imagination: A Reader.* Buckingham, U.K.: Open University Press.

Bachelard, Gaston. 1948. *La terre et les rêveries du repos.* Paris: Corti.

———. 1994. *The Poetics of Space.* Trans. Maria Jolas. Boston: Beacon.

Bal, M., and N. Bryson. 1991. "Semiotics and Art History." *Art Bulletin* 73:174–208.

Baldinucci, Filippo. [1682] 1966. *The Life of Bernini.* Trans. Catherine Enggass. University Park: Pennsylvania State University Press.

Balmond, Cecil. 1998. *Number 9: The Search for the Sigma Code.* Munich: Prestel.

Barash, David. 1980. *Sociobiology: The Whisperings Within.* London: Souvenir.

Barth, Fredrik. 1969. *Ethnic Groups and Ethnic Boundaries: The Social Organization of Cultural Difference.* Oslo: Universitetsforlaget.

Bastien, Joseph W. 1992. *Drum and Stethoscope: Integrating Ethnomedicine and Biomedicine in Bolivia.* Salt Lake City: University of Utah Press.

Bayley, David H. 1976. "Learning about Crime: The Japanese Experience." *Public Interest* 44 (Summer): 55–68.

Becker, Wayne M., Jane B. Reece, and Martin F. Poenie. 1996. *The World of the Cell.* 3d ed. Menlo Park, Calif.: Benjamin/Cummings.

Beckett, Katherine, and Theodore Sasson. 2000. *The Politics of Injustice: Crime and Punishment in America.* Thousand Oaks, Calif.: Pine Forge.

Beer, Gavin de. 1958. *Embryos and Ancestors*. Oxford: Clarendon.

Beer, Gillian. 1983. *Darwin's Plots: Evolutionary Narrative in Darwin, George Eliot, and Nineteenth-Century Fiction*. London: Routledge & Kegan Paul.

Beneke, Timothy. 1982. *Men on Rape*. New York: St. Martin's.

———. 1997. *Proving Manhood: Reflections on Men and Sexism*. Berkeley: University of California Press.

Benjamini, Eli, and Sidney Leskowitz. 1988. *Immunology: A Short Course*. New York: Wiley-Liss.

Berlin, Isaiah. 1968. "Verification." In *The Theory of Meaning*, ed. G. H. R. Parkinson. Oxford: Oxford University Press.

Bernard, Claude. 1878. *La Science expérimentale*. Paris: J. B. Baillière et fils.

Bibel, Debra Jan. 1988. *Milestones in Immunology: A Historical Exploration*. Madison, Wis.: Science Tech Publishers.

Bourdieu, Pierre. 1977. *Outline of a Theory of Practice*. Cambridge: Cambridge University Press.

Bowker, Geoffrey C. 1993. "Constructing Science, Forging Technology and Manufacturing Society." *Studies in the History and Philosophy of Science* 24, no. 1: 147–55.

Brandt, Allan M. 1987. *No Magic Bullet: A Social History of Venereal Disease in the United States since 1880*. New York: Oxford University Press.

———. 1988. "AIDS and Metaphor: Toward the Social Meaning of Epidemic Disease." *Social Research* 55, no. 3: 413–32.

Brent, Leslie. 1997. *History of Transplantation Immunology*. San Diego, Calif.: Academic.

Bristol, Michael. 1996. *Big-Time Shakespeare*. London: Routledge.

Broyard, Anatole. 1990. "Doctor Talk to Me." *New York Times Magazine*, 26 August, 32–33, 36.

Buck-Morss, Susan. 1992. "Aesthetics and Anaesthetics: Walter Benjamin's Artwork Essay Reconsidered." *October* 62 (Fall): 3–41.

Buford, Bill. 1991. *Among the Thugs*. London: Vintage.

Burgio, Roberto, and John D. Lantos, eds. 1994. *Primum non Nocere Today: A Symposium on Pediatric Bioethics*. Amsterdam: Elsevier Science.

Burnet, Sir Frank Macfarlane. 1973. *Auto-Immunity and Auto-Immune Disease: A Survey for Physician or Biologist*. Lancaster, U.K.: Medical and Technical Publishing.

Buss, Leo W. 1987. *The Evolution of Individuality*. Princeton, N.J.: Princeton University Press.

Bynum, Caroline Walker. 1982. *Jesus as Mother: Studies in the Spirituality of the High Middle Ages*. Berkeley: University of California Press.

Cajori, Florian. 1980. *A History of Mathematics*. 3d ed. New York: Chelsea Publishing.

Cambrosio, Alberto, and Peter Keating. 1995. *Exquisite Specificity: The Monoclonal Antibody*. New York: Oxford University Press.

Campbell, Joseph. 1981. "Indian Reflections in the Castle of the Grail." In *The Celtic Consciousness*, ed. Robert O'Driscoll. New York: George Braziller.

Campbell, Neil A. 1993. *Biology*. 3d ed. Redwood City, Calif.: Benjamin/Cummings.

Canguilhem, Georges. 1989. *The Normal and the Pathological*. Trans. Carolyn R. Fawcett and Robert S. Cohen. New York: Zone Books.

Cannon, Walter B. 1932. *The Wisdom of the Body*. New York: W. W. Norton.

———. 1942. "Voodoo Death." *American Anthropologist* 44:169–81.

Carlyle, Thomas. 1925. *Sartor Resartus*. Ed. Archibald MacMechan. Boston: Athenaeum.

Carroll, Lewis. 1914. *Through the Looking Glass and What Alice Found There*. New York: Macmillan.

———. 1939. *The Complete Works of Lewis Carroll*. London: Nonesuch Press.

Cassell, Joan. 1986. "Dismembering the Image of God: Surgeons, Heroes, Wimps and Miracles." *Anthropology Today* 2, no. 2 (April): 13–15.

Castaneda, Carlos. 1998. *The Active Side of Infinity*. New York: Harper Perennial Library.

Charlesworth, Max, Lyndsay Farrall, Terry Stokes, and David Turnbull. 1989. *Life among the Scientists: An Anthropological Study of an Australian Scientific Community*. Melbourne: Oxford University Press.

Chase, Allan. 1982. *Magic Shots: A Human and Scientific Account of the Long and Continuing Struggle to Eradicate Infectious Diseases by Vaccination*. New York: Morrow.

Clark, Stephen R. L. 1975. *Aristotle's Man*. London: Oxford University Press.

Coghlan, Andy. 1998. "A Plague on Arthritis: Protein from Killer Bug Could Help Bring Pain Relief." *New Scientist*, 9 May, 9.

Cohen, Irun R. 1992a. "The Cognitive Paradigm and the Immunological Homunculus." *Immunology Today* 13, no. 12 (December): 490–94.

———. 1992b. "The Cognitive Principle Challenges Clonal Selection." *Immunology Today* 13, no. 11 (November): 441–44.

———. 1999. *Tending Adam's Garden: Evolving the Cognitive Immune Self*. San Diego, Calif.: Academic.

Cohen, Irun, and D. B. Young. 1991. "Autoimmunity, Microbial Immunity and the Immunological Homunculus." *Immunology Today* 12, no. 4 (April): 105–10.

Cohn, Melvin. 1992. "The Self/Nonself Discrimination: Reconstructing a Cabbage from Sauerkraut." *Research in Immunology* 143, no. 3: 323–34.

———. 1997a. "A New Concept of Specificity Emerges from a Consideration of the Self-Nonself Discrimination." *Cellular Immunology* 181:103–8.

———. 1997b. "Some Thoughts on the Response to Antigens That Are Effector T-Helper Independent ('Thymus Independence')." *Scandinavian Journal of Immunology* 46:565–71.

———. 1998a. "The Self-Nonself Discrimination in the Context of Function." *Theoretical Medicine and Bioethics* 19:475–84.

———. 1998b. "A Reply to Tauber." *Theoretical Medicine and Bioethics* 19:495–504.

———. 1998c. "At the Feet of the Master: The Search for Universalities. Divining the Evolutionary Selection Pressures That Resulted in an Immune System." *Cytogenetics and Cell Genetics* 80:54–60.

Cohn, Melvin, R. Langman, and W. Geckeler. 1980. "Diversity." *Progress in Immunology* 4: 153–201.

Comaroff, John, and Jean Comaroff. 1992. *Ethnography and the Historical Imagination*. Boulder, Colo.: Westview.

Cone, Richard A., and Emily Martin. 1998. "Corporeal Flows: The Immune System and the Political Economy of Food." In *The Visible Woman*, ed. P. Treichler and C. Penley. New York: New York University Press.

Connerton, Paul. 1989. *How Societies Remember*. Cambridge: Cambridge University Press.

Corin, Ellen E. 1990. "Facts and Meaning in Psychiatry: An Anthropological Approach to the Lifeworld of Schizophrenics." *Culture, Medicine, and Psychiatry* 14:153–88.

Crick, Francis. 1981. *Life Itself: Its Origin and Nature*. New York: Simon and Schuster.

Currie, Elliot. 1985. *Confronting Crime: An American Challenge*. New York: Pantheon.

Danforth, Loring M. 1989. *Firewalking and Religious Healing: The Anastenaria of Greece and the American Firewalking Movement*. Princeton, N.J.: Princeton University Press.

Darwin, Charles. 1859. *On the Origin of the Species by Means of Natural Selection; or, The Preservation of Favoured Races in the Struggle for Life*. London: J. Murray.

———. [1859] 1964. *On the Origin of Species*. Cambridge, Mass.: Harvard University Press.

———. 1871. *The Descent of Man, and Selection in Relation to Sex*. London: J. Murray.

Dawkins, Richard. 1976. *The Selfish Gene*. Oxford: Oxford University Press.

Deren, Maya. 1953. *Divine Horsemen: The Living Gods of Haiti*. New York: Thames and Hudson.

Descartes, René. 1964. *Oeuvres de Descartes*. Ed. Charles Adam and Paul Tannery. Paris: J. Vrin.

Devlin, Keith. 1997. *Goodbye, Descartes: The End of Logic and a Search for a New Cosmology of the Mind*. New York: Wiley.

DiGiacomo, Susan M. 1987. "Biomedicine as a Cultural System: An Anthropologist in the Kingdom of the Sick." In *Encounters with Biomedicine: Case Studies in Medical Anthropology*, ed. Hans A. Baer, 315–46. New York: Gordon and Breach Science Publishers.

Dodge, Theodore Ayrault. 1892. *Caesar: A History of the Art of War among the Romans down to the End of the Roman Empire*. 2 vols. Boston: Houghton, Mifflin.

Douglas, Mary. 1966. *Purity and Danger: An Analysis of the Concepts of Pollution and Taboo*. London: Routledge and Kegan Paul.

Dowling, Harry F. 1977. *Fighting Infection: Conquests of the Twentieth Century*. Cambridge, Mass.: Harvard University Press.

Dreifus, Claudia. 1998. "Blazing an Unconventional Trail to a New Theory of Immunity." *New York Times*, 16 June, B15, F4.

Duerr, Hans Peter. 1985. *Dreamtime: Concerning the Boundary between Wilderness and Civilization*. Trans. Felicitas D. Goodman. Oxford: Oxford University Press.

Dumont, Louis. 1970. *Homo Hierarchicus: An Essay on the Caste System*. Trans. Mark Sainsbury. Chicago: University of Chicago Press.

Dwyer, John. 1995. "Why the Germs Are Winning." *Times Literary Supplement*, 13 January, 7–8.

Edinger, Edward F. 1994. *The Mystery of the Coniunctio: Alchemical Image of Individuation*. Toronto: Inner City Books.

Eguchi, Shigeyuki. 1991. "Between Folk Concepts of Illness and Psychiatric Diagnosis: *Kitsune-tsuki* (Fox Possession) in a Mountain Village of Western Japan." *Culture, Medicine, and Psychiatry* 15:421–51.

Eigen, Manfred, and Ruthild Winkler-Oswatitsch. 1992. *Steps towards Life: A Perspective on Evolution*. Trans. Paul Woolley. Oxford: Oxford University Press.

Eldredge, Niles, and Stephen Jay Gould. 1972. "Punctuated Equilibria: An Alternative to Phyletic Gradualism." In *Models in Paleobiology*, ed. T. J. M. Schopf, 82–115. San Francisco: Freeman and Cooper.

Fanon, Frantz. 1966. "On National Culture." From *The Wretched of the Earth*. Trans. Constance Farrington. Harmondsworth: Penguin. Reprinted in *Colonial Discourse and Postcolonial Theory*, ed. Patrick Williams and Laura Chrisman. New York: Columbia University Press, 1994.

Farmer, Paul. 1990. "Sending Sickness: Sorcery, Politics, and Changing Concepts of AIDS in Haiti." *Medical Anthropology Quarterly* 4, no. 1: 6–27.

Farmer, Paul, and Arthur Kleinman. 1989. "AIDS as Human Suffering." *Daedalus* 118, no. 2: 135–60.

Feyerabend, Paul K. 1975. *Against Method: Outline of an Anarchistic Theory of Knowledge*. Atlantic Highlands, N.J.: Humanities Press.

Forgacs, David, ed. 1988. *An Antonio Gramsci Reader: Selected Writings, 1916–1935*. New York: Schocken.

Fort, Charles. 1941. *The Books of Charles Fort*. New York: H. Holt.

Fox, James, ed. 1980. *The Flow of Life: Essays on Eastern Indonesia*. Cambridge, Mass.: Harvard University Press.

Fraser, Steven, ed. 1995. *The Bell Curve Wars: Race, Intelligence, and the Future of America*. New York: Basic Books.

Fulcanelli [pseud.]. 1960. *Les Demeures philosophales et le symbolisme hermétique dans ses rapports avec l'art sacré et l'ésotérisme du grand oeuvre*. Paris: Jean-Jaques Pauvert.

Genette, Gérard. 1966. *Figures: essais*. Paris: Editions du Seuil.

Geracioti, Thomas D., et al. 1987. "The Onset of Munchausen's Syndrome." *General Hospital Psychiatry* 9:405–9.

Germain, Ronald N. 2001. "The Art of the Probable: System Control in the Adaptive Immune System." *Science* 293, no. 5528: 240–45.

Ghyka, Matila. [1946] 1977. *The Geometry of Art and Life*. New York: Dover.

Goffman, Erving. 1961. *Asylums: Essays on the Social Situation of Mental Patients and Other Inmates*. Garden City, N.Y.: Anchor.

———. 1963. *Stigma: Notes on the Management of Spoiled Identity*. Englewood Cliffs, N.J.: Prentice Hall.

———. 1967. *Interaction Ritual: Essays on Face-to-Face Behavior*. Garden City, N.Y.: Anchor.

Goldman, Irving. 1975. *The Mouth of Heaven: An Introduction to Kwakiutl Religious Thought*. New York: Wiley.

Good, Byron J. 1994. *Medicine, Rationality, and Experience: An Anthropological Perspective*. Cambridge: Cambridge University Press.

Good, Mary-Jo D., Byron J. Good, Cynthia Schaffer, and Stuart E. Lind. 1990. "American Oncology and the Discourse of Hope." *Culture, Medicine, and Psychiatry* 14:59–79.

Goodfield, June. 1981. *An Imagined World: A Story of Scientific Discovery*. New York: Harper and Row.

Gould, Stephen Jay. 1997. *Dinosaur in a Haystack: Reflections in Natural History*. London: Penguin.

Gould, Stephen Jay, and Niles Eldredge. 1977. "Punctuated Equilibria: The Tempo and Mode of Evolution Reconsidered." *Paleobiology* 3:115–51.

Griaule, Marcel. 1965. *Conversations with Ogotemmêli: An Introduction to Dogon Religious Ideas*. Oxford: Oxford University Press.

Gross, Alan G. 1990. *The Rhetoric of Science*. Cambridge, Mass.: Harvard University Press.

Gunn, Spence. 1997. "Natural Mathematicians." *Kew* (Summer): 23–25.

Gutmann, Matthew C. 1993. "Rituals of Resistance: A Critique of the Theory of Everyday Forms of Resistance." *Latin American Perspectives* 20, no. 2 (Spring): 74–92. Issue 77.

Hallowell, A. Irving. 1955. *Culture and Experience*. Philadelphia: University of Pennsylvania Press.

Hammersly, Martyn. 1992. *What's Wrong with Ethnography?* London: Routledge.

Hampshire, Stuart. 1965. *Freedom of the Individual*. New York: Harper and Row.

———. 1970. *Thought and Action*. London: Chatto and Windus.

Haraway, Donna. 1989. "The Biopolitics of Postmodern Bodies: Determinations of Self in Immune System Discourse." *Differences* 1, no. 1: 3–43.

———. 1991. *Simians, Cyborgs, and Women: The Reinvention of Nature*. New York: Routledge.

———. 1997. Modest_Witness@Second_Millennium.FemaleMan©_Meets_OncoMouse™: *Feminism and Technoscience*. New York: Routledge.

Harré, Rom. 1984. *Personal Being: A Theory for Individual Psychology*. Cambridge, Mass.: Harvard University Press.

Harris, Daniel. 1994. "Making Kitsch from AIDS." *Harper's*, July, 55–60.

Harris, Zellig, et al. 1989. *The Form of Information in Science: Analysis of an Immunology Sublanguage*. Dordrecht: Kluwer Academic.

Hausman, Carl R. 1989. *Metaphor and Art: Interactionism and Reference in the Verbal and Nonverbal Arts*. Cambridge: Cambridge University Press.

Hawley, Katherine. 1996. "Thomas S. Kuhn's Mysterious Worlds." *Studies in History and Philosophy of Science* 27, no. 2: 291–300.

Heckscher, William S. 1947. "Bernini's Elephant and Obelisk." *Art Bulletin* 29:155–82.

Herbst, Edward. 1997. *Voices in Bali: Energies and Perceptions in Vocal Music and Dance Theater*. Hanover, N.H.: University Press of New England.

Herrnstein, Richard, and Charles Murray. 1994. *The Bell Curve: Intelligence and Class Structure in American Life*. New York: Free Press.

Hesse, Mary. 1987. "Tropical Talk: The Myth of the Literal." In "Unfamiliar Noises," by Richard Rorty and Mary Hesse. *The Aristotelian Society*, supplementary vol. 61:297–311.

Hirst, P. Q. Durkheim. 1975. *Bernard and Epistemology*. London: Routledge and Kegan Paul.

HIV & AIDS: A Guide for Journalists. 1993. London: Health Education Authority.

Hoffmann, Roald, and Shira Leibowitz. 1991. "Molecular Mimicry, Rachel and Leah, the Israeli Male, and the Inescapable Metaphor in Science." *Michigan Quarterly Review* 30, no. 3: 383–98.

Homan, Roger. 1991. *The Ethics of Social Research*. London: Longman.

hooks, bell. 1994. *Outlaw Culture: Resisting Representations*. New York: Routledge.

Hubbard, Ruth, and Elijah Wald. 1997. *Exploding the Gene Myth: How Genetic Information Is Produced and Manipulated by Scientists, Physicians, Employers, Insurance Companies, Educators, and Law Enforcers*. Boston: Beacon.

Hughes, Thomas Parke. 1983. *Networks of Power: Electrification in Western Society, 1880–1930*. Baltimore: Johns Hopkins University Press.

Huxley, Francis. 1956. *Affable Savages: An Anthropologist among the Urubu Indians of Brazil*. London: Hart-Davis.

Huxley, Julian. [1932] 1972. *Problems of Relative Growth*. New York: Dover.

James, C. L. R. [1963] 1983. *Beyond a Boundary*. New York: Pantheon.

Janeway, C. A. 1992. "The Immune System Evolved to Discriminate Infectious Nonself from Noninfectious Self." *Immunology Today* 13:11–16.

Jardine, Nicholas. 1987. "Exploiting the Facts." *Times Literary Supplement*, 20–26 November, 1291.

Jerne, Niels K. 1973. "The Immune System." *Scientific American*, July, 52–60.

———. 1984. "Idiotypic Networks and Other Preconceived Ideas." *Immunological Reviews* 79:5–24.

Johnson, Mark. 1987. *The Body in the Mind: The Bodily Basis of Meaning, Imagination, and Reason.* Chicago: University of Chicago Press.

Joneja, Janice Vickerstaff, and Leonard Bielory. 1990. *Understanding Allergy, Sensitivity and Immunity: A Comprehensive Guide.* New Brunswick, N.J.: Rutgers University Press.

Jung, C. G. 1933. *Modern Man in Search of a Soul.* Trans. W. S. Dell and Cary F. Baynes. San Diego, Calif.: Harcourt Brace.

———. 1977. *Mysterium Coniunctionis: An Inquiry into the Separation and Synthesis of Physic Opposites in Alchemy.* Collected Works, vol. 14. Trans. R. F. C. Hull. Princeton, N.J.: Princeton University Press.

———. 1990. *The Undiscovered Self: With Symbols and the Interpretation of Dreams.* Trans. R. F. C. Hull. Princeton, N.J.: Princeton University Press.

Kak, Subhash C. 1996. "The Three Languages of the Brain: Quantum, Reorganization, and Associative." In *Learning as Self-Organization*, ed. Karl Pribram and Joseph King, 185–219. Mahwah, N.J.: L. Erlbaum Associates.

———. 2002. *Gods Within: Mind, Consciousness, and the Vedic Tradition.* New Delhi: Munshiram Manoharlal.

Keller, Evelyn Fox. 1983. *A Feeling for the Organism: The Life and Work of Barbara McClintock.* San Francisco: W. H. Freeman.

———. 1995. *Refiguring Life: Metaphors of Twentieth-Century Biology.* New York: Columbia University Press.

Kirby, G. C. 1997. "Plants as a Source of Antimalarial Drugs." *Tropical Doctor* 27, suppl. 1: 7–11.

Kittay, Eva Feder. 1987. *Metaphor: Its Cognitive Force and Linguistic Structure.* Oxford: Oxford University Press.

Kleinman, Arthur. 1988a. *The Illness Narratives: Suffering, Healing, and the Human Condition.* New York: Basic Books.

———. 1988b. *Rethinking Psychiatry: From Cultural Category to Personal Experience.* New York: Free Press.

Kleinman, Arthur, and Joan Kleinman. 1991. "Suffering and Its Professional Transformation: Toward an Ethnography of Interpersonal Experience." *Culture, Medicine, and Psychiatry* 15, no. 3: 275–301.

Kohn, Alexander. 1986. *False Prophets.* New York: Basil Blackwell.

Kruif, Paul de. 1926. *Microbe Hunters.* New York: Harcourt, Brace.

Kuby, J. 1992. *Immunology.* 3d ed. New York: W. H. Freeman.

LaFond, Richard E., ed. 1978. *Cancer: The Outlaw Cell.* Washington, D.C.: American Chemical Society.

Lakoff, George. 1987. *Women, Fire, and Dangerous Things: What Categories Reveal about the Mind.* Chicago: University of Chicago Press.

Lakoff, George, and Mark Johnson. 1980. *Metaphors We Live By.* Chicago: University of Chicago Press.

Landaw, Jonathan, and Andy Weber. 1993. *Images of Enlightenment*. Ithaca, N.Y.: Snow Lion Publications.

Langman, Rodney E. 1989. *The Immune System: Evolutionary Principles Guide Our Understanding of This Complex Biological Defense System*. San Diego, Calif.: Academic.

Langman, Rodney, and Melvin Cohn. 1992. "What Is the Selective Pressure That Maintains the Gene Loci Encoding the Antigen Receptors of T and B Cells? A Hypothesis." *Immunology and Cellular Biology* 70:397–404.

———. 1996a. "A Short History of Time and Space in Immune Discrimination." *Scandinavian Journal of Immunology* 44:544–48.

———. 1996b. "Terra Firma: A Retreat from 'Danger.' " *Journal of Immunology* 4273–76.

———. 1997a. "A Short History of Time and Space in Immune Discrimination: A Reply to the Commentaries." *Scandinavian Journal of Immunology* 46:113–16.

———. 1997b. "The Essential Self: A Commentary on Silverstein and Rose 'On the Mystique of the Immunological Self.' " *Immunological Reviews* 159:214–17.

———. 1999. "Away with Words: Commentary on the Atlan-Cohen Essay 'Immune Information, Self-Organization and Meaning.' " *International Immunology* 11, no. 6: 865–70.

———, ed. 2000. *Seminars in Immunology* 12, no. 3 (June).

Lantos, John D. 1989. "The Hastings Center Project on Imperiled Newborns: Supreme Court, Jury, or Greek Chorus?" *Pediatrics* 83:615–16.

Lappé, Marc. 1994. *Evolutionary Medicine: Rethinking the Origins of Disease*. San Francisco: Sierra Club Books.

Larkin, Marilynn. 1997. "Polly Matzinger: Immunology's Dangerous Thinker." *Lancet* 350 (5 July): 38.

Lasch, Christopher. 1984. *The Minimal Self: Psychic Survival in Troubled Times*. New York: W. W. Norton.

———. 1991. *The True and Only Heaven: Progress and Its Critics*. New York: Norton.

Latour, Bruno. 1987. *Science in Action: How to Follow Scientists and Engineers through Society*. Cambridge, Mass.: Harvard University Press.

———. 1988. *The Pasteurization of France*. Trans. Alan Sheridan and John Law. Cambridge, Mass.: Harvard University Press.

———. [1992] 1996. *Aramis; or, The Love of Technology*. Trans. Catherine Porter. Cambridge, Mass.: Harvard University Press.

———. 1993. *We Have Never Been Modern*. Trans. Catherine Porter. Cambridge, Mass.: Harvard University Press.

———. 1996. *Petite réflexion sur le culte moderne des dieux faitiches*. Paris: Le Plessis-Robinson, Synthélabo groupe.

Latour, Bruno, and Steve Woolgar. 1986. *Laboratory Life: The Construction of Scientific Facts*. 2d ed. Princeton, N.J.: Princeton University Press.

Leach, Edmund R. 1961. *Rethinking Anthropology*. London: Athlone.

———. 1964. "Anthropological Aspects of Language: Animal Categories and Verbal Abuse." In *New Directions in the Study of Language*, ed. Eric H. Lenneberg. Cambridge, Mass.: MIT Press.

Leenhardt, Maurice. 1930. *Notes d'ethnoligie néo-calédonienne*. Paris: Institut d'ethnologie.

———. 1937. *Gens de la Grande Terre*. Paris: Gallimard.

———. [1947] 1979. *Do Kamo: Person and Myth in the Melanesian World*. Chicago: University of Chicago Press.

Lemert, Charles. 1997. *Postmodernism Is Not What You Think*. Oxford: Blackwell.

Lenoir, Timothy. 1998. *Inscribing Science: Scientific Texts and the Materiality of Communication*. Stanford, Calif.: Stanford University Press.

Lévy-Bruhl, Lucien. [1949] 1975. *The Notebooks on Primitive Mentality*. Trans. Peter Rivière. Oxford: Blackwell.

Lewis, Paul. 1998. "Too Late to Say 'Extinct' in Ubykh, Eyak, or Ona; Thousands of Languages Are Endangered." *New York Times*, 15 August, B7.

Lewontin, Richard. 1992. "The Dream of the Human Genome." *New York Review of Books*, 28 May, 31–40.

Liang, Matthew, et al. 1984. "The Psychosocial Impact of Systemic Lupus Erythematosus and Rheumatoid Arthritis." *Arthritis and Rheumatism* 27, no. 1: 13–19.

Lloyd, G. E. R. 1966. *Polarity and Analogy: Two Types of Argument in Early Greek Thought*. Cambridge: Cambridge University Press.

Lovelock, James. 1988. *The Ages of Gaia: A Biography of Our Living Earth*. New York: Norton.

Luria, A. R. 1987. *The Mind of a Mnemonist: A Little Book about a Vast Memory*. Cambridge, Mass.: Harvard University Press.

Lydyard, Peter M., and Jonathan Brostoff, eds. 1994. *Autoimmune Diseases: Aetiopathogenesis, Diagnosis, and Treatment*. Cambridge, Mass.: Blackwell Science.

Magagna, Victor V. 1991. *Communities of Grain: Rural Rebellion in Comparative Perspective*. Ithaca, N.Y.: Cornell University Press.

Marchand, Roland. 1998. *Creating the Corporate Soul: The Rise of Public Relations and Corporate Imagery in American Big Business*. Berkeley and Los Angeles: University of California Press.

Margolis, Howard. 1993. *Paradigms and Barriers: How Habits of Mind Govern Scientific Belief*. Chicago: University of Chicago Press.

Margulis, Lynn. 1998. *Symbiotic Planet: A New Look at Evolution*. New York: Basic Books.

Markale, Jean. 1995. *Merlin: Priest of Nature*. Trans. Belle N. Burke. Rochester, Vt.: Inner Traditions International.

Markides, Kyriacos C. 1985. *The Magus of Strovolos: The Extraordinary World of a Spiritual Healer*. London: Routledge and Kegan Paul.

Marshall, Tim. 1995. *Murdering to Dissect: Grave-Robbing, Frankenstein and the Anatomy of Literature*. Manchester, U.K.: Manchester University Press.

Martin, Emily. 1989. "The Cultural Construction of Gendered Bodies: Biology and Metaphors of Production and Destruction." *Ethnos* 54, nos. 3–4: 143–60.

———. 1990. "Towards an Anthropology of Immunology: The Body as Nation State." *Medical Anthropology Quarterly* 4:410–26.

———. 1994. *Flexible Bodies: Tracking Immunity in American Culture from the Days of Polio to the Age of AIDS*. Boston: Beacon.

Matzinger, Polly. 1994. "Tolerance, Danger and the Extended Family." *Annual Review of Immunology* 12:991–1045.

———. 2002. "The Danger Model: A Renewed Sense of Self." *Science* 296, no. 5566 (12 April): 301–5.

Matzinger, Polly, M. Flajnik, H. G. Rammensee, G. Stockinger, T. Rolinck, and L. Nicklin, eds. 1987. *The Tolerance Workshop, 1–3*. Basel: Editiones Roche.

Matzinger, Polly, and E. J. Fuchs. 1996. "Beyond 'Self' and 'Nonself': Immunity Is a Conversation Not a War." *Journal of NIH Research* 8:35.

Mayr, Ernst. 1976. "Teleological and Teleonomic: A New Analysis." In *Evolution and the Diversity of Life: Selected Essays*, 383–404. Cambridge, Mass.: Harvard University Press.

———. 2000. "Darwin's Influence on Modern Thought." *Scientific American* 283, no. 1: 79–83.

Mazumdar, Pauline M. H., ed. 1989. *Immunology 1930–1980: Essays on the History of Immunology*. Toronto: Wall and Thompson.

McCaughey, Martha, and Neal King. 1995. "Rape Education Videos: Presenting Mean Women Instead of Dangerous Men." *Teaching Sociology* 23 (October): 374–88.

McClintock, Peter, and Dmitri Luchinsky. 1999. "Glorious Noise." *New Scientist*, 9 January, 36–39.

McFarland, Thomas. 1987. *Shapes of Culture*. Iowa City: University of Iowa Press.

McRoy, R. G. 1989. "An Organizational Dilemma: The Case of Transracial Adoptions." *Journal of Applied Behavioral Science* 25, no. 2: 145–60.

Medawar, Peter. 1982. *Pluto's Republic*. New York: Oxford University Press.

———. 1984. *The Limits of Science*. New York: Harper and Row.

Meier, C. A. 1989. *Healing Dream and Ritual*. Einsiedeln, Switzerland: Daimon.

Meštrović, Stjepan G. 1992. *Durkheim and Postmodern Culture*. New York: Aldine de Gruyter.

Midgley, Mary. 1994. "Darwinism and Ethics." In *Medicine and Moral Reasoning*, ed. K. W. M. Fulford, G. Gillett, and J. M. Soskice. Cambridge: Cambridge University Press.

Morowitz, Harold J. 1985. *Mayonnaise and the Origin of Life: Thoughts of Minds and Molecules*. New York: Scribner.

———. 1992. *Beginning of Cellular Life: Metabolism Recapitulates Biogenesis*. New Haven, Conn.: Yale University Press.

Moulin, Anne-Marie. 1989. "The Immune System: A Key Concept for the History of Immunology." *History and Philosophy of the Life Sciences* 11:221–36.

———. 1990. "La Métaphore du soi et le tabou de l'auto-immunité." In *Soi et non-soi: Des biologistes, médecins, philosophes, et théologiens s'interrogent*, ed. J. Bernard et al. Paris: Seuil.

———. 1991. *Le Dernier Language de la médecine: Histoire de l'immunologie de Pasteur au Sida*. Paris: Presses Universitaires de France.

———. 1996. *L'Aventure de la vaccination*. Paris: Penser la Medecine, Fayard.

Napier, A. David. 1986. *Masks, Transformation, and Paradox*. Berkeley and Los Angeles: University of California Press.

———. 1992. *Foreign Bodies: Performance, Art, and Symbolic Anthropology*. Berkeley and Los Angeles: University of California Press.

———. 1996. "Unnatural Selection: Social Models of the Microbial World." In *Vaccinia, Vaccination, and Vaccinology: Jenner, Pasteur and Their Successors*, ed. S. Plotkin and B. Fantini. Proceedings, International Meeting on the History of Vaccinology, Marnes-la-Coquette, France. New York: Elsevier.

———. 2001. "Masks and Metaphysics in the Ancient World: An Anthropological View." In *Rūpa-Pratirūpa: Mind, Man, and Mask*, ed. S. C. Malik. New Delhi: Indira Gandhi National Centre for the Arts.

———. 2002. "Our Own Way: On Anthropology and Intellectual Property." In *Exotic No More: Anthropology on the Front Line*, ed. Jeremy MacClancy. Chicago: University of Chicago Press.

———. Forthcoming a. "Self and Other in an 'Amodern' World." In *A Companion to Psycholog-*

ical Anthropology: Modernity and Psychocultural Change, ed. Conerly Casey and Robert Edgerton. Oxford: Blackwell.

———. Forthcoming b. "Metaphor and Immunology." In *The Cultural Lives of Immune Systems*, ed. James Wilce. New York: Routledge.

———. Forthcoming c. "The Writing of Passage: Illness and Representation in Medical Anthropology." In *The Wounded Ethnographer*, ed. Susan B. DiGiacomo. New York: Routledge.

Needham, Rodney. 1967. "Percussion and Transition." *Man*, n.s., 2:606–14.

———. 1972. *Belief, Language, and Experience*. Chicago: University of Chicago Press.

———. 1975. "Polythetic Classification: Convergence and Consequences." *Man*, n.s., 10:349–69.

———. 1978. *Primordial Characters*. Charlottesville: University Press of Virginia.

———. 1979. *Symbolic Classification*. Santa Monica, Calif.: Goodyear Publishing.

———. 1980. *Reconnaissances*. Toronto: University of Toronto Press.

———. 1983. "Tarzan of the Apes: A Re-appreciation." *Foundation* 28:20–28.

Newman, Andy. 1999. "In Pursuit of Autoimmune Worm Cure." *New York Times*, 31 August.

Nossal, G. J. V. 1969. *Antibodies and Immunity*. New York: Basic Books.

Ochert, Ayala. 1998. "Deconstructing DNA." *New Scientist*, 16 May, 32–35.

Ohno, Susumu. 1976. "Promethean Evolution as the Biological Basis of Human Freedom and Equality." *Perspectives in Biology and Medicine* 19 (Summer): 527–32.

Ohno, Susumu, J. T. Epplen, T. Matsunaga, and T. Hozumi. 1982. "The Curse of Prometheus Is Laid upon the Immune System." In *Progress in Allergy*, vol. 39, ed. P. Kallós, 8–39. Basel: S. Karger.

Olds, Linda E. 1992. *Metaphors of Interrelatedness: Toward a Systems Theory of Psychology*. Albany: State University of New York Press.

Oldstone, Michael B. A. 1998. *Viruses, Plagues, and History*. New York: Oxford University Press.

Onians, R. B. 1951. *The Origins of European Thought: About the Body, the Mind, the Soul, the World, Time, and Fate*. Cambridge: Cambridge University Press.

Ortner, Sherry. 1984. "Theory in Anthropology since the Sixties." *Comparative Studies in Society and History* 26, no. 1: 126–66. Reprinted in *Culture/Power/History: A Reader in Contemporary Social and Cultural Theory*, ed. Nicholas B. Dirks, Geoff Eley, and Sherry B. Ortner. Princeton, N.J.: Princeton University Press, 1994.

Payer, Cheryl. 1991. *Lent and Lost: Foreign Credit and Third World Development*. London: Zed Books.

Payer, Lynn. 1988. *Medicine and Culture: Varieties of Treatment in the United States, England, West Germany, and France*. New York: Penguin.

Peacock, James L. 1986. *The Anthropological Lens: Harsh Light, Soft Focus*. Cambridge: Cambridge University Press.

Peirce, Charles S. 1991. *Peirce on Signs: Writings on Semiotic*. Chapel Hill: University of North Carolina Press.

Pennisi, Elizabeth. 1994. "Number 12 Steps Up to Bat: Will This Immune System Messenger Hit a Grand Slam?" *Science News* 146, no. 8 (20 August): 120–21, 124.

———. 1996. "Teetering on the Brink of Danger." *Science* 27, no. 5256 (22 March): 1665–67.

Perkins, Harold. 1999. "Soul Food for the Boardroom." *Times Literary Supplement*, 22 January, 6.

Pfeiffer, John, et al. 1964. *The Cell.* New York: Harper.

Phillips, Adam. 1994. *On Flirtation.* Cambridge, Mass.: Harvard University Press.

Pleydell-Bouverie, Jasper. 1993. "Convenience Shipping." *Geographical Magazine* 65, no. 6 (June): 16–20.

Pope, Carl. 1996. "Corporate Citizens." *Sierra,* November/December, 14.

Porter, Roy. 1992. "History of the Body." In *New Perspectives on Historical Writing,* ed. Peter Burke. University Park: Pennsylvania State University Press.

Poundstone, William, and Robert T. Wainwright. 1985. *The Recursive Universe: Cosmic Complexity and the Limits of Scientific Knowledge.* New York: William Morrow.

———. 1988. *Labyrinths of Reason: Paradox, Puzzles, and the Frailty of Knowledge.* New York: Doubleday.

Powers, William K. 1986. *Sacred Language: The Nature of Supernatural Discourse in Lakota.* Norman: University of Oklahoma Press.

Progoff, Ira. 1956. *The Death and Rebirth of Psychology.* New York: Julian Press.

———. 1973. *Jung, Synchronicity and Human Destiny: Noncausal Dimensions of Human Experiences.* New York: Julian Press.

Purves, William K., Gordon H. Orians, and H. Craig Heller. 1995. *Life: The Science of Biology.* 4th ed. Sunderland, Mass.: Sinauer Associates.

Rabinow, Paul. 1996a. *Making PCR.* Chicago: University of Chicago Press.

———. 1996b. *Essays on Anthropological Reason.* Princeton, N.J.: Princeton University Press.

Raglan, FitzRoy Richard Somerset, Baron. [1936] 1979. *The Hero.* New York: Meridian.

Rao, T. R. N., and Subhash Kak. 1998. *Computing Science in Ancient India.* Lafayette, La.: Center for Advanced Computer Studies, University of Southwestern Louisiana.

Rhodes, Richard. 1997. *Deadly Feasts: Tracking the Secrets of a Terrifying New Plague.* New York: Simon and Schuster.

Richardson, Sarah. 1996. "The End of the Self." *Discover* 17, no. 4 (April): 80–87.

Ricoeur, Paul. 1994. *Oneself as Another.* Trans. Kathleen Blamey. Chicago: University of Chicago Press.

Ridley, Mark. 1995. "The Microbe's Opportunity." *Times Literary Supplement,* 13 January, 6–7.

Roberts, Royston M. 1989. *Serendipity: Accidental Discoveries in Science.* New York: Wiley.

Roitt, Ivan M. [1977] 1980. *Essential Immunology.* Oxford: Blackwell Scientific.

Roitt, Ivan M., and Peter J. Delves. 1995. *Essential Immunology Review.* Cambridge, Mass.: Blackwell Science.

Rosen, Robert. 1991. *Life Itself: A Comprehensive Inquiry into the Nature, Origin, and Fabrication of Life.* New York: Columbia University Press.

Ross, Doran H. 1993. "Carnaval Masquerades in Guinea-Bissau." *African Arts* 26, no. 3 (July): 64–71.

Rothenberg, Albert. 1988. "Creativity and the Homospatial Process: Experimental Studies." *Psychiatric Clinics of North America* 11, no. 3: 443–59.

Roustang, François. 1982. *Dire Mastery: Discipleship from Freud to Lacan.* Trans. Ned Lukacher. Baltimore: Johns Hopkins University Press.

Sabogal, F., and B. Faigeles. 1993. "Multiple Sexual Partners among Hispanics in High-Risk Cities." *Family Planning Perspectives* 25, no. 6: 257–62.

Sacks, Oliver. 1985. *The Man Who Mistook His Wife for a Hat and Other Clinical Tales.* New York: Summit.

Sacks, Sheldon, ed. 1997. *On Metaphor.* Chicago: University of Chicago Press.

Sahlins, Marshall David. 1976. *The Use and Abuse of Biology: An Anthropological Critique of Sociobiology.* Ann Arbor: University of Michigan Press.

——. 1995. *How "Natives" Think: About Captain Cook, For Example.* Chicago: University of Chicago Press.

Sayre, Anne. 1975. *Rosalind Franklin and DNA.* New York: Norton.

Schaffner, Kenneth F., Internet moderator. 1997. "Sense of Self: Models of Immunologic Tolerance. Synopsis of the Debate on Self-Nonself, Danger, Integrity, and Beyond." *HMS Beagle 11*, 27 June, 1–5.

Scheper-Hughes, Nancy. 1990. "Three Propositions for a Critically Applied Medical Anthropology." *Social Science and Medicine* 30:189–97.

Schindler, Lydia S. 1990. *Understanding the Immune System.* NIH, no. 90–529. Rev. ed. Bethesda, Md.: National Institutes of Health.

Schrödinger, Erwin. [1925] 1961. *Meine Weltansicht.* Vienna: Paul Zsolnay.

——. 1944. *What Is Life?* New York: Macmillan.

Schwartz, Robert S. 1995. Review of Alfred I. Tauber, *The Immune Self: Theory or Metaphor? The New England Journal of Medicine* 332:17, 1176–77.

Schwartz, Robert S., and Noel R. Rose, eds. 1986. *Autoimmunity: Experimental and Clinical Aspects.* New York: New York Academy of Sciences.

Scott, James C. 1985. *Weapons of the Weak: Everyday Forms of Peasant Resistance.* New Haven, Conn.: Yale University Press.

Segal, Lee A., and Irun R. Cohen, eds. 2001. *Design Principles for the Immune System and Other Distributed Autonomous Systems.* Oxford: Oxford University Press.

Seidenberg, A. 1962. "The Ritual Origin of Geometry." *Archive for History of Exact Sciences* 1:488–527.

——. 1978. "The Origin of Mathematics." *Archive for History of Exact Sciences* 18:301–42.

Shah, Idries. 1970. *Tales of the Dervishes.* New York: Dutton.

Shapiro, Andrew L. 1992. *We're Number One! Where America Stands and Falls in the New World Order.* New York: Vintage.

Shattuck, Roger. 1996. *Forbidden Knowledge: From Prometheus to Pornography.* New York: St. Martin's.

Sherley-Price, Leo, trans. 1959. *The Little Flowers of Saint Francis: With Five Considerations on the Sacred Stigmata.* Harmondsworth, U.K.: Penguin.

Silverstein, Arthur M. 1989. *A History of Immunology.* San Diego, Calif.: Academic.

Singer, Jerome L. 1990. *Repression and Dissociation: Implications for Personality Theory, Psychopathology, and Health.* Chicago: University of Chicago Press.

Smith, Crosbie, and M. Norton Wise. 1989. *Energy and Empire: A Biographical Study of Lord Kelvin.* Cambridge: Cambridge University Press.

Smith, John Maynard, and Eörs Szathmáry. 1999. *The Origins of Life: From the Birth of Life to the Origin of Language.* Oxford: Oxford University Press.

Sontag, Susan. 1978. *Illness as Metaphor.* New York: Farrar, Straus and Giroux.

——. 1990. *Illness as Metaphor; and AIDS and Its Metaphors.* New York: Doubleday.

Spencer, Jonathan. 1989. "Anthropology as a Kind of Writing." *Man*, n.s., 24 (March): 145–64.

Spini, Tito, and Sandro Spini. 1976. *Togu na: The African Dogon "House of Men, House of Words."* Trans. Verna Kaye-Ciappini. New York: Rizzoli.

Spock, Benjamin. 1994. *A Better World for Our Children: Rebuilding American Family Values.* Bethesda, Md.: National Press Books.

Steele, Edward J., Robyn A. Lindley, and Robert V. Blanden. 1998. *Lamarck's Signature: How Retrogenes Are Changing Darwin's Natural Selection Paradigm.* Reading, Mass.: Perseus.

Stein, Gertrude. 1933. *The Autobiography of Alice B. Toklas.* New York: Literary Guild.

Stewart, Ian. 1998. *Life's Other Secret: The New Mathematics of the Living World.* New York: Wiley.

Stites, Daniel P., et al. 1994. *Basic and Clinical Immunology.* 8th ed. Stamford, Conn.: Appleton and Lange.

Stoller, Paul. 1986. "Bad Sauce, Good Ethnography." *Cultural Anthropology* 1:336–52.

———. 1989. *Fusion of the Worlds: An Ethnography of Possession among the Songhay of Niger.* Chicago: University of Chicago Press.

———. 1997. *Sensuous Scholarship.* Philadelphia: University of Pennsylvania Press.

Stoller, Paul, and Cheryl Olkes. 1987. *In Sorcery's Shadow: A Memoir of Apprenticeship among the Songhay of Niger.* Chicago: University of Chicago Press.

Szasz, Thomas S. [1961] 1974. *The Myth of Mental Illness: Foundations of a Theory of Personal Conduct.* Rev. ed. New York: Harper and Row.

Szilard, L. 1929. "On the Decrease of Entropy in a Thermodynamic System by the Intervention of Intelligent Beings." *Behavioral Science* 9:301–10.

Tan, E. M., et al. 1982. "The 1982 Revised Criteria for the Classification of SLE." *Arthritis and Rheumatism* 25:1271–77.

Tauber, Alfred I. 1991. *Organism and the Origins of Self.* Dordrecht: Kluwer Academic.

———. 1994. *The Immune Self: Theory or Metaphor?* Cambridge: Cambridge University Press.

Tauber, Alfred I., and Leon Chernyak. 1991. *Metchnikoff and the Origins of Immunology: From Metaphor to Theory.* New York: Oxford University Press.

Taylor, F. Kräupl. 1979. *The Concepts of Illness, Disease and Morbus.* Cambridge: Cambridge University Press.

Thompson, D'Arcy Wentworth. 1961. *On Growth and Form.* Abridged ed. Ed. John Tyler Bonner. Cambridge: Cambridge University Press.

Vaucher, Andréa R., ed. 1993. *Muses from Chaos and Ashes.* New York: Grove Press.

Vidal, Gore. 1987. "Armageddon?" In *At Home: Essays 1982–1988,* 92–104. New York: Random House.

von Baeyer, Hans Christian. 1998. *Maxwell's Demon: Why Warmth Disperses and Time Passes.* New York: Random House.

Waelhens, Alphonse de. 1967. *Une Philosophie de l'ambiguïté: L'existentialisme de Maurice Merleau-Ponty.* 2d ed. Louvain, Belgium: Nauwelaerts.

Walker, Matt. 1999. "Back from the Dead: Ancient Viruses Lurking in the Polar Ice Could Cause Lethal Epidemics." *New Scientist* 4, no. 2202: 4.

Walpole, Brenda. 1995. *Counting.* Milwaukee, Wis.: Gareth Stevens Publishing.

Watson, Richard A. 1987. *The Breakdown of Cartesian Metaphysics.* Atlantic Highlands, N.J.: Humanities Press.

Weiner, Annette. 1988. *The Trobrianders of Papua New Guinea.* New York: Holt, Rinehart and Winston.

———. 1992. *Inalienable Possessions.* Berkeley: University of California Press.

Werth, Barry. 1991. "How Short Is Too Short? Marketing Human Growth Hormone." *New York Times Magazine*, 16 June, 14–17, 28–29, 47.

———. 1994. *The Billion-Dollar Molecule: One Company's Quest for the Perfect Drug.* New York: Simon and Schuster.

Wikan, Unni. 1990. *Managing Turbulent Hearts: A Balinese Formula for Living.* Chicago: University of Chicago Press.

Wilson, Adrian. 1990. "The Politics of Medical Improvement in Early Hanoverian London." In *The Medical Enlightenment of the Eighteenth Century,* ed. Andrew Cunningham and Roger French. Cambridge: Cambridge University Press.

Wilson, Edward O. 1975. *Sociobiology: The New Synthesis.* Cambridge, Mass.: Harvard University Press.

———. 1978. *On Human Nature.* Cambridge, Mass.: Harvard University Press.

Witherspoon, Gary. 1977. *Language and Art in the Navajo Universe.* Ann Arbor: University of Michigan Press.

———. 1978. *On Human Nature.* Cambridge, Mass.: Harvard University Press.

Zaner, Richard M. 1964. *The Problem of Embodiment: Some Contributions to a Phenomenology of the Body.* The Hague: M. Nijhoff.

Zimring, Franklin, and Gordon Hawkins. 1995. *The Scale of Imprisonment.* Chicago: University of Chicago Press.

———. 1997. *Crime Is Not the Problem: Lethal Violence in America.* New York: Oxford University Press.

Index